HIKE

Continued on next page

60 HIKES
WITHIN 60 MILES

HARRISBURG

INCLUDING
CUMBERLAND, DAUPHIN,
LEBANON, LANCASTER, PERRY,
AND YORK COUNTIES

MENASHA RIDGE PRESS
Birmingham, Alabama

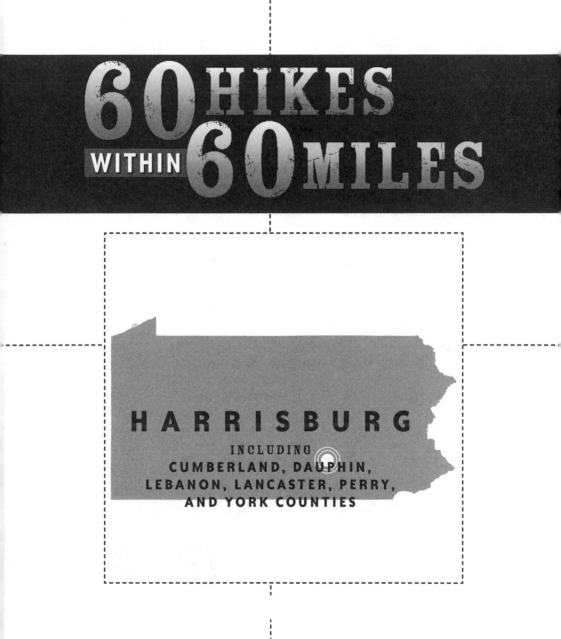

60 HIKES WITHIN 60 MILES

HARRISBURG

INCLUDING
CUMBERLAND, DAUPHIN,
LEBANON, LANCASTER, PERRY,
AND YORK COUNTIES

MATT WILLEN

DISCLAIMER

This book is meant only as a guide to select trails in the Harrisburg area and does not guarantee hiker safety in any way—you hike at your own risk. Neither Menasha Ridge Press nor Matt Willen is liable for property loss or damage, personal injury, or death that result in any way from accessing or hiking the trails described in the following pages. Please be aware that hikers have been injured in the Harrisburg area. Be especially cautious when walking on or near boulders, steep inclines, and drop-offs, and do not attempt to explore terrain that may be beyond your abilities. To help ensure an uneventful hike, please read carefully the introduction to this book, and perhaps get further safety information and guidance from other sources. Familiarize yourself thoroughly with the areas you intend to visit before venturing out. Ask questions, and prepare for the unforeseen. Also stay informed regarding weather reports, maps of the area you intend to visit, and any relevant park regulations.

Copyright © 2008 by Matt Willen
All rights reserved
Printed in the United States of America
Published by Menasha Ridge Press
Distributed by Publishers Group West
First edition, third printing 2014

Library of Congress Cataloging-in-Publication Data

Willen, Matthew.
  60 hikes within 60 miles, Harrisburg: including Cumberland, Dauphin, Lebanon, Lancaster, Perry, and York counties/Matt Willen.
        p. cm.
  ISBN-13: 978-0-89732-042-9
  ISBN-10: 0-89732-042-5
      1. Hiking—Pennsylvania—Harrisburg Region—Guidebooks. 2. Harrisburg Region (Pa.)—Guidebooks. I. Title. II. Title: Sixty hikes within sixty miles, Harrisburg.
GV199.42.P42H379 2008
917.48'1804—dc22

                                    2007038253

Cover and text design by Steveco International
Cover and interior photographs © Matt Willen
Author photograph by Cynthia Kasales
Cartography and elevation profiles by Scott McGrew, Lohnes+Wright, and Matt Willen

Menasha Ridge Press
P.O. Box 43673
Birmingham, AL 35243
www.menasharidge.com

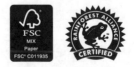

FOR JOE NOLD AND HERB KINCEY—
LONGTIME FRIENDS AND INSPIRATION

—MATT WILLEN

TABLE OF CONTENTS

ACKNOWLEDGMENTS

Anyone who does any of these hikes owes a great debt of gratitude to all of the volunteers and employees of the state, county, local, public, and private organizations and foundations who have worked to construct and maintain the numerous trails in this area. Without their efforts, this book and the wonderful experiences I had while writing it would not have been possible.

So many people assisted me in many ways as I wrote this book. I am indebted to their kindness and wisdom. I would like to thank all of the folks who work for the Pennsylvania Bureau of Forestry, Pennsylvania Department of Conservation and Natural Resources, and the Pennsylvania Fish and Game Commission for answering my endless questions with kindness and courtesy, and for pointing me in the right direction (figuratively and literally). In particular, I would like to thank Beth Kepley and Gavin Smith for providing me with the opportunity to share what I have learned with campers at Gifford Pinchot State Park and Pine Grove Furnace State Park; Susan Crosby at the Strawberry Hill Nature Center and Preserve provided me with invaluable information on the center and on South Mountain more generally; Gina Padilla at Kings Gap told me all about gypsy moths and the history of the environmental education center there; and Kathy Watts at Wildware Backcountry in Harrisburg, the best outdoor store in the region, has been very supportive of this project. I also owe many thanks to Ad Crable with the *Lancaster New Era* for his support of my tent camping book, and for pointing me in the direction of the hikes along the lower Susquehanna River.

I met so many people on the trails over the past year with whom I walked for a short distance or who simply engaged me in conversation for a few minutes. These interactions are extremely memorable and often provided me with insight into other trails and terrain. To all of these people, I appreciate your taking the time to talk and walk with me.

I am indebted to the folks at Menasha Ridge Press for allowing me to write this book. Russell Helms has been a saint in working with me and helping me to understand the business of writing books. Many thanks also go out to Molly Merkle, Tricia Parks, and Travis Bryant for all of their assistance with various parts of this and my tent-camping project. Thank you so much, all of you, for this opportunity.

Finally, this book would have been impossible without the assistance of a couple of key individuals. The first of these is my ex-wife, Cynthia, who, regardless of our differences, has been very supportive in providing me with the time to get out and do the hikes and allowing me to get the writing done. She has been a good friend. Rick San Severino has been a bulwark of support over the years. I truly appreciate the interest he has taken in this project and his patience in listening to me rattle on about it and other sundry topics. And finally, I owe so many thanks to my sons, Jackson, who is about the best hiking partner a father can hope for, and Ian, who has loved to listen to my stories about tramping around the woods. Without them, nothing would be possible.

—MATT WILLEN

FOREWORD

Welcome to Menasha Ridge Press's *60 Hikes within 60 Miles,* a series designed to provide hikers with the information they need to find and hike the very best trails surrounding metropolitan areas.

Our strategy is simple: First, find a hiker who knows the area and loves to hike. Second, ask that person to spend a year researching the most popular and very best trails around. And third, have that person describe each trail in terms of difficulty, scenery, condition, elevation change, and other categories of information that are important to hikers. "Pretend you've just completed a hike and met up with other hikers at the trailhead," we told each author. "Imagine their questions, and be clear in your answers."

An experienced hiker and writer, Matt Willen has selected 60 of the best hikes in and around the Harrisburg metropolitan area. From Rocky Knob to the Gold Mine Trail, Willen provides hikers (and walkers) with a great variety of outings—and all within roughly 60 miles of Harrisburg.

You'll get more out of this book if you take a moment to read the Introduction explaining how to read the trail listings. The "Topographic Maps" section will help you understand how useful topos are on a hike, and will also tell you where to get them. And though this is a "where-to," not a "how-to" guide, readers who have not hiked extensively will find the Introduction of particular value.

As much for the opportunity to free the spirit as well as to free the body, let these hikes elevate you above the urban hurry.

All the best,
The Editors at Menasha Ridge Press

ABOUT THE AUTHOR

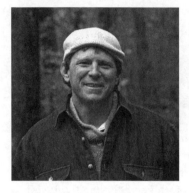

MATT WILLEN is currently an associate professor in the English department at Elizabethtown College, where he teaches courses in writing. He spends much of his time out of the classroom exploring the backcountry of central Pennsylvania, typically with a pack full of camera gear in tow. This book is Willen's second for Menasha Ridge Press, his first being *The Best in Tent Camping: Pennsylvania*. When he isn't hiking, writing, or teaching, he can be found messing around with his two sons, Jackson and Ian, or playing music. He lives on a farm just outside of Hershey, Pennsylvania.

PREFACE

When I began working on this book a little more than a year ago and I told my friends what I was doing, the first thing that everyone seemed to ask was, "*Are* there 60 hikes within 60 miles of Harrisburg?" The question demonstrates the need for this book. In fact, my greatest difficulty in writing this book was limiting the number of hikes to 60. I could have done 100 within 60 miles and still had many more to choose from.

My objective in selecting hikes was to aim for variety. I wanted to provide hikes of various lengths and difficulties, that provided access to different types of terrain and wildlife, and that would be accessible to all sorts of travelers, from seasoned hikers to families to people with special needs. Mostly, though, I have tried to provide hikes that help people get outdoors and into nature. I think going out for walks is the best therapy for and antidote to the crazy lives that we live these days. We are so plagued by information, by multitasking, by cell phones, e-mail, MPEGs, DVDs, and the like, that we tend to live more like extensions of machines rather than as human beings. People need to put that stuff aside for a while. A good hike helps us to slow down and notice what we have around us. Doing so makes us feel better. It helps keep people sensible and it helps to keep people from getting mean (in every sense of the word).

The area covered in this guidebook is all part of the lower Susquehanna River basin. All streams that you'll pass on these hikes eventually flow to the Susquehanna and then south to the Chesapeake Bay. The region can be divided into four major physiographic provinces, each of which offers a different kind of hiking experience. If you draw a circle around Harrisburg, with a perimeter extending 60 miles from the center of the city, most of the northern half of that circle is home to the Valley and Ridge Province, which extends from the Maryland state line north and east toward Scranton and Wilkes-Barre.

Characterized by long, level, rocky ridgetops separated by valleys of fertile farm land, the origins of these mountains date back 200 to 300 million years, from the major Allegheny mountain building period. Because the rocks on the ridgetops are so hard, they are quite resistant to erosion. The exceptions to this rule, however, are the numerous water gaps which bisect the ridges at several points. The most prominent of these gaps are those along the Susquehanna River north of Harrisburg, where the river cuts directly through five different ridges as it makes its way south. Other smaller gaps are located throughout the region. The gaps are something of a geological anomaly: after all, the water should theoretically follow the path of least resistance and make its way around a ridge rather than directly through it. Their origins are still contested by geologists, though current thought suggests that changes in the direction of flow of the Susquehanna River caused by periods of uplift of bedrock allowed river currents to capitalize on weaknesses in the upper strata.

The Valley and Ridge Province is home to several major hiking trails that pass through the region. The Appalachian Trail (A.T.) cuts through a long segment of the province, entering from the south just west of Harrisburg and then angling east and passing just north of Harrisburg parallel to Interstate 81. The Tuscarora Trail in Perry County is part of a 248-mile trail that extends from the A.T. in Shenandoah National Park to Pennsylvania. It was constructed as an alternate route to the busy A.T. corridor. Many people say that it offers more wilderness and solitude than the A.T., and I would agree with that assessment. The trail extends 110 miles from the Maryland state line through the Valley and Ridge Province to Deans Gap on Blue Mountain, where it joins the A.T. west of Harrisburg. You'll also find the Darlington Trail, the Horse-Shoe Trail, and many side trails in these mountains, making for nearly limitless hiking opportunities. Large tracts of public land can be found in these mountains, administrated by either the Pennsylvania Bureau of Forestry, the Department of Conservation and Natural Resources, or the Fish and Game Commission.

The hiking in this region is characteristically rugged and remote. Many trails follow the paths of old haul roads built for moving coal and timber during the 19th century. They tend to be rather rocky, and almost inevitably entail a steep climb from a valley to the top of a ridge. A good pair of sturdy hiking boots is a wise investment for exploring this terrain. The area is home to black bear, white-tailed deer, bobcats, foxes, coyotes, and other woodland mammals. The abundance of birdlife, as throughout the entire region, is remarkable. The forest is typically hardwood and you'll find an enormous diversity of tree and plant life in the area.

To the south of the Valley and Ridge Province runs the Great Valley Province. The Great Valley (also referred to as the Cumberland Valley west of the Susquehanna and Lebanon Valley to the east) extends from New Jersey west and south along the east side of the Appalachian mountains all the way to Georgia. The geology of this province is characterized by large areas of limestone, the origins of which date back to when the region was once under water millions of years ago.

Much of the development in the central Pennsylvania region has taken place in the Great Valley. Harrisburg, Carlisle, Lancaster, and York are all located in it or on its edge. The area is home to many farms and is traversed by small tributaries of the Susquehanna River. The hikes in the Great Valley tend to be comparatively gentle, often following the paths of old railroad grades converted to rail-trails. The Appalachian Trail cuts directly north through it just east of Carlisle. This region is home to an abundance of birdlife, particularly waterfowl and riparian birds along the rivers and creeks, and owls and hawks around the farm country. You'll also find many animals that prefer open range to the deep woods, including red fox, muskrat, opossum, groundhogs, and shrews, as well as turtles and other reptiles and amphibians near water sources.

Much of the southeastern section of the circle consists of the Piedmont Province, where you will find large outcroppings of quartzite, mica, and schist. Perhaps the most distinctive part of this province is the lower Susquehanna River gorge, which begins in the area around Chickies Rock just north of Columbia at US 30. To the south, the river is fed by streams that have their headwaters in the Great Valley. As the streams have made their way to the river over the years they have carved wonderful ravines, glens, and small gorges through weaknesses in the underlying strata. Several of the hikes in Lancaster County explore these hemlock- and rhododendron-filled steep hollows. One of these, Kelly's Run, in my eyes, is a national treasure. The Piedmont Province provides excellent opportunities for birding, with the Susquehanna River in this area being home to bald eagle, osprey, and many other birds that prefer a riparian environment.

Finally, the fourth and smallest physiographic province is South Mountain, which straddles the Pennsylvania and Maryland border south and west of York County. Characterized by rolling hills, many of which are capped with erosion-resistant white quartzite rock outcroppings, the lay of these mountains couldn't be more different than those found in the Valley and Ridge Province. Here, the mountains are much more irregular in shape and look more like one would expect a mountain range to look (some of the views in South Mountain remind me of northern New Mexico or New England). Unlike the hikes in the Valley and Ridge area, where you tend to have one big mile-long hill, the hikes in South Mountain tend to be rolling, with plenty of ups and downs. The region is thick with mountain laurel, the Pennsylvania state flower, and the foliage can be breathtaking in late May or early June.

All of the hikes in this book are on public lands that are administrated by several different state and local agencies. Many of the hikes make use of state game lands. Although there are no regulations concerning opening and closing hours for game lands, typically camping is not allowed except by thru-hikers on the Appalachian Trail corridor. Most important, when hiking on game lands, respect the rights of hunters. Exercise extra caution during hunting season and consider hiking on Sundays, when hunting is not allowed. From November 15 through December 15, you must wear at least 250 square inches of blaze orange (a vest and hat are adequate). As the signs say at many of the game-land entrances, "Hunters Wear Orange, So Should You!"

Many of the trails traversed by the hikes described in this book are marked with blazes, painted marks on trees indicating the path of the trail. A single named trail uses a blaze of one color. When you see blazes of multiple colors, that typically means that two or more trails are sharing a common path. Typically, a tree (or sometimes a rock) will be marked with a single blaze indicating that the trail continues basically straight. Double blazes of the same color indicate a change of direction, and you should take care to stay on track. Currently, no consistent system for blaze colors is used throughout this part of the state, with the exception of the Appalachian Trail, which is always marked with white blazes. So some hikes may have orange blazes, some red, some orange that look like red, some blue, pink, lavender, and so forth (I am not exaggerating). I have been told that Pennsylvania parks and public lands will be making a transition to the Appalachian Trail system over the next few years, meaning (I believe) that main trails will be blazed with white and side trails with blue. I am not sure how much confusion that will create and how much it will alleviate. Nonetheless, please beware that the trail markings may change over time (indeed, the trails themselves are often rerouted) and that in spite of how good the guidebook is, travel in the backcountry still requires sound judgment and making decisions.

The area covered by this book is extremely rich in both natural and cultural history, more than one can hope to learn in a lifetime. As I worked on this guide, I found the following three books indispensable for helping me to learn about the area:

The Geological Story of Pennsylvania, John H. Barnes and W. D. Sevon (The Pennsylvania Geological Survey, Harrisburg, PA, 2002).

Susquehanna: River of Dreams, Susan Q. Stranahan (Johns Hopkins University Press, Baltimore and London, 1993).

Wildlife of Pennsylvania and the Northeast, Charles Fergus and Amelia Hansen (Stackpole Books, Harrisburg, PA, 2000).

I also relied extensively on many of the nature and wildlife guides available in bookstores for helping me to identify and learn about the flora and fauna of the region.

I have tried to be as accurate as possible in my collection of information and data for this book, and in identifying what I have seen. I'm not a professional naturalist, so I may have misnamed things (the identification of trees beyond simple classifications of oak, maple, pine, spruce, hemlock, etc. continues to escape me). If you notice any errors, omissions, or changes in routes, or have suggestions for other hikes or comments, please contact me at **willenm@etown.edu.**

RECOMMENDED HIKES

HIKES 1–3 MILES

HIKES 3–6 MILES

HIKES 3–6 MILES *(continued)*

HIKES 6–9 MILES

HIKES > 9 MILES

HIKES ALONG CREEKS

HIKES GOOD FOR KIDS

HIKES WITH GOOD VIEWS

HIKES WITH GOOD VIEWS *(continued)*

HIKES GOOD FOR BIRD-WATCHING

HIKES GOOD FOR SEEING WILDLIFE

HIKES NEAR LAKES

HIKES WITH SPECIAL NATURAL OR HISTORICAL INTEREST

INTRODUCTION

Welcome to *60 Hikes within 60 Miles: Harrisburg*! If you're new to hiking or even if you're a seasoned trailsmith, take a few minutes to read the following introduction. We explain how this book is organized and how to use it.

HOW TO USE THIS GUIDEBOOK

THE OVERVIEW MAP AND OVERVIEW-MAP KEY

Use the overview map on the inside front cover to assess the exact locations of each hike's primary trailhead. Each hike's number appears on the overview map, on the map key facing the overview map, and in the table of contents. As you flip through the body of the book, a hike's full profile is easy to locate by watching for the hike number at the top of most right-hand pages. The book is organized by region, as indicated in the table of contents. A map legend that details the symbols found on trail maps appears on the inside back cover.

REGIONAL MAPS

The book is divided into regions, and prefacing each regional section is an overview map of that region. The regional provides more detail than the overview map, bringing you closer to the hike.

TRAIL MAPS

Each hike contains a detailed map that shows the trailhead, the route, significant features, facilities, and topographic landmarks such as creeks, overlooks, and peaks. The author gathered map data by carrying a GPS unit while hiking. This data was downloaded into a digital-mapping program, Topo USA, and processed by expert cartographers to produce the highly accurate maps found in this book. Each trailhead's GPS coordinates are included with each profile (see next page).

ELEVATION PROFILES

Corresponding directly to the trail map, each hike contains a detailed elevation profile. The elevation profile provides a quick look at the trail from the side, enabling you to visualize how the trail rises and falls. Key points along the way are labeled. Note the number of feet between each tick mark on the vertical axis (the height scale). To avoid making flat hikes look steep and steep hikes appear flat, height scales are used throughout the book to provide an accurate image of the hike's climbing difficulty.

GPS TRAILHEAD COORDINATES

To collect accurate map data, each trail was hiked with a handheld GPS unit (Garmin eTrex series). Data collected was then downloaded and plotted onto a digital U.S. Geological Survey (USGS) topographic map. In addition to rendering a highly specific trail outline, this book also includes the GPS coordinates for each trailhead in two formats: latitude–longitude and Universal Transverse Mercator (UTM). Latitude and longitude coordinates tell you where you are by locating a point west (latitude) of the 0° meridian line that passes through Greenwich, England, and north or south of the 0° (longitude) line that belts the earth, aka the equator.

Topographic maps show latitude–longitude as well as UTM grid lines. Known as UTM coordinates, the numbers index a specific point using a grid method. The survey datum used to arrive at the coordinates in this book is WGS84 (versus NAD27 or WGS83). For readers who own a GPS unit, whether handheld or onboard a vehicle, the latitude–longitude or UTM coordinates provided on the first page of each hike may be entered into the GPS unit. Just make sure your GPS unit is set to navigate using WGS84 datum. Now you can navigate directly to the trailhead.

Most trailheads, which begin in parking areas, can be reached by car, but some hikes still require a short walk to reach the trailhead from a parking area. In those cases, a handheld unit is necessary to continue the GPS navigation process. That said, however, readers can easily access all trailheads in this book by using the directions given, the overview map, and the trail map, which shows at least one major road leading into the area. But for those who enjoy using the latest GPS technology to navigate, the necessary data has been provided. A brief explanation of the UTM coordinates from Hike 7, Greenland Road Loop (page 42), follows.

UTM Zone	18T
Easting	0356918
Northing	4486658

The UTM zone number 18 refers to one of the 60 vertical zones of the UTM projection. Each zone is 6 degrees wide. The UTM zone letter T refers to one of the 20 horizontal zones that span from 80 degrees south to 84 degrees north. The easting number 0356918 indicates in meters how far east or west a point is from the central meridian of the zone. Increasing easting coordinates on a topo map or on your GPS screen indicate that you are moving east; decreasing easting coordinates indicate you are moving west. The northing number 4486658 references in meters how far you are from the equator. Above and below the equator, increasing northing coordinates indicate you are traveling north; decreasing northing coordinates indicate you are traveling south. To learn more about how to enhance your outdoor experiences with GPS technology, refer to *GPS Outdoors: A Practical Guide For Outdoor Enthusiasts* (Menasha Ridge Press).

HIKE DESCRIPTIONS

Each hike contains seven key items: an In Brief description of the trail, a Key At-a-Glance Information box, directions to the trail, GPS trailhead coordinates, a trail map, an elevation profile, and a trail description. Many hike profiles also include notes on nearby activities. Combined, the maps and information provide a clear method to assess each trail from the comfort of your favorite reading chair.

IN BRIEF

A "taste of the trail." Think of this section as a snapshot focused on the historical landmarks, beautiful vistas, and other sights you may encounter on the hike.

KEY AT-A-GLANCE INFORMATION

The information in the key at-a-glance boxes gives you a quick idea of the statistics and specifics of each hike.

LENGTH The length of the trail from start to finish (total distance traveled). There may be options to shorten or extend the hikes, but the mileage corresponds to the described hike. Consult the hike description to help decide how to customize the hike for your ability or time constraints.

CONFIGURATION A description of what the trail might look like from overhead. Trails can be loops, out-and-backs (trails on which one enters and leaves along the same path), figure eights, or a combination of shapes.

DIFFICULTY The degree of effort an "average" hiker should expect on a given hike. For simplicity, the trails are rated as "easy," "moderate," or "difficult."

SCENERY A short summary of the attractions offered by the hike and what to expect in terms of plant life, wildlife, natural wonders, and historic features.

EXPOSURE A quick check of how much sun you can expect on your shoulders during the hike.

TRAIL TRAFFIC Indicates how busy the trail might be on an average day. Trail traffic, of course, varies from day to day and season to season. Weekend days typically see the most visitors. Other trail users that may be encountered on the trail are also noted here.

TRAIL SURFACE Indicates whether the trail surface is paved, rocky, gravel, dirt, boardwalk, or a mixture of elements.

HIKING TIME How long it takes to hike the trail. A slow but steady hiker will average 2 to 3 miles an hour, depending on the terrain.

DRIVING DISTANCE Listed in miles.

ACCESS A notation of any fees or permits necessary to hike or park at the trailhead.

MAPS Here, you'll find a list of maps that show the topography of the trail, including Appalachian Trail maps, state-forest maps, and USGS topo maps.

FACILITIES What to expect in terms of restrooms and water at the trailhead or nearby.

WHEELCHAIR TRAVERSABLE Indicates whether all or part of the hike can be enjoyed by persons with disabilities.

SPECIAL COMMENTS Any extra details that don't fit into the categories above.

DIRECTIONS

Used in conjunction with the overview map, the driving directions will help you locate each trailhead. Once at the trailhead, park only in designated areas.

GPS TRAILHEAD COORDINATES

These can be used in addition to the driving directions if you enter the coordinates into your GPS unit before you set out. See page 2 for more information.

DESCRIPTION

The heart of each hike. Here, the authors provide a summary of the trail's essence and highlight any special traits the hike has to offer. The route is clearly outlined, including landmarks, side trips, and possible alternate routes along the way. Ultimately, the hike description will help you choose which hikes are best for you.

NEARBY ACTIVITIES

Look here for information on things to do or points of interest: nearby parks, museums, restaurants, and the like. Note that not every hike has a listing.

WEATHER

With the exception of rather short-lived extremes in weather, hiking can be done year-round in south-central Pennsylvania. Each season brings its own distinctive and pleasant features, all of which are worth exploring. My favorite time of year for getting out is the fall, which tends to offer many clear and crisp days, and, for a couple of weeks, the colorful foliage. If you spend enough time trekking around, you'll notice that fall brings other events, such as the seasonal hawk migrations, the shortening of the days, and a lot of hustle and bustle around the forest as the animals prepare for winter. The fall is also accompanied by the constant crunching of leaves beneath your feet, making it very difficult to be silent as you walk. Fall can also bring wet, cold rain—perfect conditions for hypothermia—so be prepared for sudden weather changes when you go out.

Winter brings the short days, rather stark lighting as the leaves have fallen from the trees, and occasional snowfalls. A snowpack of a couple of feet is not uncommon in the high country, but my experience shows that it tends to be rather short-lived. This is an especially good time of year for seeing fox, and for watching birds because it is more difficult for them to hide with the absence of foliage. Some of my nicest days out have been during the winter, though you do want to be prepared for sudden changes in weather and dips in temperature. At this time of year, you want to take special care around stream crossings, which are often icy, as a slip could have very unpleasant consequences.

Spring in south-central Pennsylvania can be a little muddy and wet, but this part of the state is home to many species of surprising and beautiful wildflowers. The bird and animal life becomes more active as they begin raising young, and the seasonal migrations can be extraordinary. Take a trip out to the Middle Creek Wildlife Management Area to view the snow geese migration. Again, be prepared for sudden changes in weather, particularly in March and April when cold rains are not atypical. This is also the time of year when streams run high, making some hikes impassable or more hazardous.

Finally, summers are characteristically warm and can be rather humid, especially getting into August. This is a great time of year to hike along the high ridges north of Harrisburg, but take care to hike early to avoid afternoon thunderstorms and the heat of midday. Be sure to carry plenty of water with you as the humidity can deplete your strength very quickly.

Average Temperatures by Month: Harrisburg

	Jan	Feb	Mar	Apr	May	Jun
High	38	41	51	63	73	81
Low	23	25	33	42	51	61

	Jul	Aug	Sep	Oct	Nov	Dec
High	86	84	76	64	53	42
Low	66	64	57	45	36	28

WATER

How much is enough? Well, one simple physiological fact should persuade you to err on the side of excess when deciding how much water to pack: A hiker working hard in 90-degree heat needs approximately 10 quarts of fluid per day. That's 2.5 gallons—12 large water bottles or 16 small ones. In other words, pack along one or two bottles even for short hikes.

Some hikers and backpackers hit the trail prepared to purify water found along the route. This method, while less dangerous than drinking it untreated, comes with risks. Purifiers with ceramic filters are the safest. Many hikers pack along the slightly distasteful tetraglycine–hydroperiodide tablets to de-bug water (sold under the names Potable Aqua, Coughlan's, and others).

Probably the most common waterborne "bug" that hikers face is giardia, which may not hit until one to four weeks after ingestion. It will have you living in the bathroom, passing noxious rotten-egg gas, vomiting, and shivering with chills. Other parasites to worry about include E. coli and cryptosporidium, both of which are harder to kill than giardia.

For most people, the pleasures of hiking make carrying water a relatively minor price to pay to remain healthy. If you're tempted to drink "found water," do so only if you understand the risks involved. Better yet, hydrate prior to your hike, carry (and drink) 6 ounces of water for every mile you plan to hike, and hydrate after the hike.

CLOTHING

Use common sense when dressing for a hike and be prepared for sudden changes in weather. I always check the forecast before I go out for a hike, and then I always count on it being worse than predicted. Getting caught without the appropriate clothes can be both dangerous and uncomfortable.

In the summertime, I tend to hike in shorts and T-shirt. In my pack, however, I carry rain gear (both a jacket and pants) and a wool sweater or some type of synthetic pullover (polypropylene, Capilene, Thermax, etc.). I also wear a broad-brimmed hat during the summer as the sun can be very strong. In the winter, I dress in layers, and carry a GORE-TEX jacket and wind pants. I wear gloves, a wool hat, and wool socks. Because I hike alone quite often, I always ask myself, "What if?" I typically pack so that I have enough clothes to spend a night if doing so should become necessary. In the winter, I always carry an extra set of dry pile pants and top with me. Pennsylvania winters can be notoriously damp and stream crossings can be troublesome.

Footwear is something that needs to be taken rather seriously when hiking around south-central Pennsylvania. For most of the rail-trails, you can get away with a good pair of sneakers or lightweight pair of hiking books. When you get into the backcountry, you would be foolhardy not to wear a good, sturdy pair of boots. Many of the trails are extremely rocky and rugged. By wearing lightweight boots, not only do you risk a sprained ankle, but you can also develop some very painful foot injuries (such as heel spurs) that take a long time to heal. I typically wear a traditional pair of one-piece leather hiking boots, and I don't have problems.

THE TEN ESSENTIALS

One of the first rules of hiking is to be prepared for anything. The simplest way to be prepared is to carry the "Ten Essentials." In addition to carrying the items listed below, you need to know how to use them, especially navigation items. Always consider worst-case scenarios like getting lost, hiking back in the dark, broken gear (for example, a broken hip strap on your pack or a water filter getting plugged), twisting an ankle, or a brutal thunderstorm. The items listed below don't cost a lot of money, don't take up much room in a pack, and don't weigh much, but they might just save your life.

Water: durable bottles, and water treatment like iodine or a filter
Map: preferably a topo map and a trail map with a route description
Compass: a high-quality compass
First-aid kit: a good-quality kit including first-aid instructions
Knife: a multitool device with pliers is best
Light: flashlight or headlamp with extra bulbs and batteries
Fire: windproof matches or lighter and fire starter
Extra food: you should always have food in your pack when you've finished hiking
Extra clothes: rain protection, warm layers, gloves, warm hat
Sun protection: sunglasses, lip balm, sunblock, sun hat

FIRST-AID KIT

A typical first-aid kit may contain more items than you might think necessary. These are just the basics. Prepackaged kits in waterproof bags (Atwater Carey and Adventure Medical make a variety of kits) are available. Even though there are quite a few items listed here, they pack down into a small space:

Ace bandages or Spenco joint wraps
Antibiotic ointment (Neosporin or the generic equivalent)
Aspirin or acetaminophen
Band-Aids
Benadryl or the generic equivalent, diphenhydramine (in case of allergic reactions)
Butterfly-closure bandages
Epinephrine in a prefilled syringe (for people known to have severe allergic reactions to such things as bee stings)
Gauze (one roll)
Gauze compress pads (a half-dozen 4 x 4-inch pads)
Hydrogen peroxide or iodine
Insect repellent
Matches or pocket lighter
Moleskin or Spenco "Second Skin"
Sunscreen
Whistle (it's more effective in signaling rescuers than your voice)

HIKING WITH CHILDREN

No one is too young for a hike in the outdoors. Be mindful, though. Flat, short, and shaded trails are best with an infant. Toddlers who have not quite mastered walking can still tag along, riding on an adult's back in a child carrier. Use common sense to judge a child's capacity to hike a particular trail, and always count that the child will tire quickly and need to be carried.

When packing for the hike, remember the child's needs as well as your own. Make sure children are adequately clothed for the weather, have proper shoes, and are protected from the sun with sunscreen. Kids dehydrate quickly, so make sure you have plenty of fluid for everyone. To assist an adult with determining which trails are suitable for children, a list of hike recommendations for children is provided on page xxi.

GENERAL SAFETY

In addition to the wonderful places you come across in the backcountry, much of the excitement of going for a hike stems from having to make decisions and having to be somewhat self-reliant. There is no reason why exploring the woods should not be as safe as or safer than traveling around an urban area. Yet, being safe requires a certain presence of mind. When I go out into the woods, whether for a couple of hours or a couple of weeks, I try to adopt what I call an "expedition mentality," something that I learned many years ago when I spent a lot of time climbing mountains. That is to say, I always behave and make decisions as if rescue or assistance were days away. Getting hurt or lost isn't an option from this mindset, and rather than do something foolhardy, it is best to just turn back. Here are some things that you can do to help make your excursions safe and enjoyable.

- **Always let someone know your itinerary. Leave word about where you are going, when you will return, and what should be done if you are overdue. No matter how careful you are, things do happen. Someone knowing your plans can be critical if an emergency arises. That said, always let the person know when you have returned.**

- **Always carry food and water whether you are planning to go overnight or not. Food will give you energy, help keep you warm, and sustain you in an emergency situation until help arrives. You never know if you will have a stream nearby when you become thirsty. Bring potable water or treat water before drinking it from a stream. Boil or filter all found water before drinking it.**

- **Stay on designated trails. Most hikers get lost when they leave the path. Even on the most clearly marked trails, there is usually a point where you have to stop and consider which direction to head. If you become disoriented, don't panic. As soon as you think you may be off-track, stop, assess your current direction, and then retrace your steps back to the point where you went awry. Using map, compass, and this book, and keeping in mind what you have passed thus far, reorient yourself, and trust your judgment on which way to continue. If you become absolutely unsure of how to continue, return to your vehicle the way you came in. Should you become completely lost and have no idea of how to return to the trailhead, remaining in place along the** trail and waiting for help is most often the best option for adults and always the best option for children.

- Be especially careful when crossing streams. Whether you are fording the stream or crossing on a log, make every step count. If you have any doubt about maintaining your balance on a foot log, go ahead and ford the stream instead. When fording a stream, use a trekking pole or stout stick for balance and face upstream as you cross. If a stream seems too deep to ford, turn back. Whatever is on the other side is not worth risking your life.

- Be careful at overlooks. While these areas may provide spectacular views, they are potentially hazardous. Stay back from the edge of outcrops and be absolutely sure of your footing; a misstep can mean a nasty and possibly fatal fall.

- Standing dead trees and storm-damaged living trees pose a real hazard to hikers and tent campers. These trees may have loose or broken limbs that could fall at any time. When choosing a spot to rest or a backcountry campsite, look up.

- Know the symptoms of hypothermia. Shivering and forgetfulness are the two most common indicators of this insidious killer. Hypothermia can occur at any elevation, even in the summer, especially when the hiker is wearing lightweight cotton clothing. If symptoms arise, get the victim shelter, hot liquids, and dry clothes or a dry sleeping bag.

- Take along your brain. A cool, calculating mind is the single most important piece of equipment you'll ever need on the trail. Think before you act. Watch your step. Plan ahead. Avoiding accidents before they happen is the best recipe for a rewarding and relaxing hike.

- Ask questions. Forest and park employees are there to help. It's a lot easier to gain advice beforehand and avoid a mishap away from civilization when it's too late to amend an error. Use your head out there and treat the place as if it were your own backyard.

ANIMAL AND PLANT HAZARDS

TICKS

Ticks like to hang out in the brush that grows along trails. Hot summer months seem to explode their numbers, but you should be tick-aware during all months of the year. Ticks, which are arthropods and not insects, need a host to feast on in order to reproduce. The ticks that light onto you while hiking will be very small, sometimes so tiny that you won't be able to spot them. Primarily of two varieties, deer ticks and dog ticks, both need a few hours of actual attachment before they can transmit any disease they may harbor. The best way to avoid getting ticks is by wearing long pants tucked into your socks. This is not always pleasant when hiking in the summer. Alternately, or in addition, use a bug spray that contains DEET, which is very effective. I typically spray my pants, socks, and boots when I go out. Ticks may settle in shoes, socks, and hats, and may take several hours to actually latch on. The best strategy is to visually check every half hour or so while hiking, do a thorough check before you get in the car, and then, when you take a posthike shower, do an even more thorough check of your entire body. Ticks that haven't attached are easily removed but not easily killed. If you pick off a tick in the woods, just toss it aside. If you find one on your body at home, dispatch it and then send it down the toilet. For ticks that have embedded, removal with tweezers is best. If you suspect that an embedded tick is a deer tick, which carries Lyme disease, put it in a plastic bag and call your doctor. Many times doctors will have the tick checked for Lyme disease, so that treatment can begin before symptoms arise.

SNAKES

South-central Pennsylvania is home to two types of poisonous snake—the timber rattler and the copperhead. In all of my travels, I have seen neither. Nonetheless, they are out there and you should bear this in mind, particularly when travel-

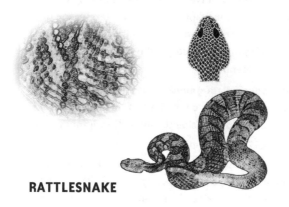

RATTLESNAKE

ing the rocky, mountainous areas. Be careful if you move rocks or when climbing around outcrops where snakes like to sun themselves. If you see any snake that has a diamond-shaped head (characteristic of many poisonous snakes) or have any doubts, give it a wide berth. There is no need to bother any wildlife you come across.

POISON IVY, OAK, AND SUMAC

Recognizing poison ivy, oak, and sumac and avoiding contact with them is the most effective way to prevent the painful, itchy rashes associated with these plants. In central Pennsylvania, poison ivy ranges from a thick, tree-hugging vine to a shaded ground cover, three leaflets to a leaf; poison oak occurs as either a vine or shrub, with three leaflets as well; and poison sumac flourishes in swampland, each leaf containing 7 to 13 leaflets. Urushiol, the oil in the sap of these plants, is responsible for the rash. Usually within 12 to 14 hours of exposure (but sometimes much later), raised lines and/or blisters will appear, accompanied by a terrible itch. Refrain from scratching because bacteria under fingernails can cause infection and you will spread the rash to other parts of your body. Wash and dry the rash thoroughly, applying calamine lotion or another product to help dry the rash. If itching or blistering is severe, seek medical attention. Remember that oil-contaminated clothes, pets, or hiking gear can easily cause an irritating rash on you or someone else, so wash not only any exposed parts of your body but also clothes, gear, and pets.

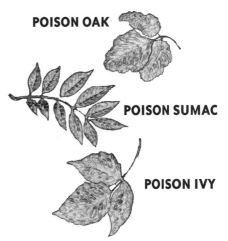

POISON OAK

POISON SUMAC

POISON IVY

MOSQUITOES

Although it's not a common occurrence, individuals can become infected with the West Nile virus by being bitten by an infected mosquito. Culex mosquitoes, the primary varieties that can transmit West Nile virus to humans, thrive in urban rather than natural areas. They lay their eggs in stagnant water and can breed in any standing water that remains for more than five days. Most people infected with West Nile virus have no symptoms of illness, but some may become ill, usually 3 to 15 days after being bitten.

In south-central Pennsylvania, late spring and summer are the times thought to be the highest risk periods for West Nile virus. At this time of year—and anytime you expect mosquitoes to be buzzing around—you may want to wear protective clothing, such as long sleeves, long pants, and socks. Loose-fitting, light-colored clothing is best. Spray clothing with insect repellent. Remember to follow the instructions on the repellent and to take extra care with children.

WILDLIFE

The mountains around central Pennsylvania are home to a wide variety of wildlife, including white-tailed deer, black bear, bobcats, foxes, raccoons, porcupines, etc. For the most part, these animals pose little danger unless they feel threatened or harassed. If you see any wildlife, it is okay to watch from a distance, but it is neither safe nor ethically sound to approach it, feed it, or engage it in any fashion. Consider yourself a guest in its home. Black bears are probably the only mammals that may pose any sort of threat. In spite of there being a fair population in the area, I've never come across one, though I have seen tracks and droppings on several occasions. If you encounter a bear in the woods, it will likely run off. If not, try to look large, make noise, and back away slowly. Don't run off or climb a tree.

TIPS FOR ENJOYING HARRISBURG

Before you go out for a hike, do some homework to make sure things go as smoothly as possible. Check the forecast to find out what the weather is going to be like so you can plan accordingly. There is no reason not to hike when it is raining, provided you're not venturing out into a hurricane or thunderstorm. Just dress appropriately. Some of nature's finest wonders reveal themselves during foul weather. If you are like me and enjoy solitude, try to hike during the week. I do most of my hiking during the week and I never see anybody, except along the Appalachian Trail.

Review the descriptions in this book to see if you are up for the hike. In particular, you might find the elevation profiles included in each chapter to be very helpful. From them, you can get a pretty good sense of how much climbing and descending you will have to do. Also, plan plenty of time for your hike. The hiking times I provided are based on a hiking speed of about 2 miles per hour. Many people may think that is somewhat slow. Personally, I am in no rush when I get out in the woods; I want to spend as much time out as possible. If you like to look at flowers or take pictures or simply sit and relax, allow more time. This area of Pennsylvania is not a place that lends itself to the sweeping view of the landscape. Many of its treasures are small and easily overlooked. You will feel more relaxed, and you will see more things if you take your time and take a closer look at the land around you. You will be surprised by what is out there.

TOPO MAPS

The maps in this book have been produced with great care and, used with the hiking directions, will direct you to the trail and help you stay on course. However, you will find superior detail and valuable information in the USGS's 7.5-minute-series topographic maps. Topo maps are available online in many locations, including a well-known free service at **terraserver.microsoft.com.** Another free service with fast click-and-drag browsing is located at **www.topofinder.com.** You can view and print topos of the entire United States from these Web sites, and view aerial photographs of the same area at terraserver. Several online services such as **www.trails.com** charge annual fees for additional features such as shaded relief, which makes the topography stand out more. If you expect to print out many topo maps each year, it might be worth paying for shaded-relief topo maps. The downside to USGS topos is that many of them are outdated, having been created 20 to 30 years ago. But they still provide excellent topographic detail.

Digital topographic-map programs such as DeLorme's Topo USA enable you to review topo maps of the entire United States on your PC. You can also gather your own data while hiking with a GPS unit, then download the data onto the software and plot your own hikes.

If you're new to hiking, you might be wondering, "What's a topographic map?" In short, a topo indicates not only linear distance but elevation as well, using contour lines. Contour lines spread across the map like dozens of intricate spider webs. Each line represents a particular elevation, and at the base of each topo, a contour's interval designation is given. If the contour interval is 20 feet, then the distance between each contour line is 20 feet. Follow five contour lines up on the same map, and the elevation has increased by 100 feet.

Let's assume that the 7.5-minute-series topo reads "Contour Interval 40 feet," that the short trail we'll be hiking is two inches in length on the map, and that it crosses five contour lines from beginning to end. What do we know? Well, because the linear scale of this series is 2,000 feet to the inch (with roughly 2¾ inches representing 1 mile), we know our trail is approximately four-fifths of a mile long (with 2 inches representing 4,000 feet). But we also know we'll be climbing or descending 200 vertical feet (five contour lines are 40 feet each) over that distance. And the elevation designations written on occasional contour lines will tell us if we're heading up or down.

In addition to the outdoor shops listed in the Appendixes, you'll find topos at major universities and some public libraries, where you might try photocopying the ones you need to avoid the cost of buying them. But if you want your own and can't find them locally, visit the USGS Web site at **topomaps.usgs.gov.**

TRAIL ETIQUETTE

Whether you're on a city, county, state, or national-park trail, always remember that great care and resources (from nature as well as from your tax dollars) have gone into creating these trails. Treat the trail, wildlife, and fellow hikers with respect.

- **Hike on open trails only. Respect trail and road closures (ask if not sure), avoid possible trespassing on private land, and obtain all permits and authorization as required. Also, leave gates as you found them or as marked.**

- **Leave only footprints. Be sensitive to the ground beneath you. This also means staying on the existing trail and not blazing any new trails. Be sure to pack out what you pack in. No one likes to see the trash someone else has left behind.**

- **Never spook animals. An unannounced approach, a sudden movement, or a loud noise startles most animals. A surprised animal can be dangerous to you, to others, and to itself. Give it plenty of space.**

- **Plan ahead. Know your equipment, your ability, and the area in which you are hiking—and prepare accordingly. Be self-sufficient at all times; carry necessary supplies for changes in weather or other conditions. A well-executed trip is a satisfaction to you and to others.**

- **Be courteous to other hikers, bikers, equestrians, and others you encounter on the trails.**

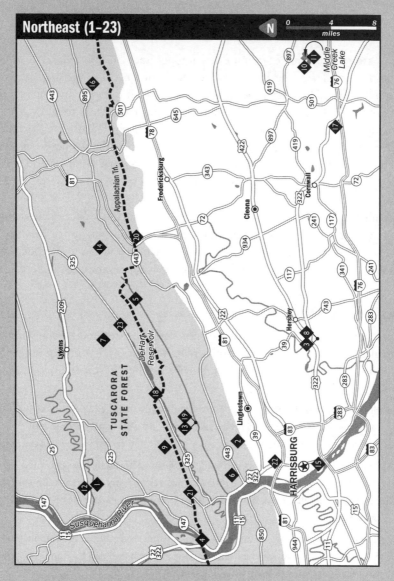

NORTHEAST

01 BERRY'S MOUNTAIN

ⓘ KEY AT-A-GLANCE INFORMATION

LENGTH: About 2.5 miles
CONFIGURATION: Balloon
DIFFICULTY: Moderate
SCENERY: Berry's Mountain
EXPOSURE: More shade than sun
TRAIL TRAFFIC: Light
TRAIL SURFACE: Dirt
HIKING TIME: About 2 hours
DRIVING DISTANCE:
ACCESS: 8 a.m.–dusk
MAPS: USGS Millersburg; Ned Smith Center for Nature and Art Trail Guide available at the center bookstore
FACILITIES: None at trail; water and restrooms available at the Ned Smith Center on Water Co. Road
WHEELCHAIR TRAVERSABLE: No
SPECIAL COMMENTS: At the time of this writing, not all of the trails were blazed. This hike therefore requires some fundamental route-finding skills.

GPS Trailhead Coordinates

UTM Zone (WGS84)   18T
Easting   337381
Northing   4487903
Latitude   N 40° 31′ 33.33″
Longitude   W 76° 55′ 11.47″

IN BRIEF

This hike begins with a straightforward walk along the ridge of Berry's Mountain to the first set of power lines. From there it descends the Powerline Trail (very steep!) to an unmarked trail heading east. Following that trail, it gradually climbs back to the ridge, along Ned's Trail. Some of the trail junctions are not easy to locate.

DESCRIPTION

This hike makes a loop on the crest and north side of Berry's Mountain just a few miles west of Millersburg. All of the trails are on land that belongs to the Ned Smith Center for Nature and Art. At the time of this writing, some the trails were still under development, meaning that the trails are there, though some of the junctions are a little difficult to find and some of the trails are not blazed. Personally, I found these facts to be quite appealing. Making the

Directions ⟶

From PA 147 in Millersburg, turn right onto PA 209 and follow it for 1.85 miles to Water Co. Road. Turn right. Follow Water Co. Road downhill past the Ned Smith Center for Nature and Art to Woodside Station Road (about 0.7 miles). Turn right and follow Woodside Station Road over the creek and make the first right after the bridge. Woodside Station Road is now dirt. In about 100 yards, you'll reach the trailhead for the Railroad Bed Trail. Woodside Station Road continues uphill to the left and climbs to the ridge of Berry's Mountain in 0.85 miles, where you will find scattered parking and the trailhead. *Note:* Beyond the Railroad Bed Trail trailhead, Woodside Station Road becomes very steep and rugged and may not be passable by vehicles with low clearance or after heavy rains.

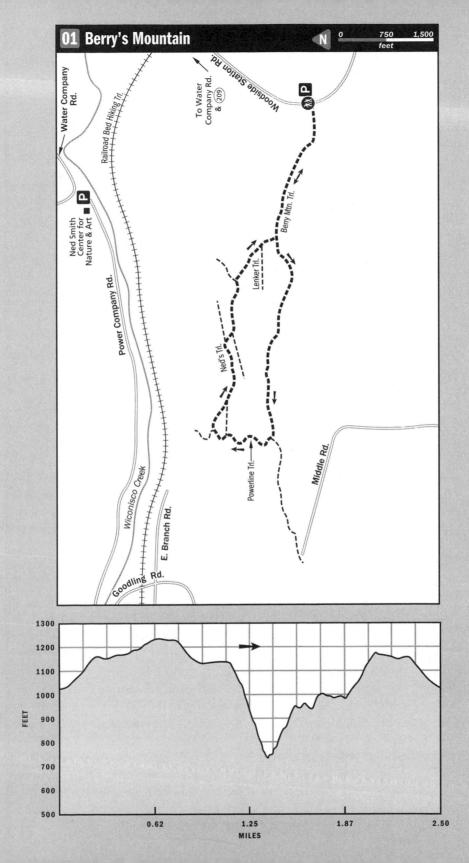

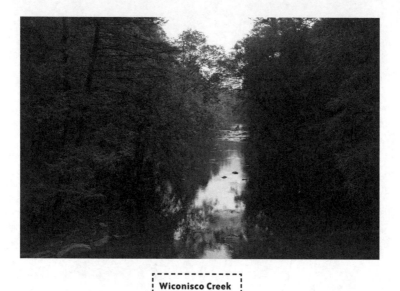

Wiconisco Creek

excursion on the lower section of the mountain required some route-finding decisions and got my attention.

Begin this hike at the crest of Woodside Station Road. Pick up the blue-blazed Berry Mountain Trail, an obvious dirt road at the ridge crest heading to the west. The trail climbs rather steeply and is somewhat washed out at first before it levels out and improves. The Berry's Mountain ridge is quite lovely, with its maple, beech, oak, and black gum trees, and pretty understory of sassafras. I found the Berry Mountain Trail, though, to be something of a disappointment, as I passed a couple of ATVs along the trail (which are not allowed to be on the trails owned by the Ned Smith Center), and I saw a lot of trash on the trail. I try to pick up bottles and cans and other garbage that I come across, and I encourage readers to do the same. A little bit of effort by each hiker makes an enormous difference.

Follow the Berry's Mountain Trail for about 1.1 miles out to where it passes beneath a power line. Along the way (about 0.5 miles), you'll pass a road descending steeply to the north by a pair of white blazes. This marks the beginning of the loop part of the hike and you will return via that trail. Don't give in to the temptation to do the loop counterclockwise and head off down that trail. Hiking up that trail may look a little tough, but it is much more pleasant than hiking up the Powerline Trail would be. Plus, locating the trails while hiking west across the north side of Berry's Mountain would be considerably more difficult than following them from the Powerline Trail east.

Another half mile or so beyond that trail you'll reach the power lines, which afford a beautiful view of the island-studded Susquehanna River to the south and to the Wiconisco Valley to the north. If you continue straight along the ridge from here, you'll come out to a gate and a parking area at the end of Middle Road in about 0.25 miles. It is not especially worth the extra walking.

Instead, head over to the north edge of the ridge and pick up the *very* steep dirt road just to the left (west) of the power lines. This is the Powerline Trail. Take your time as you hike down this trail along the north side of the ridge. If you have weak knees, you may want to bring some ski poles or a hiking stick for the descent. The path weaves back and forth beneath the power lines from one edge of the cut to the other. The second time the trail reaches the east side of the cut, you'll see a small cairn on a rock on the right, indicating that a trail heads off into the woods to the east. Reaching that trail from this point is difficult, so instead continue a little farther downhill as the trail leads over to the other side of the cut and then back to the east side again, just above a set of power line towers (1.4 miles). To be sure, this is the third time the trail reaches the woods on the east side of the power-line cut. Enter the woods to the east, heading slightly uphill along a not-so-obvious path. Soon the path becomes quite obvious and after about 200 feet joins with an old haul road. Follow the haul road to the east across the hillside, climbing gradually. The path is not blazed but is easy to follow.

The next bit of fun comes in locating the next trail junction, about 0.25 miles from the power lines. The haul road you are following levels out and then begins to descend by a large oak tree on the left. Just before reaching that tree, you'll come to a small level area along the steep hillside by a couple of saplings. At the time of this writing, a piece of orange flagging was tied to a tree marking the junction to the right. Hike up the little (5 feet) hill to the right of the haul road and the trail will be obvious. Continue east along this trail, and soon it reaches another old haul road, now covered with many saplings. Turn left and follow the path as it winds through the saplings. This is a very pretty section of the hike, and is worth the trip itself.

Soon enough you'll come to a very obvious path (1.9 miles), onto which you will turn right, heading uphill. The going is rather steep and gets a little more so near the top of the ridge, but the trail is good and the walking is pleasant. Soon you'll pass the Lenker Trail (gray blazes) on the right (2 miles). This trail is named for Harold and Thelma Lenker, who donated to the Ned Smith Center the land upon which the trail is located. Shortly beyond, attain the ridge and the Berry's Mountain Trail. Catch your breath, turn left, and walk back down to the car.

NEARBY ACTIVITIES

Be sure to visit the Ned Smith Center for Nature and Art on Water Co. Road. In Millersburg, you'll find a nice restaurant, the Wooden Nickel, at the town square. The Millersburg Ferry is also worth a visit. It is the last operational ferry on the Susquehanna River. The paddle-wheel boat has room for three cars and passengers, and the trip across the river takes about 30 minutes. Follow signs for the ferry from the town square.

02 BOYD BIG TREE PRESERVE CONSERVATION AREA

KEY AT-A-GLANCE INFORMATION

LENGTH: 5.1 miles

CONFIGURATION: Loop

DIFFICULTY: Moderate

SCENERY: Conservation area environs and nice views of the Lebanon Valley to the north from the Janie Trail

EXPOSURE: More shade than sun

TRAIL TRAFFIC: Light

TRAIL SURFACE: Dirt

HIKING TIME: 2.5–3 hours

DRIVING DISTANCE: 3 miles from junction of PA 443 and US 22/322 west of Harrisburg

ACCESS: Dawn–dusk

MAPS: USGS Harrisburg East; maps of the park are available at the parking area.

FACILITIES: Water, toilets, telephone, picnic tables

WHEELCHAIR TRAVERSABLE: No

SPECIAL COMMENTS: This hike combines several trails, all well marked, to follow the perimeter of the conservation area. A multitude of variations to it can be made with assistance from the park map.

IN BRIEF

From the parking area, this hike follows the Pond Loop Trail to the Creek Trail and the Coach Trail along the western edge of the conservation area. After a short climb, this hike joins the Janie Trail and follows it along the ridge to the eastern edge of the conservation area. A short stretch on the Upper Spring Trail takes you to the East Loop Trail and then back to the parking lot.

DESCRIPTION

Located only 8 miles or so from downtown Harrisburg, the Boyd Big Tree Conservation Area is a gem of a recreation area. The park is similar in design to the Joseph Ibberson Conservation Area located two valleys to the north, with its educational pavilion on the edge of the parking area overlooking a valley to the north (see page 50). The Boyd Big Tree area was established in 1999 thanks to Alexander Boyd of the Union Deposit Corporation, who donated the land for conservation purposes. Situated mostly on the north side of Blue Mountain, the area provides habitat to diverse species of tall trees, wildflowers, birds, and mammals. The park sports seven trails of various lengths and difficulties, providing a variety of options for exploring the terrain, viewing

GPS Trailhead Coordinates

UTM Zone (WGS84) 18T

Easting   342855

Northing   4468674

Latitude   N 40° 21′ 13.80″

Longitude   W 76° 51′ 1.81″

Directions

From US 22/322 west of Harrisburg, take the PA 443, Fishing Creek, exit. Follow 443 east for about 2.8 miles. Turn right onto the access road for the park (marked by a sign), just beyond Frog Hollow Road. The parking area is at the top of the hill.

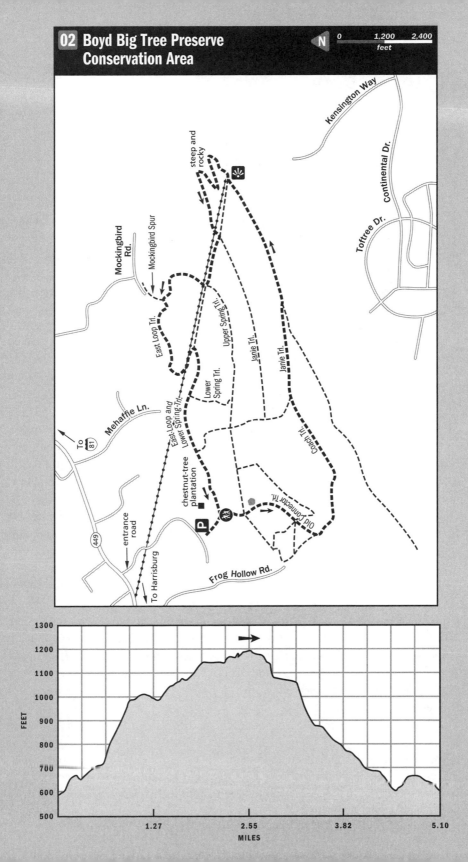

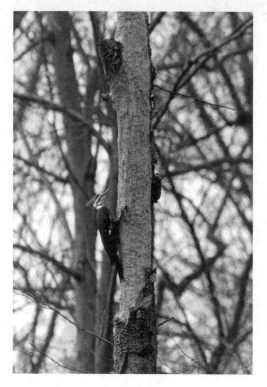

Pileated woodpecker

some of the plant and animal life, and simply getting a little bit of peace and quiet.

This hike strings together several of the park trails to create an excursion around the perimeter of the conservation area. Much of the walking is on old logging roads that have been converted to trails, so the grades are generally easy and the footing is mostly pleasant and secure. Start out by following the pink-blazed Pond Loop Trail southeast from the parking area, staying right at a junction after a couple of hundred feet. Continue uphill following the pink blazes, passing another trail junction at approximately 0.25 miles. From that junction the trail descends to the small pond, surrounded by stands of cattails and thicket on its banks. You'll find a bench at the far end of the pond and several bird boxes in the area.

As you pass the pond on the old logging road to its right, take a look off into the woods and notice the prolific signs of woodpeckers on the trees. In addition to the common downy woodpeckers, if you keep your eyes open you may also see the large pileated woodpecker, redheaded woodpeckers, and even some flickers. Follow the path uphill for a short distance to the junction with the East Creek Trail, identified by its blue blazes. The Pond Loop turns left here. Continue straight on the East Creek Trail for 200 feet or so at which point the main blue trail heads downhill and an old connector trail with blue blazes continues ahead. Go straight on the connector trail for about 0.15 miles to the main East Creek Trail again at the edge of the park and turn left, heading uphill for a short distance to a Y-intersection with the yellow-blazed Coach Trail. Turn right at the Y, and follow the Coach Trail.

The Coach Trail follows an old coach road for about 0.75 miles across the hillside through a lovely forest of mature white oak, poplar, hickory, and beech trees. At the end of the Coach Trail, you'll reach the red-blazed Janie Trail, which makes a 2.5-mile loop through the park. Turn right and follow the red blazes as the trail rises gently along the side of Blue Mountain to its ridge. At the crest, you'll get a nice view of the Lebanon Valley to the south. A major geographic feature southeast of the Valley and Ridge Province, the Lebanon Valley is one section of the

Great Valley, an unbroken valley that extends from New York to Georgia. A small meadow on the ridge provides habitat for many songbirds and bedding for white-tailed deer. From the crest, the Janie Trail makes a left turn and follows the ridge just south of the crest for 0.65 miles to some power lines. Along the way, you'll pass through sections of dense thicket, which provide cover for many songbirds. The clear-cut at the power lines is a great place to spot cardinals, bluebirds, and chickadees, and offers a nice view of the valleys to the south and to the north from the ridgetop.

At the power lines, follow the trail to the right back into the woods and along the ridge for a short distance. As you walk along, keep your eyes open to the left for a small cairn that marks the place where the Janie Trail leaves the old roadbed and heads over the ridge to the north. The junction is tough to spot, particularly in the fall. If you reach a gate across the roadbed, you've gone about 100 feet too far. From the junction, you should be able to spot a red blaze on prominent silver-barked tree to the north of the road. Follow the blazes to the north side of the ridge, where the trail leads back west toward the power lines. The trail gets rocky in this area, then makes a switchback by some tall spruce trees, and descends a steep and rugged bit before reaching another old coach road at about 2.9 miles. Turn left (west) on the road and walk out to the power lines, where you'll turn right on to the Upper Spring Trail, marked by a white blaze on a post. Head downhill beneath the power lines and turn right onto the green-blazed East Loop Trail just before you reach the second tower.

Also an old roadbed, the East Loop Trail winds through a beautiful section of forest with pine trees scattered among the hardwoods. As the trail bends back to the west, it comes to a T-intersection above a hollow on the left where you will stay to the right. At about 4.2 miles, you'll regain the power line again at a pretty area where a small creek flows beneath—yet another great place for birding here. The East Loop Trail leaves the power line and heads west for just shy of a mile to the junction with the Pond Loop Trail near the parking lot.

At the parking area, be sure to take a walk to the plantation of young chestnut trees surrounded by a fence across from the pavilion. Chestnuts were all but wiped out earlier in the 20th century by blight, and this represents an attempt at redeveloping the species. The bird boxes surrounding the plantation provide homes for eastern bluebirds, which are abundant in the area.

NEARBY ACTIVITIES

The Fort Hunter Mansion north of the Harrisburg city limits provides an interesting historical excursion, with its museum and mansion, not to mention a view of the Susquehanna River and a nice place to picnic and walk. Follow PA 443 west to Front Street and turn left. The park is about 0.5 miles ahead on the right.

03   BULLFROG VALLEY NATURE PATH

KEY AT-A-GLANCE INFORMATION

LENGTH: 3.1 miles

CONFIGURATION: Balloon

DIFFICULTY: Easy–moderate

SCENERY: Bullfrog Valley Pond and creek; Shank Park environs

EXPOSURE: Mostly shaded

TRAIL TRAFFIC: Moderately heavy

TRAIL SURFACE: Paved and dirt sections

HIKING TIME: 1.5 hours

DRIVING DISTANCE: 0.8 miles from US 322 in Hershey

ACCESS: Dawn–dusk

MAPS: USGS Hershey and Middletown

FACILITIES: Portable toilet, soda/water machines, picnic pavilion at trailhead

WHEELCHAIR TRAVERSABLE: The first 0.85 miles are paved.

SPECIAL COMMENTS: Although the trail can get busy, within Shank Park it is always possible to find some peace and privacy at one of the many benches along the hike.

IN BRIEF

This hike follows the paved Jonathan Eshenour Memorial Trail beneath a canopy of tall tulip poplars into Shank Park. Upon entering the park, the nature trail departs from the Eshenour Trail and makes a loop around the perimeter of the park.

DESCRIPTION

The Shank Park–Bullfrog Pond Nature Trail begins at the Bullfrog Valley Pond parking area and then follows a 0.85-mile section of the Jonathan Eshenour Memorial Trail south to Shank Park. At that point, the nature trail departs from the Eshenour Trail, enters the woods, and makes a 1.5-mile loop through the environs of the 90-acre Shank Park before rejoining the paved Eshenour Trail and returning to the car.

To begin this hike, walk from your car in the Bullfrog Valley Pond parking lot across the footbridge over the feeder stream to Bullfrog Valley Pond, and turn left on the Eshenour Trail. A box containing a numbered "life list" of the different flora you can spot on the hike is located on the right side of the trail. The list is impressive, with approximately 170 entries, more than 50 of which are broadleaf trees alone. The numbers on the list correspond to

GPS Trailhead Coordinates

UTM Zone (WGS84) 18T

Easting 356777

Northing 4457700

Latitude N 40° 15′ 27.06″

Longitude W 76° 41′ 3.04″

Directions ———————————→

From US 322 in Hershey, head south on Bullfrog Valley Road. This is either the first light after US 322 and US 422 split coming from the west or the last light before they join coming from the east (just beyond the Penn State Milton S. Hershey Medical Center). The parking lot for Bullfrog Valley Park is 0.82 miles ahead on the right, just past the intersection with Wood Road at the obvious duck pond.

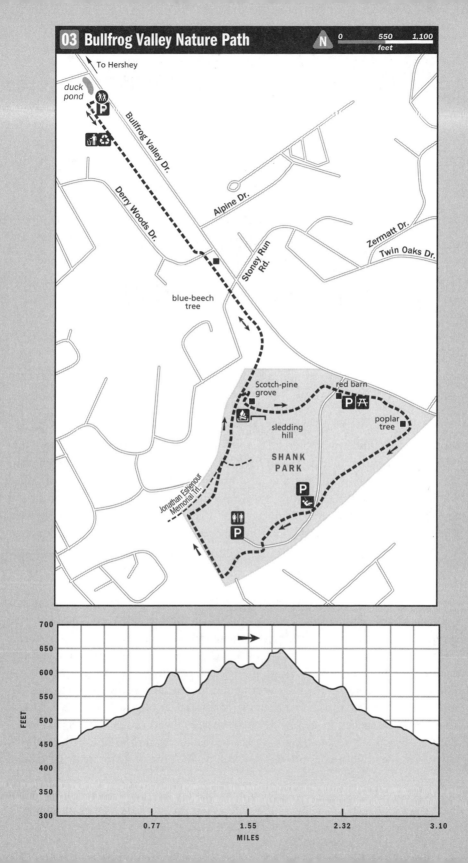

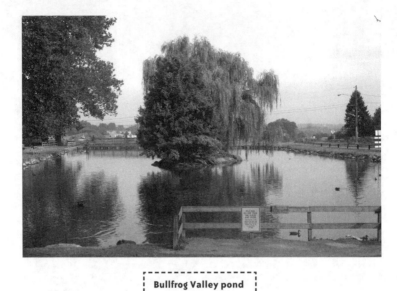

Bullfrog Valley pond

small numbered signs posted on trees or placed into the ground to make for easy identification. The variety of trees makes the hike a spectacular blaze of color during the fall.

The nature trail here follows the Eshenour Trail along the path of the old Brownstone–Middletown Railroad grade. Originally a wagon road used for transporting brownstone blocks from quarries west of Waltonville Road, the railroad was developed along this path because breakage of the stone was too common when hauled by wagon. In 1892, a standard-gauge railroad was built that hauled the stone for approximately 3 miles to the Reading Railroad in Hummelstown. The railroad was rather short-lived, ending operations in 1939 when brick became a cheaper alternative to quarried brownstone. Nonetheless, in its heyday, brownstone was a sought-after building material, and the stone quarried in Pennsylvania was shipped as far away as Tampa, Chicago, and St. Louis.

The railroad bed is now a lovely paved walking trail that climbs gently up Bullfrog Valley, parallel to the course of the small Bullfrog Creek. On this lower section of the path, you walk beneath a wonderful canopy of tall tulip poplar trees. At 0.1 mile, the trail passes by a bench, some waste and recycling baskets, and a 7.75-mile marker, indicating the distance from the beginning of the Eshenour Memorial Trail at the eastern boundary of Derry Township (see page 46 for information on Jonathan Eshenour Memorial Trail). At 0.4 miles into this hike, the trail reaches an area landscaped with a tie wall and crosses Derry Woods Road. A bench sits in an attractively landscaped area to the right of the trail. At 0.5 miles, the trail crosses Stoney Run Road, and just past this crossing have a look at the lovely wetlands area with plenty of cattails to the right of the trail. At 0.7 miles, the trail passes over a small tributary to Bullfrog Creek and through a cut in a rocky section of the valley. The creek on the right is picturesque as it tumbles over a rough angular stone bed.

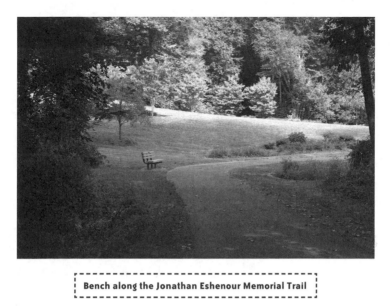

Bench along the Jonathan Eshenour Memorial Trail

At 0.85 miles, the nature trail departs from the Eshenour Trail, entering the woods and Shank Park to the left. A sign marks the intersection, and the trail surface at first is mulch. Quickly the trail passes a small bench, crosses a footbridge, turns to dirt, and climbs for a short distance into a pretty and fragrant stand of Scotch pine trees, which is a great place to spot inchworms hanging around (literally!) on a warm summer day. Leaving the pines, the trail enters a high meadow and passes by several broadly scattered conifer and deciduous trees as it crosses the top of a hill. This hill serves as the local sledding area in the winter.

At 1 mile, the trail enters the woods again at a location marked by a sign indicating that you are indeed following the nature trail. Immediately, you will come to a bench and the trail splits into three forks, all heading downhill. All of the forks take you to the same location down below, though the left option is the least steep and from my best estimation the trail proper. At the bottom of the hill, the trail turns right and shortly crosses the main Shank Park road. A large red barn with restrooms and soda machines sits uphill from the trail as it passes into an open area with several picnic tables, some tall shade trees, and a few barbecue grills. Through this open area, the trail is narrow but has an asphalt surface until it reenters the woods aside Bullfrog Creek, where it becomes dirt again. The creek here is a good place to hunt for salamanders and small crawfish.

After entering the woods, the trail meanders about the creek crossing two footbridges and passing a small bench, bends to the right and climbs gently. Just beyond the second footbridge, keep your eyes open on the right for an enormous tulip poplar, at least 80 feet tall. It is quite a sight. As the trail levels off again, it passes by soccer fields, and next to a beautiful white oak tree (#5 on the life list) and a bench. Continue along the trail a short distance until it leaves the woods, becomes paved again, and crosses the park road at a playground and pavilion (restrooms located here). The trail enters the woods next to the pavilion and in another 0.25 miles exits the woods, makes a quick left turn, crosses the park road under some power lines, and enters the woods again. Be careful here, as two trails enter the woods from beneath the power lines. Take the right-hand trail, marked by a small sign.

Shortly, the trail passes a spur that takes off to the right to a ball field. The nature trail descends gently to the left and meets up with a dirt road at the boundary of the park (1.9 miles). Turn right on the dirt road, which changes to grass, and continue walking downhill past a footbridge that exits the park on your left for another 150 feet. A manhole cover in the grass marks your next bit of route finding. Make a 90-degree right turn and cross the grassy hill under some power lines. Resist the temptation to walk directly downhill to the paved Eshenour Trail just below you as the area around that trail can be rather marshy. Just past the power lines, the trail enters the woods yet again (marked by a trail sign), and meanders gently downhill past some thick woods and berry bushes. At 2.15 miles, the trail emerges from the woods in a shaded grassy area, which you walk across to the paved Eshenour Trail. Be sure to turn right on the paved trail, and when you reach the fork just ahead, stay to the left.

In just about a mile, you will return to the Bullfrog Valley Pond parking area. As a final note, about 0.1 mile past the above-mentioned fork, a small dirt spur exits the Eshenour Trail to the right that heads back to some benches and a fire ring next to the stand of Scotch pines the trail passed through earlier. That is a pleasant and serene spot to rest for a snack or simply some solitude. The benches are visible from the Eshenour Trail.

NEARBY ACTIVITIES

Hershey Park and ZooAmerica in Hershey are destinations for families from mid-Atlantic states. The Hotel Hershey on the hill to the north of town provides some high-quality dining along with pretty views of the countryside. Across the street from the hotel are the Hershey Gardens, which in themselves make a lovely walk.

CLARKS FERRY LOOP 04

IN BRIEF

This hike follows the Appalachian Trail (A.T.) for a short distance uphill from the Susquehanna River before picking up a side trail that takes you to the top of Peters Mountain near the Clarks Ferry Shelter. Upon reaching the ridge, pick up the A.T. and walk out to the shelter and to the ridge crest just above. To return, this hike follows the A.T. back to the parking lot.

DESCRIPTION

The Appalachian Trail from Clarks Ferry on the Susquehanna River north of Harrisburg is a very popular place for area hikers. Understandably so: the route up to the crest of Peters Mountain provides several excellent views of the river and side valleys. Plus, the hiking is very pleasant. This hike offers a little variation on the typical out-and-back excursion, allowing you to make a loop hike over Peters Mountain.

This hike begins where the A.T. crosses the railroad tracks across the street from the parking area. Look for the large trail sign on the shoulder of the road, make your way over the tracks, and begin traversing the steep hillside. Although the terrain is steep, the trail climbs at a very pleasant grade generally toward the south. Not far beyond a rock outcrop,

KEY AT-A-GLANCE INFORMATION

LENGTH: 5 miles

CONFIGURATION: Loop with a stretch of out-and-back

DIFFICULTY: Moderate

SCENERY: Overlooks of Susquehanna River; nice ridge walk

EXPOSURE: Mostly shaded

TRAIL TRAFFIC: Moderately heavy

TRAIL SURFACE: Dirt and some scrambling among rocks along ridgetop

HIKING TIME: 2.5 hours

DRIVING DISTANCE: 12 miles from intersection of Interstate 81 and US 22/322 outside of Harrisburg

ACCESS: Open

MAPS: USGS Duncannon and Halifax; *Appalachian Trail in Pennsylvania, Sections 7 and 8: Susquehanna River to Swatara Gap*

FACILITIES: None

WHEELCHAIR TRAVERSABLE: No

SPECIAL COMMENTS: A fine mountain walk near Harrisburg

Directions ————————➤

Follow US 22/322 west from Harrisburg and take the PA 147/Halifax exit (just before the highway crosses the Susquehanna River). Park on the left at the end of the exit ramp.

GPS Trailhead Coordinates

UTM Zone (WGS84) 18T

Easting 329599

Northing 4473639

Latitude N 40° 23′ 45.36″

Longitude W 77° 00′ 28.24″

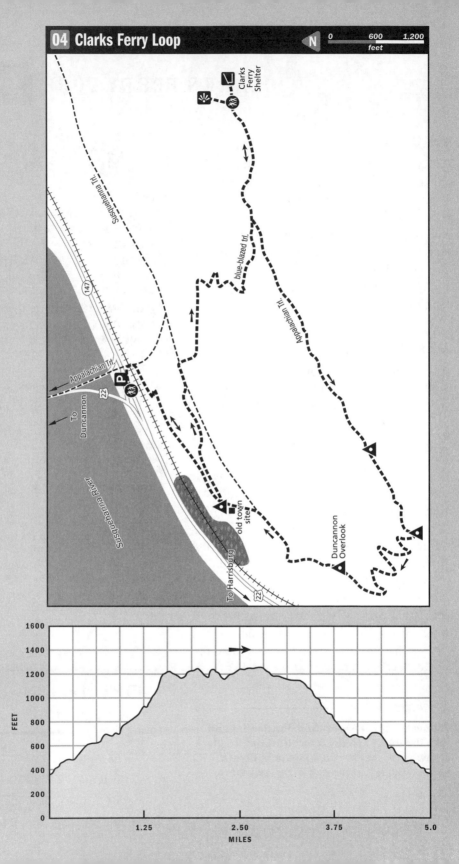

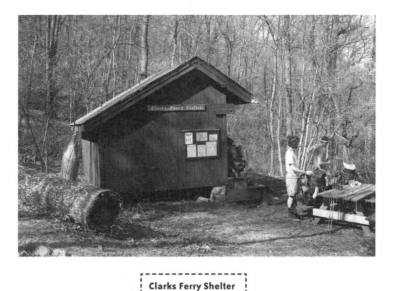

Clarks Ferry Shelter

the terrain levels out and a blue-blazed trail heads off on a northern track (about 0.5 miles). The trail departs to the left of an A.T. sign indicating that Duncannon and the Thelma Marks Shelter (now the Cove Mountain Shelter) are 2 miles and 5.5 miles south along the trail respectively, while the Clarks Ferry Shelter (our destination) is 2.6 miles to the north.

Rather than following the A.T. to the shelter, turn left and follow the blue blazes along level ground until you reach an old dirt road heading east/west and marked with blue blazes. This old road is the Susquehanna Trail, and it leads east across the north side of Peters Mountain to a power line which you can follow up to the A.T. on the ridge. That is about a 5- or 6-mile trek one-way. To reach the crest of Peters Mountain directly and the Clarks Ferry Shelter, walk across the road and follow a blue-blazed footpath as it begins to climb and switchback up the side of Peters Mountain. Although the trail gets a bit rocky in a few places, it is never excessively steep. Before you know, about a mile has passed and you have reached the ridge of Peters Mountain, where you rejoin the A.T. about 0.3 miles west of the shelter. So this little path saves slightly more than a mile of hiking up and is no steeper than following the A.T.

After joining the A.T., turn left, descend for a short distance, and just before returning to the ridge you'll reach the junction with the trail for the shelter, visible about 100 yards slightly downhill. The shelter has a nearby spring (treat the water if you drink it), a picnic table, and privy. About 100 yards from the junction, the A.T. crosses the ridge between two rock outcrops. When the leaves aren't thick on the trees, you can get a decent view to the north from this area.

The return trip follows the A.T. back along the ridge. After passing the blue-blazed side trail that you followed up, the ridge gets rather narrow in places and requires you to do a fair bit of scrambling around and over rocks. At several spots you get nice views from the rocks to the north and south, but the

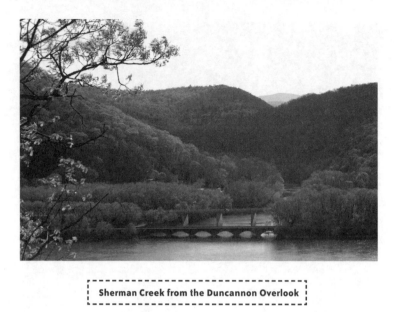

Sherman Creek from the Duncannon Overlook

granddaddy of them all is reached at about 0.75 miles beyond the junction with ascent trail. The A.T. passes an open area along the rocks, and affords a spectacular vista of the Susquehanna River and surrounding hillsides to the south.

Not far beyond the view point, the ridge widens, and the trail begins to descend to the right of a rock outcrop. For the next quarter of a mile or so, the trail hugs rocks near the ridge, which afford many good places to have a seat and look out over the river. As the rocks come to an end, the A.T. begins to switchback down the very end of the Peters Mountain ridge as it descends to the river. Just beyond the last switchback is another very pretty vantage point that affords a view of Duncannon and the mouth of Sherman Creek across the river.

From the overlook, you have about a half mile of pleasant, mostly level walking through the woods. This section of woods was home to an old settlement, the ruins of which still remain. Just before the junction with the ascent trail, you'll notice several stone foundations to the left of the trail. If you walk over to them, you can get another nice view of the river. From there, the A.T. descends for a half mile back to the parking area.

Aside from the excellent views, this hike is also a nice place for birding, especially early and late in the day when the forest is filled with birdsong. Many species common to central Pennsylvania can be found in the area, including woodpeckers, warblers, and thrushes.

NEARBY ACTIVITIES

See profile for the nearby Cove Mountain–Hawk Rock Loop (page 123).

COLD SPRINGS AND RAUSCH GAP LOOP 05

IN BRIEF

This wonderful hike follows the Cold Spring Trail north out of the old town site of Cold Springs to the ridge of Sharp Mountain, where it joins with the Appalachian Trail. From there, you follow the A.T. east into Rausch Gap and down to the Stony Creek Trail (aka the Dauphin and Susquehanna Railroad Grade). Then follow the railroad grade west back to the parking area.

DESCRIPTION

This is a great hike that is neither long nor difficult and takes you through some wild and remote country. As you descend Cold Springs Road from the top of Second Mountain, either by car or by foot, look up the valley to the east and you'll be able to see a gap in Sharp Mountain, the ridge north of the Stony Creek valley. That gap is Rausch Gap, the eastern extent of the hike.

This hike begins at the old town site of Cold Springs, a popular summer resort in the latter part of the 19th century. Reasonably

----

Directions ⟶

Take the Fort Indiantown Gap exit off Interstate 81 north of Harrisburg. Follow PA 934 north for 0.5 miles and turn left on Asher Miner Road, which eventually becomes PA 443. Follow 443 north into the water gap (Indiantown Gap). Turn left onto McClean Road (also called Ammo Road) just as you pass through the gap (there is a sign for the Second Mountain Hawk Watch on the right at the turn). Turn right on Cold Springs Road and follow it through the military reservation over the top of Second Mountain and down to the Cold Springs parking area in the Stony Creek valley. See note on page 37.

KEY AT-A-GLANCE INFORMATION

LENGTH: 6.4 miles

CONFIGURATION: Loop

DIFFICULTY: Moderate except for 1 hill climb

SCENERY: Cold Springs town site, upper Rausch Creek, Rausch Gap, Stony Creek valley

EXPOSURE: Shade

TRAIL TRAFFIC: Light

TRAIL SURFACE: Dirt

HIKING TIME: 3–4 hours

DRIVING DISTANCE: 6.4 miles from Interstate 81 and PA 934 north of Harrisburg

ACCESS: Open

MAPS: USGS Grantville, Tower City, and Indiantown Gap; *Appalachian Trail in Pennsylvania, Sections 7 and 8: Susquehanna River to Swatara Gap*; the entire hike is on PA State Game Land 211, maps 211b and 211c, which can be downloaded from www.pgc.state.pa.us/pgc/game/maps/default.asp?rgn=Southeast.

FACILITIES: None

WHEELCHAIR TRAVERSABLE: No

See additional comments at end of Description, page 37.

GPS Trailhead Coordinates

UTM Zone (WGS84) 18T

Easting 362191

Northing 4482004

Latitude N 40° 28' 38.27"

Longitude W 76° 37' 32.86"

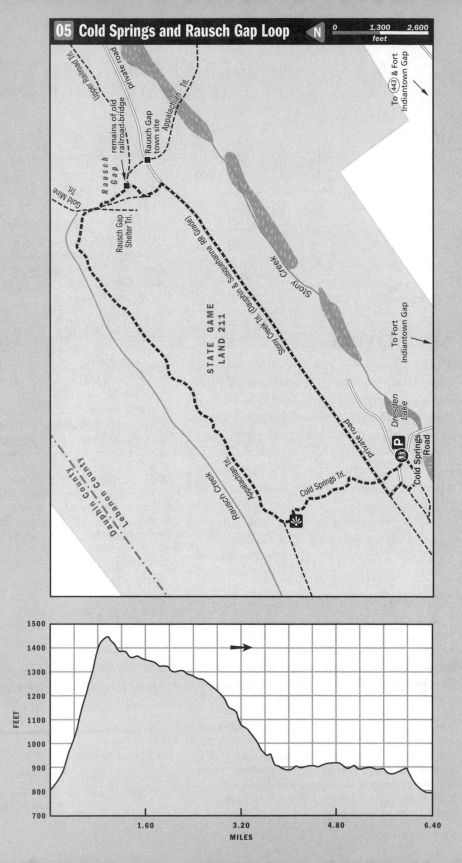

N

0   1,300   2,600
feet

To (443) & Fort
Indiantown Gap

Rausch Gap

Upper Railroad Trl.

Appalachian Trl.

remains of old
railroad.bridge

Rausch Gap
town site

Gold Mine Trl.

Rausch Gap
Shelter Trl.

Stony Creek Trl. (Dauphin & Susquehanna RR Grade)

Stony Creek

STATE GAME
LAND 211

Rausch Creek

Appalachian Trl.

Dauphin County
Lebanon County

private road

Cold Springs Trl.

Dresden
Lake

P

Cold Springs
Road

To Fort
Indiantown Gap

1500

1400

1300

1200

1100

1000

900

800

700

FEET

1.60   3.20   4.80   6.40

MILES

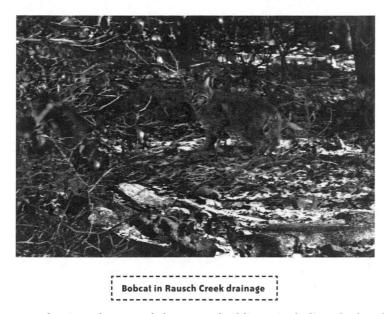

Bobcat in Rausch Creek drainage

well-preserved ruins of many of the resort buildings, including the hotel, caretaker's house, and mineral springs, still remain. After the resort closed, a water bottling company came into the area and attempted to market the spring water. And in the 1920s and '30s, a YMCA camp was located in the large meadow around what is now the parking area.

Begin this hike by walking north out of the parking lot past the large gate. After about 50 yards, turn right onto a significant (though unmarked) trail, following the path of an old logging road through a hemlock forest. This is the Cold Spring Trail. Walk uphill along the trail for about 0.25 miles and you'll reach the Stony Creek Trail. A sign marks the crossing of the Cold Spring Trail and another points in the direction of the Appalachian Trail, located just shy of a mile away on Sharp Mountain at the end of the Cold Spring Trail. Cross the rail-trail and head for the A.T. Although the trail is rather rocky and climbs the entire way, it never gets excessively steep and makes for a rather pleasant warm-up. Just below the ridge, the trail joins a significant old roadbed and makes a couple of switchbacks up to the crest. You'll find a nice place to rest there at the junction with the A.T. Enjoy the view, and take a snack.

Head east now on the A.T. At this point, you are traveling in the upper part of the Rausch Creek drainage, as wild and remote a country as you can find in this part of the state. To the right of the trail, the forest is rather open on the hillside up toward the ridge and consists of oak and hickory trees with some pines scattered about the rocky terrain. To the left, you'll see mountain laurel and thick brush because the creek is in that direction and the terrain more swampy. The forest in the area provides excellent cover for all sorts of wildlife. On a December day with a couple of inches of fresh snow on the ground, I came up here and had the good fortune of spotting a bobcat sitting on the trail.

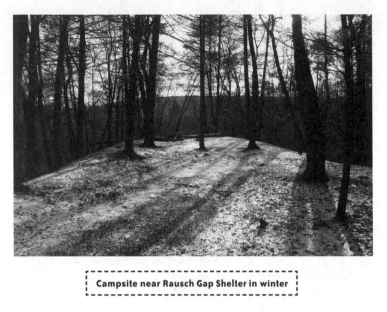

Campsite near Rausch Gap Shelter in winter

The A.T. parallels Rausch Creek for about 2 miles before both the trail and the creek make a bend to the south and cut through the Sharp Mountain ridge. This is Rausch Gap. A distinctive feature of the Valley and Ridge Physiographic Province of Pennsylvania, the origin of water gaps such as Rausch Gap (as well as others like the nearby Swatara and Indiantown gaps) is uncertain, though many geologists believe that they may have been formed by the erosive force of glacial runoff as it found its way through weak bands of rock in the ridges many millions of years ago.

Approaching Rausch Gap, about 3 miles into the hike, you'll begin to see evidence of the coal mines that were in operation in the area late in the 19th century. Piles of culm and rock waste, now covered by ferns and trees, are an integral feature of the forest landscape. As you enter the gap, the trail passes in close proximity to the creek and at 3.25 miles, the red-blazed Gold Mine Trail (see page 72) enters from the left by a large camping area. Another 0.15 miles take you to the junction with the blue-blazed Rausch Gap Shelter access trail (0.3 miles) to the right.

From the shelter trail, you can simply follow the A.T. down into the valley. I highly recommend, however, a slight deviation from that route for historic as well as aesthetic interest. At the junction with the shelter trail, look in the woods toward the creek and you'll see some red blazes. This is the lower end of the Gold Mine Trail. Although the trail is indistinct at times, the blazes are prolific as they follow the banks of Rausch Creek at its steepest and most rugged section. The creek thunders in places as it tumbles over boulders and steep drops to the Stony Creek. Follow those red blazes along the creek for about 0.5 miles to the impressive ruins of an old railroad bridge across the creek. The bridge was the crossing on the upper railroad spur that used to run between Gold Mine Run and Rausch Gap. At the bridge, turn right on the old railroad grade and follow it back out to the A.T. (about 0.1 mile). Turn left and follow the A.T. down to the Stony Creek Trail, 0.25 miles farther on.

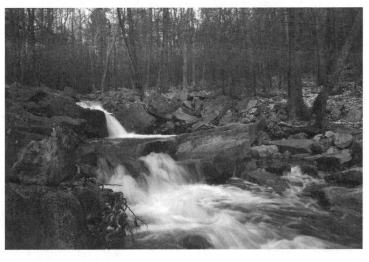

Rausch Creek

When you reach the rail-trail, take a few minutes to walk east over to the town site of Rausch Gap. The stone-arch bridge over Rausch Creek at the site is quite pretty. To complete this hike, walk 2 miles west on the rail-trail to the Cold Spring Trail. Before you head back to the car, however, be sure to visit some of the ruins of the old town site of Cold Springs. Walk another 0.2 miles west on the rail-trail and turn left onto the significant dirt road. Soon the road comes to a **T**. To the right will be the remains of the old hotel with its enormous spruce trees lined up across the front of it. On the left will be the foundation of the caretaker's house. If you turn left at the **T**, you'll come to the parking area very quickly. If you turn right and then make a quick left on the first old road, you'll come to the site of the old spring house. It is worth visiting. From there, you can pick up a red-blazed trail heading east and follow that a short distance to the parking area.

Note: Cold Springs Road from the top of Second Mountain to the parking area can be very rough. If you don't have a high-clearance vehicle, park at the top and walk down the road a short distance to see if it is passable. If not, park at the top of Second Mountain and walk down to the trailhead. Doing so will add about 1.6 miles to the round-trip, but may save you considerable aggravation.

NEARBY ACTIVITIES

Memorial Lake State Park in the town of Fort Indiantown Gap has picnic and recreational facilities. The Second Mountain Hawk Watch, accessed by car along the ridge of Second Mountain east of Cold Springs Road, is well worth a visit. During the spring hawk migration, it is a popular spot for local wildlife enthusiasts. At all times of the year, it offers excellent views of Indiantown Gap, the Stony Creek valley, and the terrain that the hike passes through.

06 FORT HUNTER CONSERVANCY AND SECOND MOUNTAIN

KEY AT-A-GLANCE INFORMATION

LENGTH: 1.4 miles. An out-and-back side trip of 1 mile can be made to the ridge of Second Mountain.

CONFIGURATION: Loop

DIFFICULTY: Moderate. The optional out-and-back up Second Mountain is very strenuous.

SCENERY: A nice walk in the woods

EXPOSURE: Mostly shade

TRAIL TRAFFIC: Light

TRAIL SURFACE: Dirt with some rocky sections

HIKING TIME: 1 hour

DRIVING DISTANCE: About 2 miles from US 22/322 and PA 443, Fishing Creek Road, west of Harrisburg

ACCESS: Dawn–dusk

MAPS: USGS Harrisburg West; *Appalachian Trail in Pennsylvania, Sections 7 and 8: Susquehanna River to Swatara Gap*

FACILITIES: None

WHEELCHAIR TRAVERSABLE: No

SPECIAL COMMENTS: This old trail is heavily eroded in places, making the walking a little rugged. The side trip to the ridge of Second Mountain is quite difficult, though it offers a great view of the city of Harrisburg.

IN BRIEF

This short hike makes a loop on the south side of Second Mountain, just a few minutes north of Harrisburg. From the halfway point, a mile-long out-and-back side trip to the ridge of Second Mountain offers a nice view of Harrisburg along the river.

DESCRIPTION

I discovered this hike one evening while poring over the myriad side trails listed on the map *Appalachian Trail in Pennsylvania, Sections 7 and 8*. I've always found the ridges north of Harrisburg to be extremely fascinating topography, and full of potential for great hikes. I was looking for a nice short loop hike not too far from town that a hiker might be able to do in a couple of hours in the evening after work. This one seemed to fit the bill.

The Fort Hunter Conservancy tract consists of 153 acres of forested land donated to the conservancy for preservation in 1986. The tract was once contiguous with the original Fort Hunter Estate, located along Front Street north of Harrisburg. The lands have been divided, and that is no longer the case. This hike follows an old trail beginning on Camp Riley Road above Fishing Creek and looping around the south flank of Second Mountain.

GPS Trailhead Coordinates

UTM Zone (WGS84) 18T

Easting 338430

Northing 4469328

Latitude N 40° 21′ 31.96″

Longitude W 76° 54′ 9.91

Directions

From Harrisburg, follow US 22/322 north to the Fishing Creek exit. Turn right on Fishing Creek Road and drive east for about 1 mile. Turn left onto Camp Riley Road and follow it to the end. Park on the right by the trailhead, identified by a large wooden platform atop a set of wooden steps. Be careful not to block the private driveways.

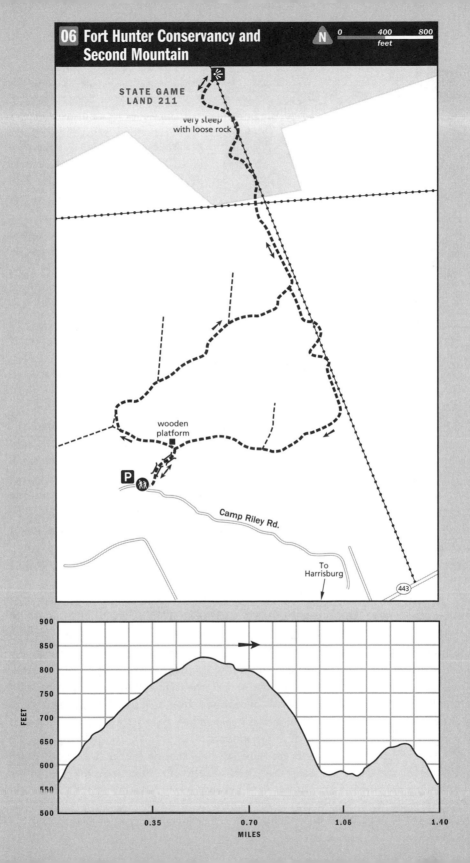

06 Fort Hunter Conservancy and Second Mountain

N

0   400   800
feet

STATE GAME
LAND 211

very steep
with loose rock

wooden
platform

P

Camp Riley Rd.

To
Harrisburg

443

FEET

900
850
800
750
700
650
600
550
500

0.35   0.70   1.05   1.40

MILES

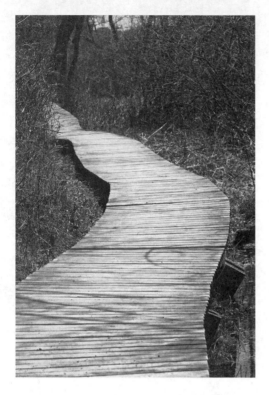

Short section of boardwalk on lower trail

It offers some nice exposure to the Valley and Ridge topography. Like Peters Mountain, two ridges to the north, Second Mountain is another of the significant ridges east of the Susquehanna River. The extent of the ridge can be traced (at least topographically if not in name) as far east as Jim Thorpe, Pennsylvania. The ridge continues across the Susquehanna River to the west as the southern flank of Cove Mountain. Second Mountain is so named because it's the second prominent ridge north of Harrisburg and the Great Valley.

From the parking area on Camp Riley Road, climb the steps to the top of the wooden platform above the road. Pick up the trail as it makes its way uphill to the right of a small creek. The trail meanders over to the left side of the creek and soon after back to the right via a couple of small bridges. In a short distance (200 yards from the car), the trail climbs to a second wooden observation platform at an old road. The road is the path of the loop hike and it walks considerably better if you follow it clockwise. The path is generally marked with red and white blazes, though you'll see many confusing markings on the trees. So you will do best simply to follow the route as explained here.

Turn left onto the roadbed, walking uphill to the west. The forest here is of hardwood trees, mostly oak and birch with several pines scattered throughout. After about 0.25 miles, you'll reach a junction with another old road. As you approach that junction, the trail becomes considerably eroded by recent heavy rains. At the junction, turn right and follow the heavily eroded path for another 0.25 miles to a fork in the trail. Again, stay to the right following the blazes. Soon you'll pass a second trail that leads off to the left and shortly beyond that you'll emerge from the woods at a significant power line near a wide (several hundred yards) flat area on the slope of the mountain.

The loop itself continues on the road beneath the power line to the right. You can, however, make a side trip from here to the crest of Second Mountain following the path beneath the power lines to the left. You can see the entire walk to the ridge from where you stand, and it is as rough and steep as it looks.

The view of the city that you'll get from the ridge is quite striking, probably the nicest view of Harrisburg in its setting along the river I have seen.

To make the side trip, turn left and head straight toward the ridge along a flat section of road. You will quickly reach a large cleared area where two power lines cross. This is a good spot for watching wildlife around dusk as the creatures that hole up in the scrub along the power-line cut (foxes, deer, bobcat, and weasels, as well as a plethora of birds) become active late in the day. From the crossing, the trail climbs up to the ridge. In effect, it makes three very steep, rugged, and rocky switchbacks up the face of Second Mountain, the second of which is the longest and most steep.

At the ridgetop, you'll find a very nice open flat area to have a sit, and a wonderful view (albeit partially obstructed by power lines) of the city of Harrisburg and the Susquehanna River to the south, and of the valleys and ridges to the north. According to the Appalachian Trail map, a trail follows the ridgetop to the west for a little more than a mile out to an overlook above the Susquehanna River. In fact, that trail is long disused and its track not obvious at best. So the hike to the river overlook, from here in any case, is a rather serious bushwhack. If you decided to go for it, allow several hours. Otherwise, retrace your steps down from the ridge. Be careful on the descent as the walking can be quite treacherous.

When you reach the junction with the main trail, continue along the power line road toward the valley below. As the road begins to descend, it bends left, beneath the power line, then right, then left again, and right again. After that second right, keep your eyes open to the right for the lower portion of the trail as it enters the woods. It is a little difficult to spot as the entrance to the woods is somewhat overgrown. You should be able to locate a blaze on a tree and at that point head into the woods picking up the significant roadbed. Follow the road as it climbs along the side of the hill for about 0.3 miles. Along the way, a couple of smaller road cuts depart heading uphill to the right. Stay to the main path, and shortly you will reach the wooden platform at the beginning of the loop.

NEARBY ACTIVITIES

Fort Hunter Park and Mansion is located 2 miles north of downtown Harrisburg on Front Street. The park is rich in regional history, and you can get a wonderful view of the river and mountains from the grounds. The park offers an interpretive walking path and tours of the mansion, and is a nice place to visit. Check **www.forthunter.org** for more information.

07 GREENLAND ROAD LOOP

KEY AT-A-GLANCE INFORMATION

LENGTH: 11.1 miles

CONFIGURATION: Loop

DIFFICULTY: Strenuous because of length

SCENERY: Beautiful fields, forests, and streams

EXPOSURE: Half sun, half shade

TRAIL TRAFFIC: Light

TRAIL SURFACE: Dirt

HIKING TIME: 5–6 hours

DRIVING DISTANCE: 22.5 miles from US22/322 and PA 225 west of Harrisburg

ACCESS: Open; state-game-land regulations apply.

MAPS: USGS Lykens and Tower City; *Appalachian Trail in Pennsylvania, Sections 7 and 8: Susquehanna River to Swatara Gap*

FACILITIES: None

WHEELCHAIR TRAVERSABLE: No

SPECIAL COMMENTS: This entire hike is on wide-open trails with the exception of about 2 miles at its most northern edge where it passes through some dense stands of mountain laurel. This is a great hike for viewing wildlife.

IN BRIEF

This hike makes a circuit through Pennsylvania State Game Land 210, following open trails to the south before heading to the north. At about 6 miles, the open trails give way to a small footpath that descends into East Branch Rattling Creek. The hike follows an old path along the creek for about a mile and then follows a good trail back south along Nine O'Clock Run. It finishes with a couple of miles of gentle walking on Greenland Road.

DESCRIPTION

I found this hike on the old "Our Favorite Hikes" list on the Web site of the Susquehanna Appalachian Trail Club (www.satc-hike.org), where it is referred to as the "Nine O'Clock Run Circle Hike." The description sounded interesting, so I figured I would give it a shot. I am glad I did. At more than 11 miles, it is a long hike; however, all of the grades are gentle, most of the hiking is on game land roads, and it is a really beautiful hike through varied terrain. This is an excellent hike for seeing wildlife and for birding.

Begin the hike from the gate on Greenland Road next to the parking areas for State Game Land 210. Pass through the gate and make an immediate right onto the Hanover Trail,

GPS Trailhead Coordinates

UTM Zone (WGS84) 18T

Easting 0356918

Northing 4486658

Latitude N 40° 31′ 5.95″

Longitude W 76° 41′ 20.47″

Directions

Take US 22/322 west from Harrisburg to the PA 225, Halifax exit. Follow PA 225 north for about 10 miles to the intersection with PA 147 (on the left). Make the first right turn north of the intersection of PA 225 and PA 147 onto Powells Valley Road (SR 4013 and some maps Enterline Road). Follow that for about 12 miles to the large parking areas located at a sharp bend in the road where it turns into Lykens Road and begins to climb the ridge to the north.

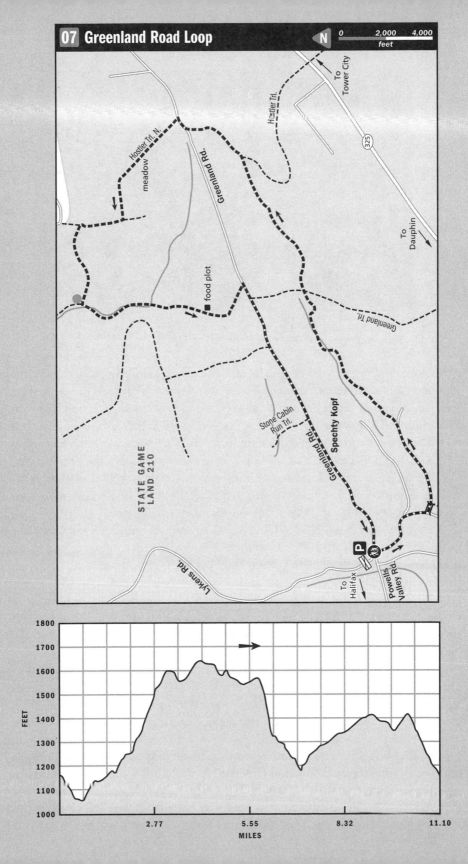

N

0   2,000   4,000
feet

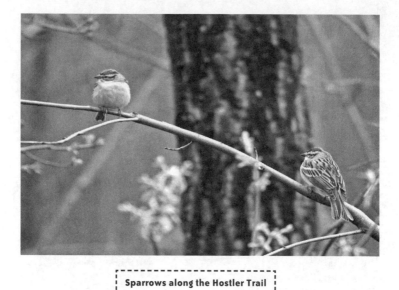

Sparrows along the Hostler Trail

a dirt road. Follow this trail downhill for about a half mile, past a couple of large food plots and then across a wooden bridge over South Fork Powell Creek. Beyond the bridge the trail bends left and climbs up to a fork near a fenced area. Turn left at the fork and follow the grassy road to east. For the first mile or so the trail heads up a hollow filled with pine and oak trees. After passing a small creek flowing across the road, the path climbs out of the hollow and passes through some lovely, generally open, high country. Plenty of low brush and mountain laurel provide cover for turkey, grouse, deer, and fox. I discovered several sets of bear tracks along this stretch of road, and I suspect that they are abundant here as well.

At just shy of 3 miles, you'll reach the crossing with the Greenland Trail, a footpath that extends from PA 325 in the south almost to Wiconisco to the north. It is identified by a small cairn on the Hanover Trail. About a mile beyond that, the Hanover Trail ends at the Hostler Trail by a very large pine tree with a very large bird box. At the junction, turn left and walk downhill for 0.6 miles to Greenland Road. The birding along this stretch of trail is excellent. Turn right on Greenland Road and follow it for 100 yards to the junction with the Hostler Trail North. Turn left and follow the grassy road as it continues its descent.

About 0.5 miles from Greenland Road, the trail passes a beautiful meadow on the left—a perfect spot for a lunch break. At 5.5 miles, the grassy road ends and the Hostler Trail becomes a small, unmarked footpath winding through thick mountain laurel. Continue straight from the end of the road. The path is obvious, and the trail a bit rocky, but after 0.2 miles, the trail comes to a T-intersection at a place that was once referred to as Carl's Crossing. Turn right and follow the north/south running trail downhill (still the Hostler Trail) for a mile to the crossing over East Branch Rattling Creek (6.25 miles). Depending on the flow, crossing the creek may require you to get your feet wet, but a large flat rock on the north side beneath a tall pine tree provides a good spot to rest and dry out.

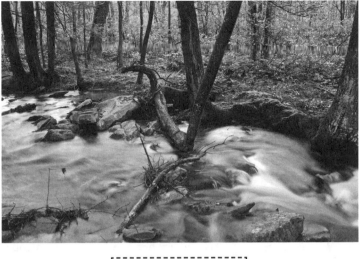

East Branch Rattling Creek

The walking for the next 0.75 miles gets rather intense. From the creek, follow the trail about 100 feet up a small incline and turn left (west) on a small, rather overgrown trail that begins just before the Hostler Trail climbs a short, steep hillside. Although the trail is not blazed, it follows East Branch Rattling Creek right along the north bank of the creek and is easy to keep track of. At times the mountain laurel is extremely dense. Plan on getting wet if you pass through this hollow after a rain. In a couple of places you'll need to negotiate some deadfall (downed trees). The trail must have been used more extensively at some time as the hollow is filled with old bird boxes.

At 6.9 miles, you'll reach a little hunting camp with benches and a fire ring on the shore of the creek. Beyond the camp the trail improves dramatically. A few minutes beyond the camp, you'll reach a small pond formed by a concrete dam. Cross the creek just downstream from the dam and pick up the Greenland Trail heading south up a hollow. Follow that trail up Nine O'Clock Run for a mile to a large clear-cut and food plot. If you have time to hang around for a while, this is a great spot for birding. I saw several scarlet tanagers and green herons here.

Follow the road through the clearings on the left side of them. It eventually makes a hard left turn and heads southeast to Greenland Road at about 8.5 miles. Turn right on Greenland Road and follow it for 2.5 miles back to the parking area, passing two significant trails that head to the north on the way. As you get closer to the trailhead, you'll see some great scenery off to the south.

NEARBY ACTIVITIES

The Carsonville Hotel has a pub with a deck and would be a good place to refresh after a long hike. It is in Carsonville on Powells Valley Road, where the road makes a 90-degree right turn.

08 JONATHAN ESHENOUR TRAIL:
Bullfrog Valley to Western Terminus

KEY AT-A-GLANCE INFORMATION

LENGTH: 3 miles

CONFIGURATION: Out-and-back

DIFFICULTY: Easy

SCENERY: Farmland and hills to the north of Harrisburg

EXPOSURE: Sunny

TRAIL TRAFFIC: Light–moderate

TRAIL SURFACE: Paved

HIKING TIME: 1 hour

DRIVING DISTANCE: 0.8 miles from US 322 in Hershey

ACCESS: Dawn–dusk

MAPS: USGS Hershey

FACILITIES: Portable toilet, soda/water machines, picnic pavilion at trailhead

WHEELCHAIR TRAVERSABLE: Yes

SPECIAL COMMENTS: A very nice hike, though it might best be avoided on hot afternoons in the summer, as there is no shade.

IN BRIEF

This pleasant hike follows the Jonathan Eshenour Memorial Trail from the Bullfrog Valley through farmland and meadows to its end west of Waltonville Road.

DESCRIPTION

The Jonathan Eshenour Memorial Trail is maintained by the Township of Derry and is named in honor of a young member of the Hershey community who was fatally injured in a bicycling accident in 1997. Funded in part by the Jonathan Eshenour Foundation, which sponsors the annual "Bike It–Hike It for Jon" event every year in May, the trail provides members of the community with safe recreational opportunities for walking, running, bicycling, inline skating, and wheelchair traveling throughout the township. Donations are accepted for development and maintenance of the trail, and interested parties can contact the Township of Derry Department of Parks and Recreation at (717) 533-7138 for information.

While estimations of its length vary depending on the source of information (the township map says the trail is 11.5 miles, while one Web site says it is 22 miles in length), my calculations show the trail to be 12.3 miles long. The primary 9-mile section extends from

GPS Trailhead Coordinates

UTM Zone (WGS84) 18T

Easting 356777

Northing 4457700

Latitude N 40° 15′ 27.06″

Longitude W 76° 41′ 3.04″

Directions

From US 322 in Hershey, head south on Bullfrog Valley Road. This is either the first light after US 322 and US 422 split coming from the west or the last light before they join coming from the east (just beyond the Penn State Milton S. Hershey Medical Center). The parking lot for Bullfrog Valley Park is 0.82 miles ahead on the right, just past the intersection with Wood Road at the obvious duck pond.

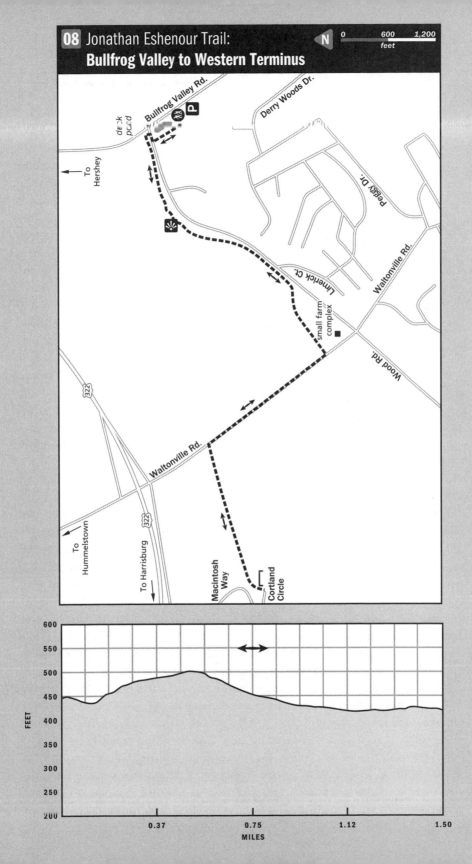

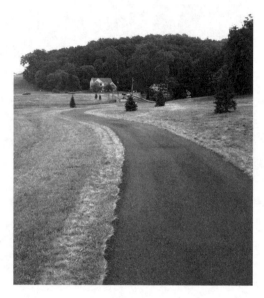

Jonathan Eshenour Memorial Trail east of Waltonville Road

the eastern boundary of Derry Township at Lingle Road near Palmyra, winding its way through commercial and residential areas, and by public parks to Waltonville Road, south and east of Shank Park. An additional 1.5-mile spur heading south from the 4.5-mile mark of the trail, along with another 1.8-mile spur, the newest section of the trail, traveling west from Bullfrog Valley Park along Wood Road, make for the rest of its mileage. Plans are under way to continue development of the trail by extending the new section west for another 3 miles to Middletown Road and the western township boundary.

This hike follows the newest leg of the trail, the 1.8-mile spur from Bullfrog Valley to the western terminus of the trail and back. I chose this section for the hike because, having hiked the entire trail many times, I think this section offers the nicest views of the farmland and hills to the north. It also does not appear to be as heavily traveled as other sections of the trail, and it tends to have less noise from traffic than other sections of the trail (especially that which follows alongside US 322 through town). The whole trail is nice, however, and is an enormous benefit to the community.

This hike begins at the parking lot at the Bullfrog Valley Park located at the corner of Bullfrog Valley Road and Wood Road. The pond here is a favorite fishing spot for young children having their first go at angling. In the past, the pond was also popular for feeding the geese and other waterfowl that visit the environs during the summer and fall. The constant supply of food, however, disrupted the migratory habits of the birds and feeding them is now prohibited.

From the parking lot, cross the small footbridge over the stream and turn right onto the trail. I was impressed by the damage to Bullfrog Creek by the heavy rains that fell earlier this summer when I visited the trail to gather information for this profile. The stream had carved a new bed around a small flood dam just upstream from the bridge. Follow the trail around Bullfrog Valley Pond to where it crosses Wood Road at a stop sign, noting the spectacular sycamore tree at the northwest corner of the pond. Cross Wood Road and turn left. The trail immediately crosses the outflow from Bullfrog Pond over a new footbridge, landscaped with black-eyed susans and ornamental grasses. From the bridge, the trail climbs up a grassy hill parallel to Wood Road on the left. At the top of the rise, 0.4 miles, you'll find a bench for sitting, with several young maple, oak, and fir trees planted behind it (aspiring shade trees). The view from this promontory to the north is outstanding, as it looks over large tracts of farmland dotted with stacked hay bales in the foreground and farther on to the hills north of Harrisburg.

From the top of the rise, the trail descends to the west and, at 0.7 miles, begins to make a long curve around a small farm complex at the intersection of Wood and Waltonville roads. At 0.9 miles, the trail meets Waltonville Road, turns sharply right (north) and follows the road for 0.3 miles, where it turns left and crosses the road. Please be sure to use caution at this crossing.

Once across Waltonville Road, the trail goes west. On the right is a large field, planted some years with corn and other years with soybeans. On the left, the trail passes by a small stand of spruce and sumac trees. This stand is undoubtedly a resting area for white-tailed deer and red fox, as I have seen droppings from both along the trail on several occasions. The stand of trees is a good place to watch for songbirds. I have spotted bluebirds and goldfinches here in the past, as well as gray jays and grackles.

The trail continues west through farmland, offering pretty views to the south, passes beneath power lines at 1.5 miles, and reaches its end at a neighborhood cul-de-sac at 1.8 miles. You'll find a bench at this end of the trail, though you won't find parking or other amenities. From here, turn around and retrace your steps back to Bullfrog Valley.

Just a final word: while this section of the trail offers a lovely hike, because it is almost entirely in the sun it can be very warm in the afternoon during the summer months.

NEARBY ACTIVITIES

Hershey Park and ZooAmerica in Hershey are destinations for families from mid-Atlantic states. The Hotel Hershey on the hill to the north of town provides some high-quality dining along with pretty views of the countryside. Across the street from the hotel are the Hershey Gardens, which in themselves make a lovely walk.

09 JOSEPH E. IBBERSON CONSERVATION AREA LOOP

 KEY AT-A-GLANCE INFORMATION

LENGTH: 3.3 miles

CONFIGURATION: Loop with a section of out-and-back

DIFFICULTY: Easy–moderate

SCENERY: Nice walk in the woods; pretty views to north

EXPOSURE: Mostly shade

TRAIL TRAFFIC: Moderate

TRAIL SURFACE: Dirt

HIKING TIME: About 2 hours

DRIVING DISTANCE: 10.75 miles from intersection of US 22/322 and PA 225 in Dauphin west of Harrisburg

ACCESS: Dawn–dusk

MAPS: USGS Enders; recreational guide and map available from PA Department of Conservation and Resources and at parking area

FACILITIES: Restrooms and water available at parking area

WHEELCHAIR TRAVERSABLE: No

SPECIAL COMMENTS: This hike is a great outing with older kids in beautiful forest. If you leave out the climb to the top of Peters Mountain, it makes a good hike for the whole family.

IN BRIEF

This hike follows the Victoria Trail from just outside the parking area up to the Peters Mountain Ridge. From the ridge, it backtracks the Victoria Trail for a half mile and then follows several easy park trails back to the parking area.

DESCRIPTION

Located about 25 minutes north of Harrisburg, the Joseph Ibberson Conservation Area hosts a network of trails along the north side of Peters Mountain. Most of the trails have been created from old forest roads, so they are generally wide open and the grades gentle. The park is, consequently, a great place for an outing with the family, and it offers hikes ranging from less than a mile to several miles in length. This hike makes use of the trails around the perimeter of the 350-acre conservation area, and includes a side trip up to the Appalachian Trail on the crest of Peters Mountain.

Originally purchased as a tree farm by forest manager Joseph Ibberson, the conservation area is home to a wide variety of trees, including oaks, pines, maples, poplars, and hemlocks. If you want to learn to identify trees, this is the place to do it. The forest

GPS Trailhead Coordinates

UTM Zone (WGS84) 18T

Easting 342319

Northing 4478521

Latitude N 40° 26′ 32.63″

Longitude W 76° 51′ 33.32″

Directions

From US 22/322 west of Harrisburg, take the PA 225/Halifax exit. Follow PA 225 north over Peters Mountain for 6 miles to Camp Hebron Road in Halifax. There is a sign for the conservation area at Camp Hebron Road. Turn right and follow Camp Hebron Road for 4.75 miles to the entrance of the park on the right.

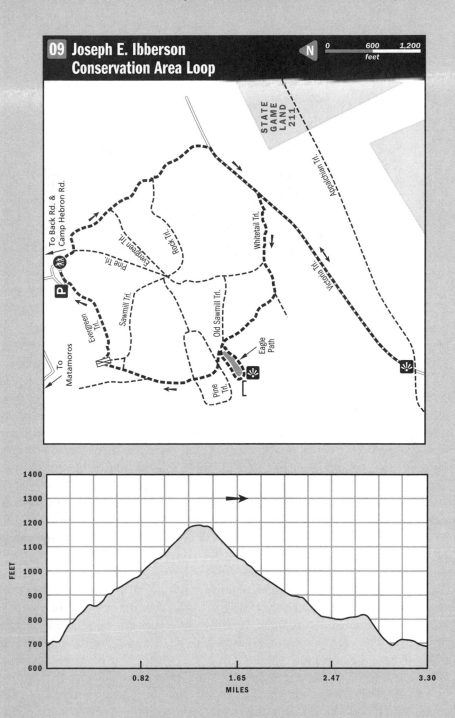

09 Joseph E. Ibberson Conservation Area Loop

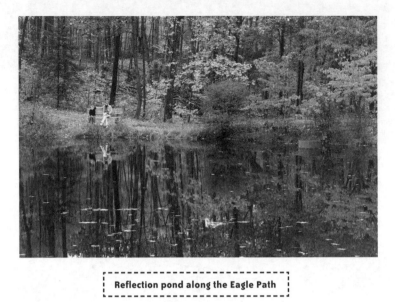

Reflection pond along the Eagle Path

provides habitat for many birds and deep-woods animals, including deer and black bear. A good time to visit the park to view wildlife is early in the day. The park is used primarily for recreational and environmental education purposes.

Begin this hike by walking out of the parking area from the main trailhead for the Evergreen Trail (by the restrooms) and turning left on the first trail, following blue blazes. This is the Victoria Trail, and it runs all the way up to the ridge of Peters Mountain and then down the other side to PA 325 at the site of the old Victoria Furnace. The original trail served as a road that provided transportation of lumber to the furnace. You'll join the old roadbed in a short distance.

As you follow the blue blazes, you will pass several trails heading off left and right. None of the junctions provide any sort of route-finding difficulties. Just continue along the path following the blazes. At 0.5 miles, the trail joins the old roadbed that was the path of the original Victoria Trail. Turn right on the road and follow it for another mile up to the ridge. As you begin walking along the road, take note of the junction with pink-blazed Whitetail Trail on the right. After visiting the ridge, you'll return to this spot and head north on that trail.

The trek along the road up to the ridge is not very difficult, though it might prove to be a bit much for young children. If that is the case, you can skip the side trip and make the hike 1 mile shorter. Older kids should have no problem with it. When the leaves are off the trees, the Victoria Trail offers some nice views of the hills to the north. At the top, you'll find a gate and the junction with the Appalachian Trail. If you follow that to the west, you'll reach the Peters Mountain Shelter in about a mile (see page 104). After visiting the ridge, walk back down to the Whitetail Trail. Turn left and follow the pink blazes along a pleasant roadbed that descends at a very gentle rate. In a short distance, a yellow-blazed trail enters

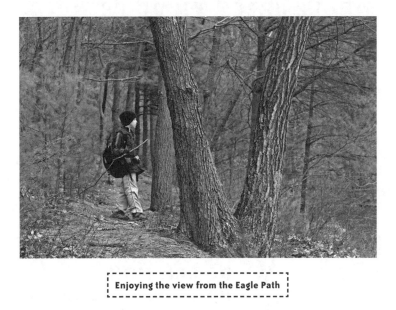

Enjoying the view from the Eagle Path

from the right (2 miles). Stay to the left following the pink blazes. After another 0.3 miles, you'll pass another junction with that yellow-blazed trail and then come to a pond on the left. A sign that says EAGLE PATH points to the short blue-blazed loop around the pond. Completing the Eagle Path loop is worth the effort. At the far end of the pond, you'll find a wonderful spot to sit and rest at a scenic bench. This pond is especially pretty in the fall when the leaves are changing.

After walking around the pond, turn left on the trail and walk up a moss-covered hill. At the top of the hill, you'll cross the green-blazed Pine Trail. Continue following the pink blazes downhill, and cross the Pine Trail yet again. In another 0.1 mile a trail with light blue blazes goes off to the left, and not far beyond that the Whitetail Trail (and the pink blazes) makes a sharp right turn uphill toward a small house in the woods. Continue downhill on the road from this point for a hundred feet or so to a gate across the road. At the gate, turn right onto the Evergreen Trail (red blazes) and follow that back to the car about 0.2 miles on.

NEARBY ACTIVITIES

Although it is not really that nearby, if you follow PA 225 north to Halifax and then pick up PA 147 north and take that to Millersburg, you can catch a ride on the Millersburg Ferry, the last operational ferry on the Susquehanna River. The paddle-wheel boat has room for three cars and passengers, and the trip across the river takes about 30 minutes.

10 MIDDLE CREEK WILDLIFE MANAGEMENT AREA:
Conservation Trail Loop

KEY AT-A-GLANCE INFORMATION

LENGTH: 1.5 miles
CONFIGURATION: Loop
DIFFICULTY: Easy
SCENERY: Views of the wildlife management area, forest, and wetlands
EXPOSURE: Mix of sun and shade
TRAIL TRAFFIC: Moderate
TRAIL SURFACE: Dirt
HIKING TIME: 1 hour
DRIVING DISTANCE: About 13 miles from US 322 and PA 419 east of Hershey
ACCESS: Dawn–dusk
MAPS: USGS Richland; a trail map and interpretive brochure are available at the visitor center.
FACILITIES: Water and restrooms available at visitor center
WHEELCHAIR TRAVERSABLE: No
SPECIAL COMMENTS: This is a great hike for kids. It can easily be done in an afternoon along with the Willow Point Trail, which ends at a wildlife viewing area by the lake. Information for the Willow Point Trail is available at the visitor center.

- -

GPS Trailhead Coordinates

UTM Zone (WGS84) 18T

Easting 393660

Northing 4458639

Latitude N 40° 16′ 17.29″

Longitude W 76° 15′ 2.66″

IN BRIEF

This short but pleasant hike begins by climbing a grassy hillside to a fence line that it follows to a trail in the forest. After a short level stretch, the trail descends, passes some food plots, and enters a wetlands area. After passing through the wetlands, it reaches a clearing for picnicking, and then climbs through a field of wildflowers back to the parking lot.

DESCRIPTION

This short hike is understandably popular with many visitors to the Middle Creek Wildlife Management Area. It provides a nice view of the management area from atop the first hill and offers the hiker exposure to various wildlife habitats including forest, wetlands, and open fields. If you walk the loop counterclockwise (recommended), you'll reach a beautiful open area for picnicking near its end.

This hike begins at the main parking lot at the visitor center for the management area. A trip to the center is something you should do before (or after) the hike. Aside from

- -

Directions ⟶

From US 322 east, turn left onto PA 419 toward Cornwall about 13 miles east of Hershey. Follow PA 419 into Cornwall, where you turn right and then make a quick left. Follow PA 419 north into Schaefferstown, where it merges with PA 897, and then turns north away from PA 897. Follow PA 897 east into Kleinfeltersville and make the first right onto Hopeland Road (11 miles from US 322). A sign for the Middle Creek Wildlife Management Area points the way. Follow Hopeland Road for 2.3 miles past the lake on the left and turn right on Museum Road into the visitor center parking lot. The trail begins from the northwest corner of the lot.

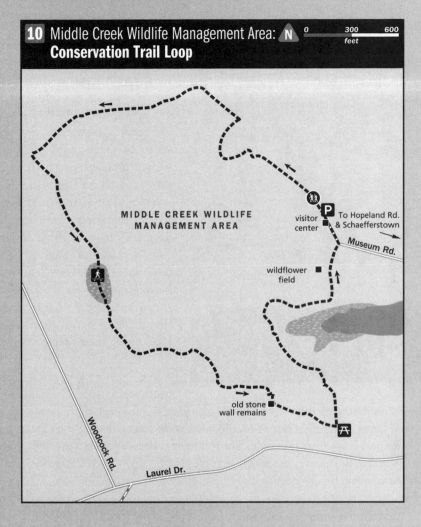

10 Middle Creek Wildlife Management Area: **N**
Conservation Trail Loop

0   300   600
feet

MIDDLE CREEK WILDLIFE
MANAGEMENT AREA

visitor
center

P

To Hopeland Rd.
& Schaefferstown

Museum Rd.

wildflower
field

old stone
wall remains

Woodcock Rd.

Laurel Dr.

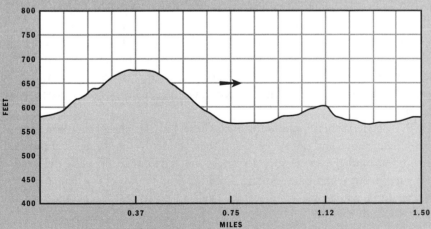

FEET

800
750
700
650
600
550
500
450
400

0.37   0.75   1.12   1.50
MILES

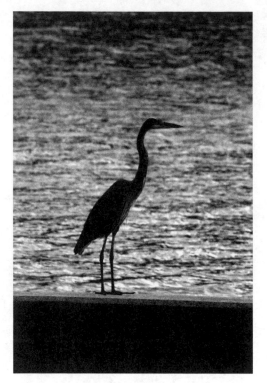

Blue heron

information about wildlife management, you will find mounted examples of many of Pennsylvania's indigenous mammals and birds. Along the back of the building is a wonderful display of owls and raptors, and a picture window that offers a great view of the songbird feeding station and the main lake. The lake is a seasonal migratory resting place for Canada geese, a large variety of ducks, as well as herons and egrets and the occasional bald eagle. In early March, thousands of snow geese visit the lake during their spring migration.

The Conservation Trail leads out of the parking area from its northwest corner. From the door of the visitor center, facing the lot, it will be to your right. A sign that indicates you are indeed going in the right direction is located in the grassy field at the base of a short hill. Yellow blazes mark the route. The trail starts out as a path cut through grass and climbs up the hill to the corner of a feed plot by the trees. Then it heads left, following the tree line before turning right up a short steep section and out to a meadow by an old fence line. The view of the wildlife-management area here is wonderful.

After stopping to soak up the scenery, follow the trail along the fence line for about 0.25 miles to where it enters the woods. The walking through the woods is pleasantly shaded on a wide-open level path that gets a little rocky in places. After another 0.25 miles or so, the trail meets an old footpath that goes off to the right. The Conservation Trail stays left and descends for about 0.1 mile. The hickory and oak trees in this area are very tall, and it is a great place to watch for birds. Nesting boxes maintained by the game commission can be found on trees throughout the hike.

I've noticed when looking for birds, here and elsewhere, that you can walk for a long distance and not see any, and then suddenly you'll see several varieties clustered around the same area. I suspect that this has to do with the available food supply. But when I am looking, I tend to listen a lot, and when I hear them I'll stop for a while, wait, and watch. I've had pretty good luck spotting some unusual species this way.

After descending the short hill, from 0.5 to 0.6 miles, the trail passes three old feed plots on the left. The right side of the trail has some dense thicket that provides

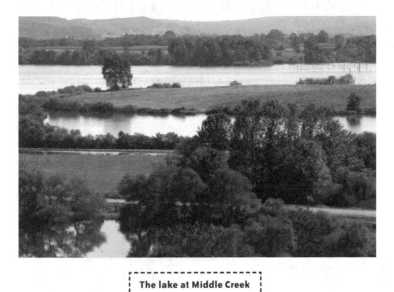

The lake at Middle Creek

good cover for chickadees and cedar waxwings. Just beyond the last of the food plots, the trail enters the wetlands area. I've always found this section of the hike rather enchanting. The trail crosses little creeks and marshy areas on bridges and short sections of boardwalk. The trees are very tall, and the lighting is rather subtle.

At 0.85 miles, the trail passes the remains of an old stone wall on the right, and another 0.1 mile takes you by a clearing, again on the right. The trail goes to the left at the clearing, not into it, and then enters a very rocky section before climbing to a large open field (the trail proper makes a sharp left where it meets the field). If you walk across the field toward the large trees, you'll find some picnic tables. Or just sit out on the grass.

To complete the hike, come back to the place where the trail meets the field and head downhill. Keep bearing left as the trail exits the woods along the side of a meadow and then back into the woods at a boardwalk through a boggy area. After passing the bog, the trail comes to a hillside of wildflowers and veers to the right along its bottom. Turn right and in a short distance the trail turns left through a cut in the field toward a large oak tree at the parking area. It's worth taking your time through this meadow, as there are several nesting boxes here that provide shelter for tree swallows, eastern bluebirds, and great crested flycatchers. This is also a great spot to see butterflies in the late summer.

NEARBY ACTIVITIES

Both Kleinfeltersville and Schaefferstown are historic villages with a few small shops that are worth some time spent looking around. Schaefferstown has the Ben Franklin Inn, where I had lunch several years ago and was quite pleased. A little farther away, the site of the old Cornwall Iron Furnace (a historic landmark) is located just south of PA 419 in Cornwall.

11   MIDDLE CREEK WILDLIFE MANAGEMENT AREA:
Middle Creek and Elder's Run Loop

KEY AT-A-GLANCE INFORMATION

LENGTH: 3.75 miles

CONFIGURATION: Loop

DIFFICULTY: Moderate

SCENERY: Middle and Elder's Creeks, ruins of CCC camp, views of Lebanon County

EXPOSURE: Mostly shaded

TRAIL TRAFFIC: Generally light

TRAIL SURFACE: Dirt, rocky in places

HIKING TIME: About 2 hours

DRIVING DISTANCE: About 14 miles from US 322 and PA 419 east of Hershey

ACCESS: Dawn–dusk

MAPS: USGS Richland and Womelsdorf; a map of trails is available at the visitor center.

FACILITIES: None on trail; water and restrooms available at visitor center

WHEELCHAIR TRAVERSABLE: No

SPECIAL COMMENTS: A good longer hike for kids, though slightly rough and rocky in places along Middle Creek. Be sure to wear blaze orange during hunting season.

GPS Trailhead Coordinates

UTM Zone (WGS84) 18T

Easting   394670

Northing   4457847

Latitude   N 40° 15′ 52.09″

Longitude   W 76° 14′ 19.44″

IN BRIEF

This hike follows the Middle Creek Trail along Middle Creek for just more than a mile to the junction with the Elder's Run Trail, which it follows for another mile up to a ridge above the wildlife-management area. There it heads east on the Horse-Shoe Trail for about 1.75 miles back down to the car.

DESCRIPTION

This is my favorite hike in the Middle Creek Wildlife Management Area. At 3.75 miles, it is a pleasant length, and it passes through some varied terrain each with its own rewards, including the pleasant scenery of the rocky Middle Creek, some old ruins, and nice views from the Horse-Shoe Trail along the ridge. This is a nice hike for kids, and for spotting birds if you are so inclined. I've seen plenty of wildlife on this hike and am always surprised by something. The loop can be done either direction, though following it clockwise makes for more pleasant walking.

Directions

From US 322 east, turn left onto PA 419 toward Cornwall about 13 miles east of Hershey. Follow PA 419 into Cornwall, where you turn right and then make a quick left. Follow PA 419 north into Schaefferstown, where it merges with PA 897 and then turns north away from PA 897. Follow PA 897 east into Kleinfeltersville and make the first right onto Hopeland Road (11 miles from US 322). A sign for the Middle Creek Wildlife Management Area points the way. Follow Hopeland Road for 3.2 miles past the lake on the left and the visitor center on the right, and park on the side of the road just before the bridge over Middle Creek at a sign that says BRIDGE MAY BE ICY. The trailhead is by the sign.

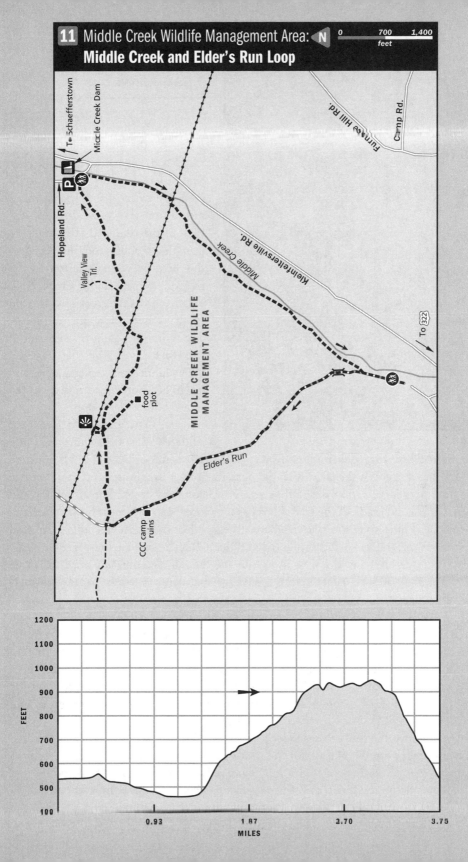

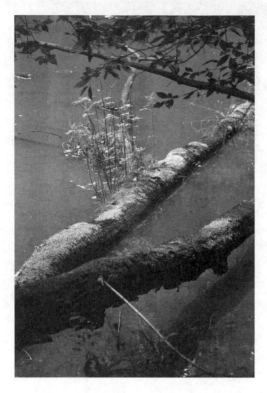

Trees across Middle Creek

The trailhead for this hike is found on the south side of Hopeland Road, just before it crosses over Middle Creek below the dam. You'll see a yellow road sign with a warning, BRIDGE MAY BE ICY, located right at the trailhead. Two trails go into the woods from here. Begin this hike by taking the left of the two trails, the Middle Creek Trail, which follows the creek downstream to the south for about 1.5 miles. The trail to the right is a segment of the Horse-Shoe Trail that traverses the wildlife-management area, and it will be your return trail from the ridge above Elder's Run.

At first, the surface of the Middle Creek Trail is dirt and mud, and it crosses over several boardwalks. The forest is full of big old birch, hickory, and beech trees in this area with the occasional huge sycamore, and you'll notice some very large recent deadfall as you walk along the creek. For all intents and purposes, the grade of the trail is level as it follows Middle Creek, but the walking can be a little tough in places where it gets rather rocky. At 1.4 miles, the trail crosses an old stone footbridge over Elder's Run, a small tributary of Middle Creek entering from the west. An ominous, though old, sign is posted on a tree to the right about 20 feet before the bridge that reads CAUTION: YELLOW JACKETS UNDER BRIDGE.

At 0.1 mile beyond the bridge, the Middle Creek Trail joins the Elder's Run Trail, a wide gravel road. Whereas the Middle Creek Trail is open to foot traffic only, Elder's Run is open to horse and bicycle travel as well. If you were to continue straight south after the junction, you would come to a parking area and a gate in another 0.1 mile. This hike, however, turns to the right and follows the Elder's Run Trail through a forest that features some very tall sycamores and tulip poplars.

Shortly, the trail crosses Elder's Run on a wide footbridge and begins to climb more steeply up the hillside for the next 0.2 miles or so before the grade becomes more gentle. In the late summer, I found a large (about six inches) spotted red salamander on the trail that I was very excited about, as I thought it was an endangered eastern mud salamander. From my photos, I determined later that it was a

Northern red salamander

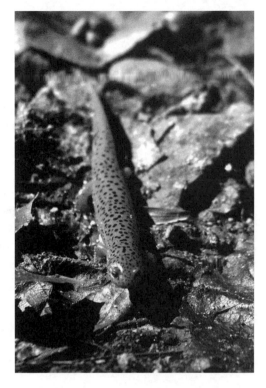

northern red salamander, which is plentiful in Pennsylvania. Nonetheless, it was an impressive and beautiful animal, especially to find just lying around on the trail.

At about 0.8 miles from the junction with the Middle Creek Trail, the Elder's Run Trail passes by the ruins of an old Civilian Conservation Corps camp in the woods to the left (west) of the trail. The foundation of an old stone house with a large chimney remains, as does the stone foundation of the spring house. In another 0.2 miles, you reach the ridge at the head of Elder's Run and the junction with the Horse-Shoe Trail, also an old roadbed at this point. A large clearing to the west provides browsing for deer, which I have seen frequently in this area, and another to the north provides a nice view toward Kleinfeltersville.

Turn right (east) here onto the Horse-Shoe Trail, and follow that for the next 2 miles or so back to the car. The path of the trail is marked with yellow blazes, and it climbs rather gently along the ridge along from the junction. After about 0.3 miles, you'll come to a fork in the trail. The Horse-Shoe Trail continues along the right track past a large food plot. The left fork heads out to a power line and an open area that offers a nice view of the conservation area to the north. The best spot for the view is about a hundred yards along this trail and it is worth the short side trip. Another worthwhile detour is to wander around the food plot to the right of the Horse-Shoe Trail just beyond the fork. It is a great area for viewing wildlife, and a grove of large trees provides a nice spot for a break.

Not far beyond the food plot, the trail comes to a clearing. The woods on the left are home to many small songbirds, and the best time of year to view them is in November after the leaves drop. The trail is a little difficult to see as it passes through the clearing. Continue keeping the woods to the left (north) until you reach the far side of the clearing. An obvious track heads left out of the northeast corner of the clearing and very quickly meets the power lines. Tempted as you may be, don't follow it. The Horse-Shoe Trail continues directly east from the same spot, although it is a little brush covered where it exits the clearing and the blazes can be a bit difficult to spot. From this point, the Horse-Shoe Trail is a single track and it descends continuously to the car. Shortly, the trail will, itself, pass beneath the power lines, and when it reenters the woods the blazes become more obvious.

At about 2.2 miles beyond the junction with the Elder's Run Trail, and about 0.4 miles from the end of the hike, the trail meets with the Valley View Trail. Marked by a sign and a yellow metallic blaze, it heads off to the left. Continue straight on the Horse-Shoe Trail, and in another 15 minutes you are back at the car.

NEARBY ACTIVITIES

Both Kleinfeltersville and Schaefferstown are historic villages with a few small shops that are worth some time spent looking around. Schaefferstown has the Ben Franklin Inn, where I had lunch several years ago and was quite pleased. A little farther away, the site of the old Cornwall Iron Furnace (a historic landmark) is located just south of PA 419 in Cornwall.

NED SMITH CENTER HIKE   12

IN BRIEF

This hike follows a brand-new trail from the Ned Smith Center parking lot downhill to the bridge over Wiconisco Creek. After crossing the bridge, it climbs up to the Railroad Bed Trail, where it turns to the right (west) or left (east). It follows the Railroad Bed Trail out to its end, and then back.

DESCRIPTION

I selected this hike because I wanted to include a nice hike that was wheelchair accessible even after a good rain and that provided reliable access to some of the beautiful Valley and Ridge scenery. I drove up to the Ned Smith Center for Nature and Art with the intention of hiking the Railroad Bed Trail, which I knew was wheelchair traversable. When I got to the center, I discovered that they were just about finished with the construction of the beginning part of this hike, which allows travelers to begin at the center and make their way across the river to the Railroad Bed Trail. I think that this makes a prettier and more varied excursion than simply following the Railroad Bed Trail, which is characteristic of a good rail-trail—well graded, mostly straight, and accessible to bikers, hikers, and horseback riders. This hike offers more varied scenery.

KEY AT-A-GLANCE INFORMATION

LENGTH: Either 2 miles or 3 miles, depending on which way you follow the Railroad Bed Trail
CONFIGURATION: Out-and-back
DIFFICULTY: Easy
SCENERY: Wiconisco Creek
EXPOSURE: More sun than shade
TRAIL TRAFFIC: Moderate
TRAIL SURFACE: Cinder and gravel
HIKING TIME: 1.5 hours
DRIVING DISTANCE: About 2 miles from PA 147 and PA 209 in Millersburg
ACCESS: 8 a.m.–dusk
MAPS: USGS Millersburg; a map of the Ned Smith Center for Nature and Art is available at the center bookstore.
FACILITIES: Water and restrooms
WHEELCHAIR TRAVERSABLE: Yes
SPECIAL COMMENTS: An excellent excursion for wheelchair users

Directions ————————————▶

From PA 147 in Millersburg, turn right onto PA 209 and follow it for 1.85 miles to Water County Road. Turn right. Follow Water County Road downhill to the Ned Smith Center on the right. Park in the lot.

GPS Trailhead Coordinates

UTM Zone (WGS84)   18T
Easting   336865
Northing   4489043
Latitude   N 40° 32′ 9.91″
Longitude   W 76° 33′ 34.43″

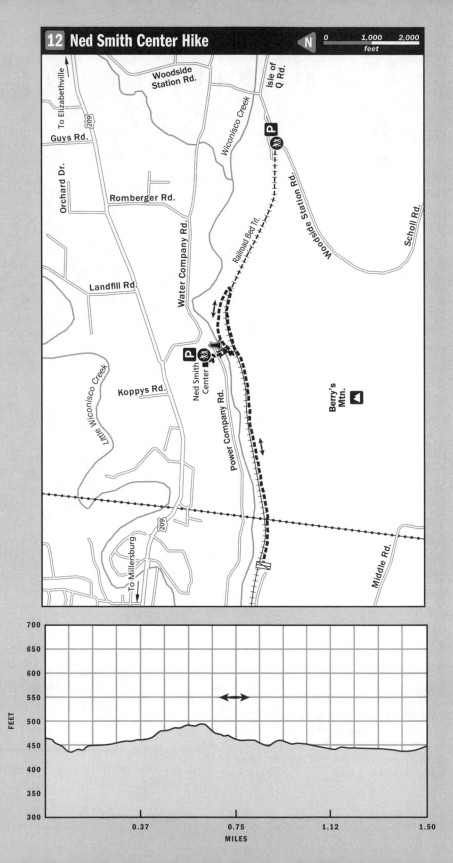

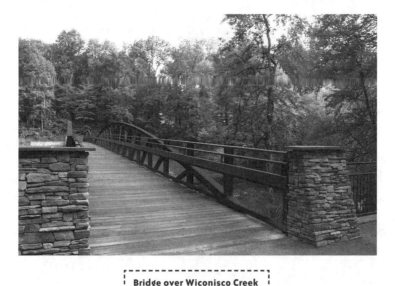

Bridge over Wiconisco Creek

The Ned Smith Center for Nature and Art is a wonderful place, and you should be sure to include a visit to its museum when you venture there to do this hike. Located just a couple of miles east of Millersburg above Wiconisco Creek at the base of Berry's Mountain, the center was founded in 1993 with the intention of promoting the relationship between nature and the arts. It is named for E. Stanley "Ned" Smith, a self-trained artist and naturalist from Millersburg, who wrote about recreation and the environment for many years. Some of his artwork is on display at the center, and it is impressive. The gallery at the center has rotating exhibits by artists of national and regional importance. It also sponsors an annual nature and arts festival and many educational programs. One of its signature programs is the Saw-Whet Owl Research Program, which allows participants to "Adopt an Owl." For more information on the center and its programs, check its Web site at **www.nedsmithcenter.org.**

Begin this hike from the upper parking area at the center. From the sidewalk along the north side of the building, pick up a crushed gravel path heading into the woods toward the west. At the time of this writing, this initial section of the trail, from the center across the creek to the Railroad Bed Trail, was being completed. The trail follows gentle grades as it winds its way downhill toward the south to the bridge over Wiconisco Creek. Cross the bridge, and stop for a moment to admire the lovely chainsaw carving of regional birds on the south side of the bridge. Once across the bridge, follow the path as it winds up gentle grades through the woods. This is a beautiful forest containing a wide variety of trees, including several species of oak, maple, hemlocks, birch, beech, and pine trees. You'll find an attractive understory of mountain laurel, some wild raspberry, and sassafras. Poison ivy is abundant in the area as well, so be cautious about what you rub up against.

The trail climbs for nearly 0.5 miles, where it makes a sharp bend to the right and joins the Railroad Bed Trail. Converted from an old rail line that used to carry

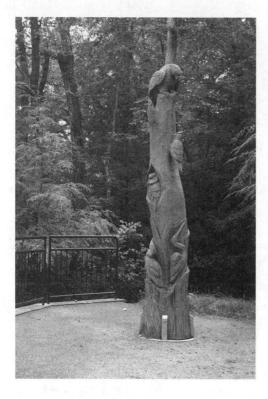

coal from up the valley in Lykens and Wiconisco to the east to Millersburg for transport along the Susquehanna River, this trail extends for 1.75 miles through the center's property along the base of Berry's Mountain. You can go either left or right on the trail. If you turn left (east), you will pass the east trailhead for the Hemlock Trail almost immediately and then pass through pretty forest until reaching the eastern terminus of the trail after about 0.5 miles. If you are traveling after or during a rain, I would advise walking in this direction, as there are one or two places where the path gets a little muddy in the other direction.

If you head west, you'll soon pass trailheads for three different paths—the Mountain Laurel and Drumming Log trails on your left, and then the western end of the Hemlock Trail on your right. Continue along the path to the west, taking in nice views of the creek and the surrounding countryside—and some raspberries if the season is right. I imagine that this would be a lovely walk in the fall. After about a mile, you'll reach a power line and the trailhead for the Powerline Trail. It is a gruesome-looking walk up the hillside. If you are at all intrigued by it, have a look at the description for the Berry's Mountain Hike (see page 16). The power line offers a pretty view of the countryside and the creek toward the north. It also makes for a good place to turn around. The trail continues for only another 0.2 miles to the west, to a gate by some private property. From the power line, turn around and retrace your path back to the parking area.

NEARBY ACTIVITIES

Be sure to visit the Ned Smith Center! In Millersburg, you'll find a nice restaurant, the Wooden Nickel, at the town square. The Millersburg Ferry is also worth a visit. It is the last operational ferry on the Susquehanna River. The paddle-wheel boat has room for three cars and passengers, and the trip across the river takes about 30 minutes. Follow signs for the ferry from the town square.

RATTLING RUN TOWN SITE 13

IN BRIEF

This beautiful hike follows the Horse-Shoe Trail from the parking area at the gate on Ellendale Road up to the abandoned town site of Rattling Run. Most of the walk is along the old railroad grade in the bottom of the Stony Creek Valley.

DESCRIPTION

I tend to refer to this hike as the "Until It Rains Hike." The day that I first did it, I was planning to do the loop hike to the Stony Creek Lookout Tower via the Water Tank Trail from the south (see page 95). On the drive to the trailhead, I listened as flood warnings were being announced for the afternoon with the arrival of Tropical Storm Ernesto. When I set out from the Ellendale gate on the Horse-Shoe Trail, I did so with an old map with misinformation, and I couldn't find the Water Tank Trail. Although I was discouraged, and was without a map of the terrain east of the Water Tank Trail, I knew that both the Appalachian Trail and the site of Rattling Run were somewhere along the trail to the east. So I figured that I would continue walking, "Until I get somewhere or until it rains." The rain started

Directions

From Harrisburg, follow US 22/322 west to Dauphin Boro/Stony Creek exit. Exit highway and cross over the creek. You are on Allegheny Street. Turn right on Schuylkill Street and then right on Erie Street (at stop sign). Signs point to Stony Creek. At the end of Erie Street, turn left on Stony Creek Road. Follow Stony Creek Road for approximately 5 miles where it turns to dirt and is called Ellendale Road. Follow for another 1.85 miles until the road ends at a gate with a large parking area.

KEY AT-A-GLANCE INFORMATION

LENGTH: 13 miles (or less)

CONFIGURATION: Out-and-back

DIFFICULTY: Easy–strenuous, depending on how far you go

SCENERY: Stony Creek valley, historic railroad, abandoned town site of Rattling Run, Kabob Hiking Club memorial

EXPOSURE: Shade

TRAIL TRAFFIC: Light

TRAIL SURFACE: Dirt and cinders

HIKING TIME: 5–6 hours

DRIVING DISTANCE: About 9 miles from US 22/322 at the Dauphin Boro/Stony Creek exit west of Harrisburg

ACCESS: Open; on state game land

MAPS: USGS Enders and Grantville; *Appalachian Trail in Pennsylvania, Sections 7 and 8: Susquehanna River to Swatara Gap;* the entire hike is on PA State Game Land 211, maps 211a and 211b, which can be downloaded from www.pgc.state.pa.us/pgc/game/maps/default.asp?rgn=Southeast.

FACILITIES: None

WHEELCHAIR TRAVERSABLE: For the first couple of miles, if dry

See additional comments at end of Description, page 71.

GPS Trailhead Coordinates

UTM Zone (WGS84) 18T

Easting 345729

Northing 4474455

Latitude N 40° 24′ 23.10″

Longitude W 76° 40′ 6.38″

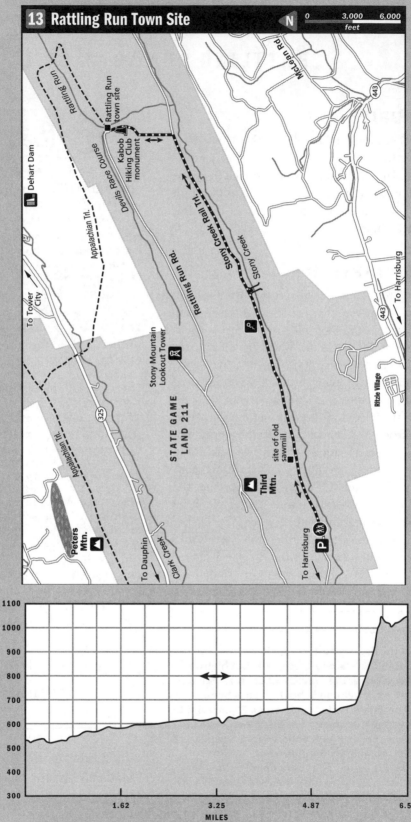

N

0   3,000   6,000
feet

Rattling Run

Dehart Dam

Appalachian Trl.

Rattling Run town site

Kabob Hiking Club monument

Devils Race Course

Rattling Run Rd.

Stony Creek Rail Trl.

Stony Creek

McLean Rd.

443

To Tower City

Stony Mountain Lookout Tower

STATE GAME LAND 211

325

To Harrisburg

443

Ritzle Village

site of old sawmill

Third Mtn.

Peters Mtn.

Appalachian Trl.

To Dauphin

Clark Creek

To Harrisburg

P

FEET

1100
1000
900
800
700
600
500
400
300

1.62   3.25   4.87   6.50

MILES

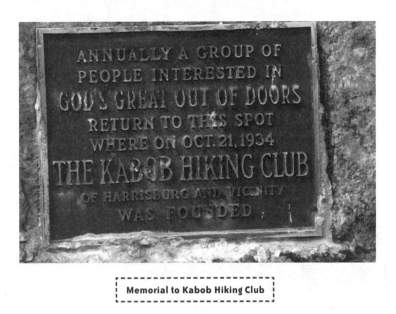

ANNUALLY A GROUP OF
PEOPLE INTERESTED IN
GOD'S GREAT OUT OF DOORS
RETURN TO THIS SPOT
WHERE ON OCT. 21, 1934
THE KABOB HIKING CLUB
OF HARRISBURG AND VICINITY
WAS FOUNDED

Memorial to Kabob Hiking Club

to fall just as I reached the monument at Rattling Run. And I'm not certain if I turned back at that point because I got somewhere or because it started to rain, though I suspect the latter.

Nonetheless, this out-and-back hike can be as long or as short as you like. It is approximately 6.5 miles from the trailhead to Rattling Run, the site of the first coal shafts in the Stony Valley (1825–1850), all but a mile of which (5 to 6 miles) is generally flat walking on a smooth cinder and dirt path. Your hike will be twice the distance you walk from the car.

The rewards of this hike are subtle. You won't find expansive views, but you'll see things such as mushrooms growing aside the trail, the contrast of fallen leaves against the brown of the trail, reflections on pools of water, shades and details and shapes of things in the woods. A few historical sites and landmarks can be found on the way. All of this against the sound of the creek flowing south of the trail.

Beginning at the Ellendale gate in the Stony Creek valley, this hike begins by following the Horse-Shoe Trail (referred to variously on some maps and locally as the Stony Creek Trail or the Stony Valley Rail Trail) along the old Dauphin and Susquehanna Railroad grade, which is suitable for bicycle and equestrian use. Although you are walking generally in an eastern direction on the railroad grade, you are actually heading toward the western terminus of the Horse-Shoe Trail as it does some meandering through and across the Stony Creek valley. The first couple of miles of this hike follow a section of the Horse-Shoe Trail intended for eastbound equestrians who forge the Stony Creek a mile or so west of the Ellendale Gate before heading south over Second Mountain. Hikers, on the other hand, are allowed to cross a logging bridge on a separate path that branches off the railroad grade a couple of miles along this hike.

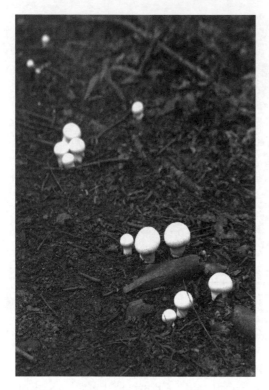

About a mile along the trail, you'll pass the site of an old sawmill on the right that operated during the late 1800s. Little remains now, with the exception of a flat area, and a disused road cut that heads back to the creek. Beyond that, at just about 2 miles into the hike, the Water Tank Trail departs uphill to the left toward Third Mountain and the Stony Mountain Lookout Tower (see page 95). This was the site of a wooden water tank that supplied engines during the days of the railroad. If you keep your eyes open to the left of the trail along these first 2 miles, you might spot pairs of T-shaped concrete posts in the ground. These were used for storing track sections for the railroad. Track damages were frequent occurrences, and these storage areas provided the railroad crews with repair materials on the spot.

Many side paths lead down to the banks of Stony Creek. Fishing in the boulder-strewn Stony is good, and it is a pleasant stream for wading in and picnicking along. An especially nice spot on the creek is located directly south of the Water Tank Trail trailhead. It is boulder strewn with large pools. I've found the area to be good for spotting common birds such as nuthatches and woodpeckers, not to mention brook trout in the creek.

At nearly 3 miles, a small spring emerges from a steel pipe in the ground north of the trail about 20 feet. It can be a little difficult to locate but is worth looking for. It is a lovely spot surrounded by lush green ferns and mosses, and plenty of mushrooms if the time of year is right. In another 0.3 miles, the trail forks with a prominent roadbed heading right and down to the creek where it crosses over a hefty wooden logging bridge. This is the hiker's crossing on the Horse-Shoe Trail. The creek is quite pretty here, and if you walk upstream along its north shore, you'll find pleasant places to relax.

Continuing straight up the valley beyond the fork, the next significant landmark is the junction of the railroad grade with the end of the Rattling Run Road, entering from the north. The railroad grade continues east for another 19 miles to the Lebanon Valley Reservoir. The Horse-Shoe Trail turns left here and climbs uphill to the Rattling Run site, 1.5 miles along the road. The first 0.8 miles provide a stiff climb before the grade becomes gentle again. If you decide to go the rest of the way, take note of the hillside to the left of the road as you climb. It is an expansive and rugged talus field in the forest all the way up.

As you approach the town site, you'll notice some ruins (mostly foundations) of old buildings on the right. Soon you'll find the monument commemorating the founding of the Kabob Hiking Club of Harrisburg and Vicinity here on October 21, 1934. I understand the club still exists, but information on their activities is difficult to come by. The turnaround for this hike is about 100 yards beyond the monument, where the Horse-Shoe Trail departs from Rattling Run Road and turns right across the Devils Race Course, the name of the drainage entering from the west. The terrain is extremely rugged and the stream here flows beneath the rocks. After a good rain, you can hear it coursing below. This boulder field is a geological formation created by the effects of erosion and freeze–thaw cycles.

If you are into very long hikes, this trek can be combined with sections of both Stony Mountain Lookout Tower hikes in this book to create a loop of about 16 miles or so back to the parking area in Ellendale (see pages 90 and 95). I've walked it, and it takes about eight or nine hours. It is a popular excursion for mountain-bike riders.

Note: This hike can be made as long or as short as you like because it is out-and-back. The walk through the woods along the Stony Creek valley is beautiful for the entire distance. A monument that commemorates the founding (in 1934) of the Kabob Hiking Club of Harrisburg is erected on the trail near Rattling Run. Because this hike crosses state game land, care should be taken during hunting season. From November 15 through December 15, you must wear at least 250 square inches of blaze orange.

NEARBY ACTIVITIES

Stony Creek is a very good fishing creek, especially in the area of the trailhead. The Stoney Creek Restaurant and Lounge at the intersection of Erie Street and Stony Creek Road in Dauphin Boro is a nice place to grab a bite after the hike.

14   RAUSCH GAP VIA GOLD MINE TRAIL

KEY AT-A-GLANCE INFORMATION

LENGTH: 10 miles

CONFIGURATION: Loop

DIFFICULTY: Strenuous

SCENERY: Gold Mine Creek, Rausch Gap Shelter on the Appalachian Trail, Rausch Gap town site and cemetery, remnants of old coal mines

EXPOSURE: Shady for first 7 miles, mostly sunny for last 3 miles

TRAIL TRAFFIC: Light

TRAIL SURFACE: Dirt

HIKING TIME: 5–6 hours

DRIVING DISTANCE: About 8 miles from the intersection of Interstate 81 and PA 72 north of Harrisburg

ACCESS: Open; on state game land

MAPS: USGS Tower City and Indiantown Gap quads; *Appalachian Trail in Pennsylvania, Sections 7 and 8: Susquehanna River to Swatara Gap;* the entire hike is on PA State Game Land 211, maps 211b and 211 c, which can be downloaded from www.pgc.state.pa.us/pgc/game/maps/default.asp?rgn=Southeast.

FACILITIES: None

WHEELCHAIR TRAVERSABLE: No, although the Susquehanna Railroad Grade would be when dry.

See additional comments at end of Description, page 76.

GPS Trailhead Coordinates

UTM Zone (WGS84) 18T

Easting 369467

Northing 4487089

Latitude N 40° 31′ 27.35″

Longitude W 76° 32′ 27.72″

IN BRIEF

This wonderful hike follows the Gold Mine Run drainage and makes a circuit around Sharp Mountain to its north. From the head of Gold Mine Run, descend into Rausch Gap, a water gap through Sharp Mountain, and join the Appalachian Trail (A.T.) near the Rausch Gap Shelter. From the shelter trail, follow the A.T. down to the Susquehanna Railroad Grade at the old town site of Rausch Gap, and then follow the grade east for 3 miles back to the car.

DESCRIPTION

This hike is one of my favorite outings in central Pennsylvania. It is a rather long hike in the mountains, but with the exception of a few short rocky sections, the trails are smooth and pleasant to walk on. All along this hike you pass through remote terrain, featuring fair populations of bear and deer, as well as wild turkeys and the occasional grouse. In the fall, when the leaves are changing, it can't be beat. In the winter, the light is stark and the scenery enchanting.

Begin this hike at the large parking area for the rail-trail along the old Dauphin and Susquehanna Railroad grade on the west side

---

Directions ⟶

From Interstate 81 north of Harrisburg, exit at Lickdale and follow PA 72 north for 3.3 miles to PA 443. Turn right on PA 443 and follow it north for 1.75 miles to Gold Mine Road. Turn left and follow Gold Mine Road for 2.8 miles over the top of South Mountain to the parking area for the Susquehanna Railroad Grade on the left. A large cement slab is visible on the right across the road from the entrance to the parking area. Park near the gate across the railroad grade.

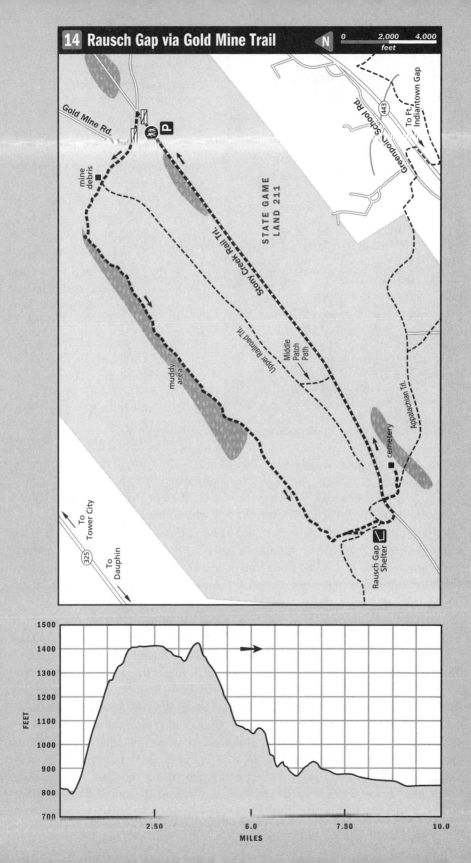

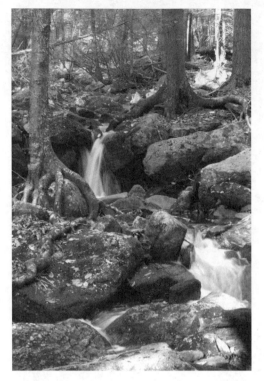

Rausch Creek in Rausch Gap

of Gold Mine Road. The trail stretches 24 miles from the Lebanon Reservoir to the east along the Stony Creek all the way to the Ellendale trailhead in the west. From the parking area, walk back out to Gold Mine Road, turn left and follow the shoulder of the road across the bridge over a creek. Just beyond the bridge, you will see a prominent gate on the left with an old dirt track behind it. Walk around the gate and follow the track as it climbs gently through an open forest of hemlock and oak for about a half mile to the junction of the Gold Mine and Upper Railroad trails.

The Upper Railroad Trail heads to the left (west), traversing the south face of Sharp Mountain to the A.T. just below Rausch Gap. That trail provides a shorter alternative (about 8 miles) to this hike, though I think not as nice. This hike on the Gold Mine Trail goes around Sharp Mountain to the north and joins with the A.T. above Rausch Gap.

From the junction, follow the Gold Mine Trail, an old haul road, as it heads north through a gap on Sharp Mountain. After 0.1 mile, a road cut enters from the right. Stay left and cross Gold Mine Run over a log crossing that demands care and attention to keep from getting dunked. The woods in this area consist of many young hemlocks interspersed with oak, hickory, and the occasional maple tree.

At 1.1 miles into the hike, you'll see some old mine shafts and piles of mine debris in the woods not far from the trail. This area was heavily mined in the late 19th century, though as far as I am able to ascertain the mining was only for coal and not gold, as the name of the creek and trail might suggest. Deposits of gold have been found in streams in Pennsylvania, notably in York County, but mostly in the form of flakes rather than the nuggets that will make anyone wealthy.

Just beyond the mine remnants, the trail reaches a flat area and turns left passing through a beautiful stand of pine trees. The path is marked by red blazes that become more abundant at this point. After passing the pine grove, continue in a southwest direction along a quiet and secluded old road, through beautiful forest for several miles. You are walking now along the north flank of Sharp Mountain, the crest of which is not far above you on the left. If you start early in the morning, the sun coming over the ridge is quite striking.

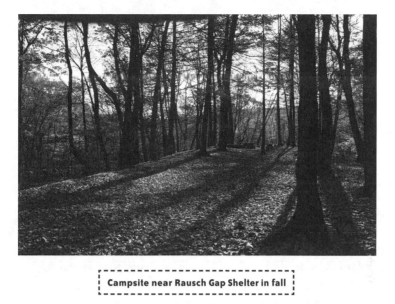

Campsite near Rausch Gap Shelter in fall

At approximately 3 miles into the hike, the trail gets rather muddy and at places less distinct as it passes through hemlocks (the state tree) and mountain laurel (the state flower). At this point, you have reached the wetlands forming the headwaters of Gold Mine Run, flowing east, and East Branch, flowing west. Shortly the trail becomes more distinct as it descends to the southwest. At 3.8 miles, it reaches a cut in the forest, a path for a pipeline. This is a nice spot for a break. From here you can see the ridge of Sharp Mountain just uphill to the south, and Stony Mountain to the north. The trail goes directly across the cut and enters the woods at a spot marked by several red blazes on the trunks of a few small maple trees.

After entering the woods, the trail becomes more of a footpath as it drops into Rausch Gap. Some attention to route finding is necessary as the trail gets closer to the A.T. The blazes are plentiful for some distance and then become less so. The trail, though, is obvious, following an old logging track to the south and west as it descends into the gap. As the hemlock trees become more abundant, the trail reaches a flat spot with the remains of an old fire ring and then drops down a very short steep section. At the bottom, the trail appears to continue left across the hillside, but the red blazes call you directly downhill. Follow the blazes down to the creek. The red blazes guide you into an area where Rausch Creek is braided, and rather than making one big crossing you'll cross several small tributaries over rocks.

If you should miss the blazes, don't worry. Ultimately, whatever way you go, you'll end up at Rausch Creek rather quickly and the A.T. is just on the other side of it. The issue, however, is getting across the creek. The farther downstream you go, the more difficult it is to cross because its banks get steeper as it flows into the gap. If you find that's the case, head upstream until you find a suitable place to cross.

In the area of the braided stream, the blazes become more difficult to follow. But if you simply continue straight across the creek at the most convenient spot, and then veer to your left when you reach the far bank, you'll shortly reach a spot with lots of campsites above the creek. Here, the Gold Mine Trail joins the A.T., with its ubiquitous white blazes that you follow south through the gap.

Not far past the junction of the two trails, a side trail marked by blue blazes heads off to the Rausch Gap Shelter. It is 0.3 miles out to the shelter along a broad, flat old railroad grade. The side trip is worth the effort. The shelter is actually built into an outcropping of rocks on the hillside. You'll find an outhouse and a spring at the shelter, plus a nice view to the east about halfway down the path.

From the junction with the shelter, follow the A.T. south down to the obvious Dauphin and Susquehanna Railroad (referred to variously on some maps and locally as the Stony Creek Trail or the Stony Valley Rail Trail) grade at 5.75 miles. Along the way, you will pass the junction with the Upper Railroad Trail, which began back at the east end of Sharp Mountain. Turn left (east) on the Susquehanna Railroad Grade, and follow the A.T. along it until the old stone arch bridge (built in 1850) over Rausch Creek. Just beyond the bridge, the A.T. leaves the railroad grade and heads south into the woods.

Historically, this is a very interesting area. Just north of the bridge you'll see the first limestone diversion well built in the United States (1986), which serves to reduce the acidity of Rausch Creek caused by drainage from old mines and acid rain. Upstream from the bridge, there are no fish; while downstream you'll find healthy native brook trout. Because Rausch Creek is the largest tributary of Stony Creek, the effect of the diversion well is significant for the pH levels as well as fish populations all the way down to the Susquehanna River.

Additionally, a sign on the south side of the trail at the bridge marks this as the site of the village of Rausch Run (1828–1910), whose major industries were coal mining and railroad repair. Although little remains of the town today, a side trip to the site of the Rausch Run cemetery is worthwhile. Follow the A.T. south from the railroad grade for 0.3 miles to a trail junction marked by a wooden sign that reads CEMETERY. Turn left on the trail and follow it to the old cemetery among hemlock trees. There are several marked resting places of townspeople, and likely several other unmarked interments.

From the stone arch bridge, the remainder of the hike follows the railroad grade for another 3.5 miles back to the parking area. It is a wonderful walk with long sections through pine and hemlock forest that has a very intense bluish green color to it.

Note: Because this hike crosses state game land, care should be taken during hunting season. From November 15 through December 15, you must wear at least 250 square inches of blaze orange.

RIVERFRONT PARK IN HARRISBURG

15

IN BRIEF

This hike begins by crossing the Susquehanna River on the Walnut Street Bridge (no motor vehicles) and then descends to the river walk at the level of the river. It follows the paved walk north to the first paved ramp beyond the Harvey Taylor Bridge. It ascends the ramp, makes a loop around Sunken Garden, and follows the paved path through Riverfront Park back to and over the Walnut Street Bridge.

DESCRIPTION

This pleasant hike in downtown Harrisburg is an ideal excursion for after work or during a long lunch break. It generally follows a route used by different organizations (the ALS Foundation and the Leukemia/Lymphoma Society, for instance) for their fund-raising walks. It is a good outing for the whole family. This trip makes a loop on one section of the Capital Area Greenbelt, a system of parks and open spaces around the city of Harrisburg joined by a 20-mile trail system accessible for hiking and biking. Although I don't know anybody who has walked the entire Greenbelt, sections of it make for some great outings. The Greenbelt stretches north to the Wildwood Nature Sanctuary (see page 108) and south to the Cameron Parkway south of Interstate 83. Along the way, it visits, among other places, Italian Lake, the Five Senses Garden, and Reservoir Park, several of the Harrisburg city parks. And it takes

KEY AT-A-GLANCE INFORMATION

LENGTH: 2.5 miles
CONFIGURATION: Loop
DIFFICULTY: Easy
SCENERY: Historic downtown Harrisburg; City Island and the Susquehanna River
EXPOSURE: Sunny
TRAIL TRAFFIC: Heavy
TRAIL SURFACE: Paved
HIKING TIME: 1–1.5 hours
DRIVING DISTANCE: About 1.25 miles from the 2nd Street exit on Interstate 83
ACCESS: 6 a.m.–10 p.m.
MAPS: USGS Harrisburg West
FACILITIES: Seasonal restrooms, water, and snacks available near parking area on City Island
WHEELCHAIR TRAVERSABLE: Yes
SPECIAL COMMENTS: If the Susquehanna River is running high, the river walk may be flooded. In this case, you can stay on the paved path above the level of the river.

Directions ————————➤

Take the Second Street exit off Interstate 83 and follow Second Street north to Market Street. Turn left onto Market, drive across the bridge, and turn right into the parking area on City Island (identified by a large sign).

GPS Trailhead Coordinates

UTM Zone (WGS84) 18T
Easting 339471
Northing 4457785
Latitude N 40° 15′ 18.50″
Longitude W 76° 53′ 15.38″

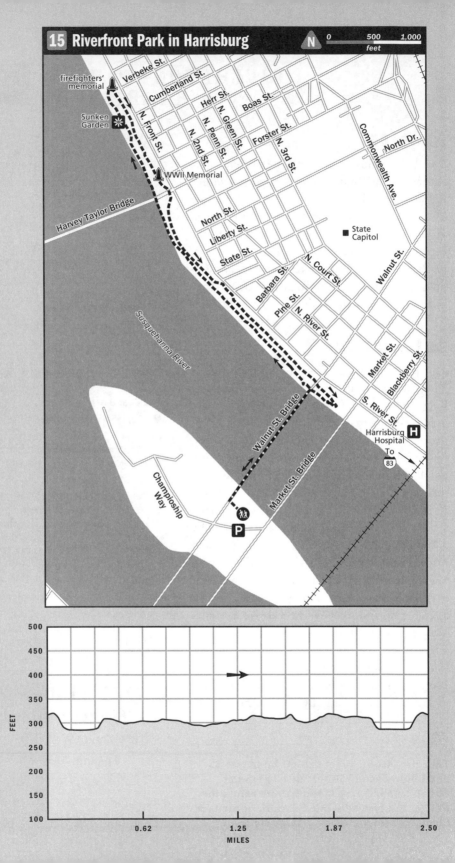

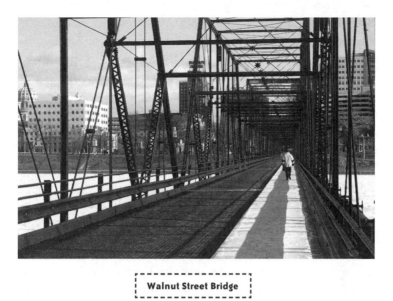

Walnut Street Bridge

the walker in proximity of the Governor's Mansion, the Farm Show Arena, and the Civil War Museum. This hike takes you through the Riverfront Park area of the Greenbelt.

Begin hiking from the parking area on City Island, a 63-acre recreational park located on an island in the Susquehanna River. It is home to the Commerce Bank Park (aka Riverside Park) where the minor-league baseball team, the Harrisburg Senators, play; Riverside Village Park; a carousel; three marinas; and the Skyline Sports Complex with its volleyball courts and ball fields. In the summer, you can hop on a paddleboat for a tour of the river. If you arrive here to begin hiking before 11 a.m. during the week, you'll have to pay $3 to park in the lot. Walk out of the parking lot directly toward the old steel bridge, the Walnut Street Bridge. Opened in 1890 by the Peoples Bridge Company, this is the oldest surviving bridge over the Susquehanna River and the oldest metal span bridge in the United States. Also known as "Old Shakey," the structure was a toll bridge until 1957. Ultimately it was closed to vehicular traffic in 1972 as a result of flood damage from Hurricane Agnes. The bridge offers a great view of the Harrisburg skyline as well as the Susquehanna River, which is about 0.25 miles wide at this point.

At the end of the bridge, you enter Riverfront Park. The park was designed by architect Warren Manning during the early 20th century and constructed as part of the City Beautiful Movement (1901–1930). Prior to the construction of the park, the area along the river was a dumping ground. From the end of the bridge, turn right and walk down the concrete path to the level of the river and turn right again to head north along the river walk. The river walk extends for several miles from the Shipoke section of town, just south of Center City, up to McClay Street near the Governor's Mansion. During periods of heavy rain or spring runoff, the level of the river will rise above the path, in which case you can stay high and follow the asphalt path through the park above the river. In the summer, you'll see plenty of people hanging out along the river. If you venture out during the winter, you can be in for a cold excursion as the river will often freeze over and an icy wind howls along it.

Follow the paved path along the level of the river for about 0.8 miles, at which point you will pass beneath the Harvey Taylor Bridge, the next span to the north of the Walnut Street Bridge. Just beyond that bridge, another path climbs to the upper level from the river walk. Follow that path and continue north above the river for a short distance to the entrance of the Sunken Garden. A public garden with a small gazebo and a sun dial, this facility was built on the excavated foundations of dwellings occupied by migrant river coal dredgers who worked the Susquehanna River bottom in the 19th and early 20th centuries.

After visiting Sunken Garden, walk around its north end and then loop back south through the park next to Front Street. You are walking now along the historic district of Harrisburg, which extends another mile or so north to McClay Street and the Governor's Mansion. Riverfront Park on the level of Front Street is formed by a wide grassy area with many bushes, tall oak trees, several sculptures, and benches every 100 feet or so, all at a level about 30 feet above the river. As you continue south, the trail winds past several monuments including a firefighters' memorial, a World War I memorial, and one dedicated to soldiers who lost their lives on submarines during World War II.

Cross over Forster Street at the Harvey Taylor Bridge, and follow the path past the old waterworks building. Prior to Hurricane Agnes in 1972, the waterworks complex provided water to the city. At State Street, you get a great view of the State Capitol. On the southeast corner of State Street is the Cameron Mansion. An impressive piece of architecture, it was the home of politician James Donald Cameron, who served as a Pennsylvania senator for 20 years beginning in 1877. Next to that is the William McClay Mansion (now owned by the Pennsylvania Bar Association). McClay was one of the country's first U.S. senators. He and John Harris laid out the city of Harrisburg in 1785. John Harris is now buried in the park across from the Governor's Mansion.

From State Street, you'll pass several stairways leading down to the level of the river, and then you will reach the Walnut Street Bridge. Cross the bridge to return to your car.

NEARBY ACTIVITIES

In addition to the amenities at City Island, Second Street in the historic section of downtown Harrisburg (one block east of Riverfront Park) is teeming with pubs and restaurants. The Whitaker Center for Science and the Arts is just a couple of blocks east of Front Street, on Market Street. In addition to being a performance venue, it shares the location with the Harsco Science Center and its IMAX Theater. Strawberry Square, with small shops and a food court, is adjacent to the science center.

ROUND HEAD 16

IN BRIEF

Beginning at the game lands parking area south of Rock, follow the Werts Path up and over Blue Mountain to the junction with the Pavement Path. Follow the Pavement Path west through dense terrain to an old section of the Appalachian Trail (now relocated). Turn left, pick up the present A.T. and follow it west to the boulder field near the Hertlein campsite. Follow an old trail north back to the junction of the Pavement Path and Werts Path, the latter of which you will follow over Blue Mountain and back to your car.

DESCRIPTION

I pieced together this hike after perusing my A.T. map for several hours. Though not especially long, it is a challenging and rugged hike. The "trail" in the first mile has some especially rocky sections. The loop requires route-finding abilities and a willingness to push through trails overgrown by blueberry and mountain laurel. The A.T. map is somewhat misleading as it doesn't have all of the trails in the area on it, making some critical junctions difficult to find, and the trail that is on the map doesn't quite square with the lay

Directions

From Interstate 81 north of Harrisburg, take the Pine Grove (PA 443) exit. Follow PA 443 east for 2 miles into Pine Grove. Turn right onto PA 895 and follow it east for 5.2 miles into the town of Rock. Turn right on the *second* Loop Road, directly across from New Swanger Road. Turn left onto Hunter Drive, which becomes Love's Road. Follow the road uphill as it turns into a dirt track and passes private property. Park at the game-land parking area at the end of the road.

---

i KEY AT-A-GLANCE INFORMATION

LENGTH: 8 miles

CONFIGURATION: Balloon

DIFFICULTY: Very difficult

SCENERY: Excellent views of the Great Valley, Shower Steps, remote terrain

EXPOSURE: Shade

TRAIL TRAFFIC: Light

TRAIL SURFACE: Dirt

HIKING TIME: 5–6 hours

DRIVING DISTANCE: 8.25 miles from Interstate 81 and PA 443 north of Harrisburg

ACCESS: Dawn–dusk

MAPS: USGS Swatara Hill; *Appalachian Trail in Pennsylvania, Sections 1 through 6: Delaware Water Gap to Swatara Gap*

FACILITIES: None

WHEELCHAIR TRAVERSABLE: No

SPECIAL COMMENTS: This is a very difficult hike that requires sturdy boots, the willingness to push through some tough terrain, and good route-finding skills. A GPS unit and the ability to use it are advisable.

GPS Trailhead Coordinates

UTM Zone (WGS84) 18T

Easting 391407

Northing 4487680

Latitude N 40° 31′ 57.90″

Longitude W 76° 16′ 55.86″

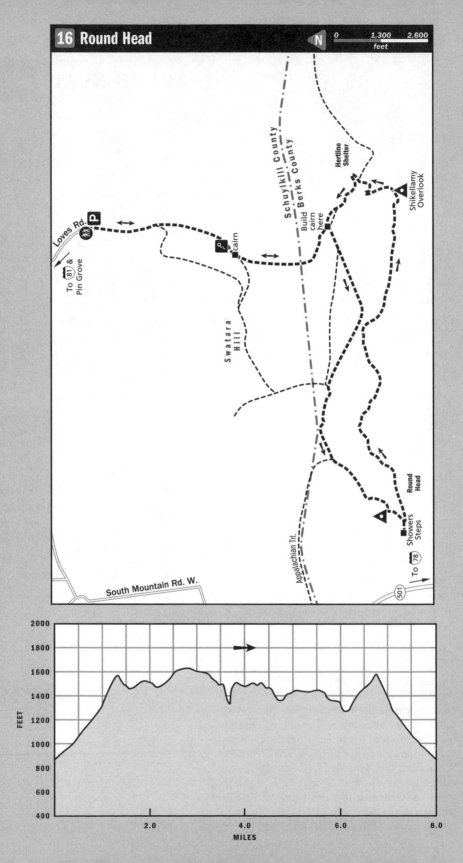

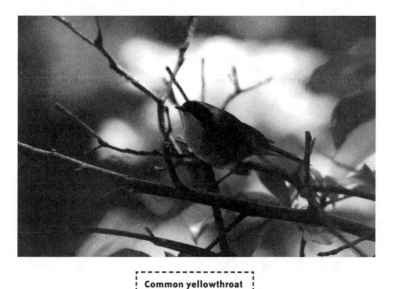

Common yellowthroat

of the land. The payoff of enduring the difficulties is a loop hike in remote terrain, several outstanding views, a nice boulder field view, and a view of the Shower Steps. I highly recommend using a GPS unit to mark waypoints on this hike. If you don't have one, you would be prudent to build cairns at all major navigation points to help complete the route or retrace your route if you are unsuccessful.

Begin at the game lands parking lot and follow the pleasant grassy road uphill past some scrub oak and sassafras trees and plenty of raspberry bushes. Don't get suckered into believing that this will be the character of the entire hike. Soon the trail passes a food plot and just beyond that the grassy road gives way to a rocky footpath entering the woods. Follow the orange blazes as the trail gets even rockier and shares the path with a creek bed. Use caution in this area; it is a likely place to sprain an ankle. At about 0.5 miles, you'll reach a gas line cut at a low spot between two steep ridges. Walk across the clearing angling slightly to the left and enter the woods at an orange blaze on a rock. Continue up the rugged trail into a marshy area to a spring marked by a sign. The water comes out the ground from underneath a small rock box, and a wooden box on a tree just above it contains two plastic cups. Don't drink the water without treating it.

Beyond the spring, pass through some marshy terrain, through ferns and past deadfall, up the steep-sided hollow for about 100 yards. Keep your eyes open for a prominent cairn on the trail. When you reach the cairn, follow the unblazed trail that goes off to the left. (Don't continue up the creek.) Although the path is not blazed, it makes a rather direct line up a moderate hillside and is easy to follow. The condition of the trail also improves dramatically once beyond the cairn.

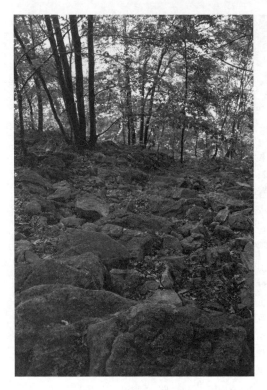

Follow the path up to the ridge (at 1.1 miles or so) and over it into another hollow. The trail gets rather overgrown with mountain laurel, and at about 1.6 miles you'll reach a trail junction of the Werts Path (which you have been following since the cairn) and the Pavement Path at a very old sign. This is a critical junction; if you have a GPS unit, be sure to create a waypoint. It can be a difficult place to find on return.

From here, you will be following the Pavement Path through the high hollow to the west along the edge of the state game lands. At times the path is quite thick with blueberry bushes and mountain laurel. The oak forest it takes you through is quite beautiful and extremely secluded. You'll have plenty of opportunity for bird-watching and a high probability of seeing some larger wildlife.

Head onto the Pavement Path, which is initially rather dense. In a short distance, the path cuts directly across a considerably more distinct (though not blazed) path (possibly an old route of the A.T.). Stop here and build a cairn or tie a bandanna to a tree. Given the thick understory of mountain laurel, missing the Pavement Path on your return is quite likely. Although rather overgrown in places, the Pavement Path beyond is a straight and level trail with occasional white blazes spray-painted on trees and is pretty easy to navigate.

About 0.5 miles from the crossing, you'll reach a trail post spray-painted white and the trail angles off to the right into a hollow. Continue through the hollow and as the terrain flattens out, the overgrowth becomes unpleasantly thick. Push through for about 200 feet to an obvious path tending north–south. This is an old route of the A.T., and here you want to turn left and follow it out to the current route of the A.T.. The understory is still a little dense at times, but not nearly as thick as what you've been through.

When you reach the main A.T., turn left and follow it out along the ridge to Round Head. In about 0.5 miles, you'll pass a campsite on the left of the trail. A side trail departs to the right from there, taking you out to a wonderful overlook at the top of a boulder field. Beyond the campsite, the A.T. descends for a short distance and then comes out to splendid overlook above the Great Valley. The A.T. makes a sharp left here, which is the route of the hike. However, before turning left, hike a couple of hundred feet downhill on the blue-blazed trail that descends to the right to see the Showers Steps—approximately 500 stone steps set into the hillside by Lloyd Showers.

Follow the A.T. to the north for 2 miles to the Shikellamy Overlook, where you'll get another splendid view of the Great Valley. After soaking up the scenery, continue along the A.T. as it descends into a hollow, making one switchback. Entering the hollow, you'll reach a junction with an old disused trail and a sign for the boulder field. Drop your pack, walk over to the boulder field for a look, and then come back to this spot.

From the boulder-field sign, follow the disused trail north and uphill through a creek bed.

If you are using the A.T. map, you'd assume that this trail will take you right to the junction of the Werts and Pavement paths, just about 0.25 miles away. It doesn't. In fact, this trail passes by the junction about 200 feet to the west. With the thick understory, all the terrain tends to look the same through here, and you can end up wandering around for hours. This is where you need to start looking for the cairn that you built earlier (which should be on this path), or checking your GPS coordinates. Find your cairn, turn right, and walk over to the junction and then back along the Werts Path to your car.

17 STATE GAME LAND 156

KEY AT-A-GLANCE INFORMATION

LENGTH: 9.7 miles

CONFIGURATION: Balloon

DIFFICULTY: Difficult because of length

SCENERY: Furnace Hills environs; nice views of Lancaster County to southwest; pretty forest of mature white ash

EXPOSURE: About half sun and half shade

TRAIL TRAFFIC: Generally light

TRAIL SURFACE: Dirt, trail follows old roadbeds

HIKING TIME: 5–6 hours

DRIVING DISTANCE: About 8 miles from the PA 72, Lancaster/Lebanon exit off Interstate 76, the PA Turnpike

ACCESS: Open; on state game land

MAPS: USGS Manheim and Lititz; the entire hike is on PA State Game Land 256, a map of which can be downloaded from www.pgc.state .pa.us/pgc/game/maps/default .asp?rgn=Southeast.

FACILITIES: None

WHEELCHAIR TRAVERSABLE: Some sections if trail is dry

SPECIAL COMMENTS: The entire hike is on state game land. Wear blaze orange during hunting season and consider hiking on Sundays.

IN BRIEF

This hike follows the main state game lands road (snowmobiles and ATVs ridden by handicapped hunters are the only motorized vehicles allowed) west into the heart of the game lands. At the second major **T**-intersection next to a large clearing on the left, the route goes to the north (right) and makes a 3-mile loop descending down to the level of the turnpike before climbing back to the clearing.

DESCRIPTION

At nearly 10 miles in length, this is a rather long hike. Yet the entire excursion follows good dirt roads that are closed to vehicular traffic. The grades are all very reasonable, so the walking is pleasant. This excursion provides a wonderful outing through the Furnace Hills area of Lancaster County, the largest tract of forested land in the county. The region was so named because of the numerous coal furnaces and forges in operation in the area during the 19th century. Just 3 miles to the south, Speedwell Forge in Lancaster County is the closest coal forge to this hike. The Cornwall Iron Furnace in Lebanon County is also located nearby.

This entire hike is on state game lands that provide habitat for white-tailed deer,

GPS Trailhead Coordinates

UTM Zone (WGS84)   18T

Easting   385216

Northing   4454593

Latitude   N 40° 14′ 2.09″

Longitude   W 76° 20′ 57.50″

Directions ⟶

From the PA Turnpike, follow PA 72 north to US 322. Take 322 east for about 5.75 miles. Turn right on Speedwell Forge Road and just before the turnpike overpass turn right on Dead End Road, very obviously marked with a sign. Follow for about 0.75 miles to the large state game lands parking lot on the right marked by a sign on the road.

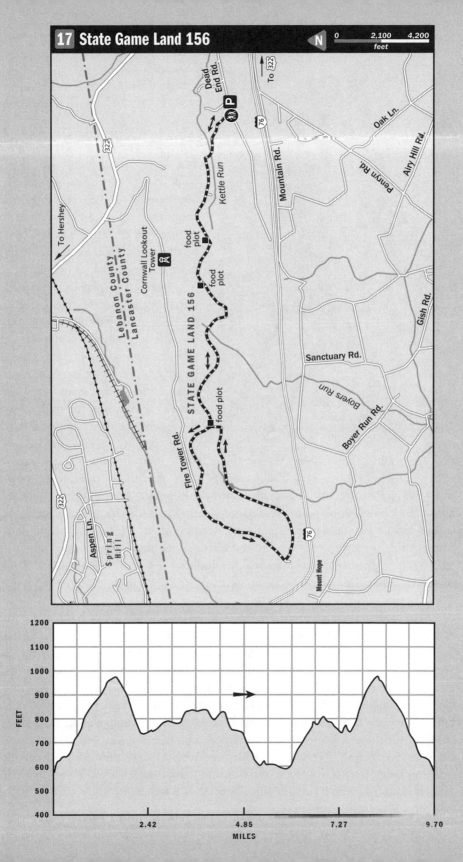

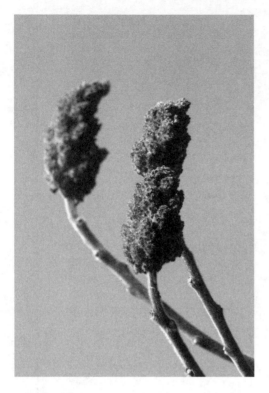

Staghorn sumac

red fox, rabbit, ruffed grouse, wild turkey, migrating warblers, wrens, and vireos among other species of wildlife. One of the most interesting aspects of the terrain is the abundance of mature white ash throughout the area. You will also find butternut trees along the lower, most distant stretch of the path.

Begin the hike by following the dirt road past the access gate in the back of the parking area. Climb a gentle grade through the woods and into an open area with quite a bit of thicket with several bird-houses along the road. After it passes the clearing, the trail enters the woods and then climbs a steady grade, passing several small clear-ings for about a mile. Along the way, you'll pass many staghorn sumac trees, which in the winter present a stocky scarlet cluster of seedpods pointing upward. They are quite attractive, especially against a blue sky. At the top of the rise, about 1.25 miles, you'll come to a large clearing identified by a small stand of spruce trees near a junction with a road heading off to a food plot on the left. The clearing offers a pretty view to the north of the main ridge line of the Fur-nace Hills, topped by radio towers and a lookout tower. The Horse-Shoe Trail traverses that ridge, and it may be accessed from Pumping Station Road by US 322 to the north.

The walking is flat for the next 0.25 miles and then the trail begins to descend by another food plot. The expansive view of Lancaster County to the southwest from here is quite lovely. Soon you enter the woods and shortly there-after (2 miles) you reach a significant T-intersection in the road. The road to the left is marked by a small, triangular, green equestrian sign and several large game lands signs indicating that the area is closed to all motor vehicles and snowmo-biles. Turn right here and descend into a large hollow, crossing a concrete bridge/culvert over the creek after a short distance. The forest consists of mature birch trees and white ash. White ash is identified best by its thin seedpods about 2 inches long. They cover the ground during the fall and winter. Taller than the related black ash, which reaches only about 40 feet in height, white ash can reach 80 feet. Many of the trees in this area are in that range.

At approximately 3.2 miles, you come to another T-intersection at a large food plot on the left that lies in a valley between two ridges. This is the beginning of a 3-mile loop through the lower, western section of the preserve. The food plot on the left provides a wonderful location for a break before and after completing the loop. Pull up a seat on an old log near the edge of the plot, and watch for birds in the bushes here. Turn to the right and traverse the hillside for another 0.75 miles past the access road to the radio towers on the north ridge. Continue walking straight along the road as it follows the ridgetop to the southwest. As you proceed you'll pass some timber sale areas that have been recently clear-cut.

At about 5 miles, the trail curves back to the east and descends for a little distance farther before beginning the climb back to the end of the loop. The Pennsylvania Turnpike is nearby, just a couple of hundred yards through the woods to the south, and its din is omnipresent. Before reaching the lowest elevation of the hike, you'll pass some ash saplings as well as some mature trees. Along the road are butternut trees, identified by the straggly branches and their bunches of seed-pods. They are distinct from the other trees, and the contrast is enough to make them easily recognizable.

Continue along the road heading up a small valley, passing a tiny pond surrounded by cattails on the right. A birdhouse and a waterfowl box have been constructed here, though neither was occupied when I passed through in the winter. The remaining 0.4 miles from the pond back to the food plot and the end of the loop passes through a very scenic area, with the road rising ahead of you beneath a tree-covered ridge. As you enter the food plot, take notice of the propagation area on the right defined by a wire fence. A forest management site, the fence is designed to keep deer from browsing on the bark of young trees within the area.

From the end of the loop, you have another 3 miles of walking back to the car, much of which is downhill. With the trek being mostly on good dirt roads, I imagine that this route would make for a nice mountain-biking trip.

NEARBY ACTIVITIES

Speedwell Forge County Park is about a mile south on Speedwell Forge Road from Dead End Road. The parking area is on the right just over Hammer Creek at a bend in the road. A short walk takes you to the site of the old forge. If you don't feel like hiking anymore (which wouldn't be surprising) but are still interested in taking in some of the history, the Cornwall Furnace in Cornwall is less than 6 miles away. It has a museum with several exhibits and informative programs. The grounds are also nice for picnicking. From Pumping Station Road, head east on US 322 for about 2.9 miles. Turn right on Granite Road and follow it for another 2 miles to the furnace.

18 STONY MOUNTAIN FROM THE NORTH

i KEY AT-A-GLANCE INFORMATION

LENGTH: 11.5 miles
CONFIGURATION: Loop
DIFFICULTY: Very strenuous
SCENERY: Appalachian Trail; Rattling Run town site; Devils Race Course
EXPOSURE: Mostly shaded
TRAIL TRAFFIC: Light
TRAIL SURFACE: Dirt and rocky
HIKING TIME: 6 hours
DRIVING DISTANCE: About 12.5 from the intersection of US 22/322 and PA 225 west of Harrisburg
ACCESS: Open; on state game land
MAPS: USGS Enders and Grantville; *Appalachian Trail in Pennsylvania, Sections 7 and 8: Susquehanna River to Swatara Gap;* entire hike is on PA State Game Land 211, maps 211a and 211b, which can be downloaded from www.pgc.state.pa.us/pgc/game/maps/defaultasp?rgn=Southeast.
FACILITIES: None
WHEELCHAIR TRAVERSABLE: No
SPECIAL COMMENTS: A beautiful long walk in the woods, though best to allow a full day. The descent could be a little treacherous if wet. Because this hike crosses state game land, care should be taken during hunting season. From November 15 to December 15, you must wear at least 250 square inches of blaze orange.

GPS Trailhead Coordinates

UTM Zone (WGS84) 18T
Easting   349385
Northing 4479406
Latitude   N 40° 27' 6.03"
Longitude   W 76° 46' 34.25"

IN BRIEF

This wonderful hike follows the Appalachian Trail as it traverses the north side of Stony Mountain to the ridge line, where it joins the Horse-Shoe Trail at its western terminus. After descending the Horse-Shoe Trail for 0.6 miles, it joins Rattling Run Road at the Devils Race Course and the old town site of Rattling Run. From here, the hike follows Rattling Run Road up to Third Mountain, where it picks up the northern extension of the Water Tank Trail and descends the mountain, concluding the loop. A short (1.2 miles round-trip) side trip brings you to the site of the Stony Mountain Lookout Tower.

DESCRIPTION

The first 3 miles of this long and beautiful hike follow the Appalachian Trail up to Stony Mountain on Pennsylvania State Game Land 211. From the parking area, cross Clark Creek over a good bridge, passing a gate. Just beyond the bridge, you'll see two blue blazes marking a forest road. That is the end of the Water Tank Trail and the end of the loop hike. The junction with the A.T. is marked at this spot by two white blazes indicating that the trail turns left.

At first the A.T. follows a small tributary of Clark Creek along an old roadbed. The forest here is one of the prettiest places I have been in Pennsylvania, with hemlock trees along

----

Directions ————————————————→

Follow US 22/322 West from Harrisburg to PA 225/Halifax exit. Follow PA 225 north 2.5 miles to PA 325. Turn right on PA 325 and follow for 9.9 miles to Appalachian Trail crossing. The A.T. is well marked. Park on the right behind the little hill next to the road.

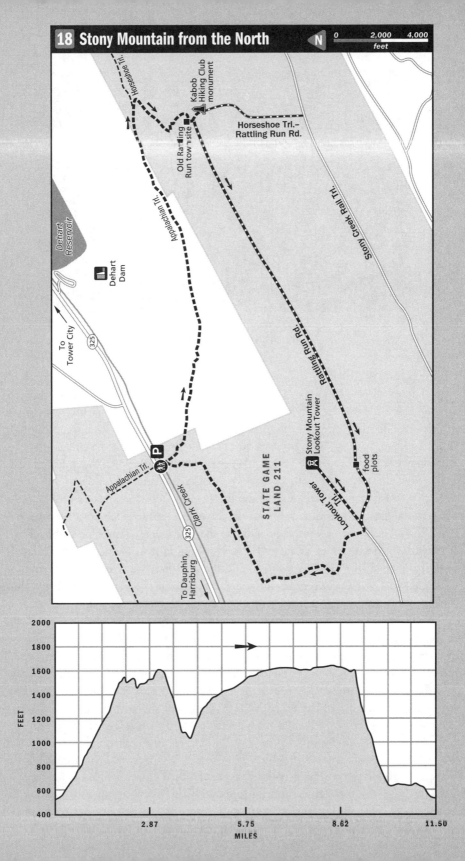

N

0   2,000   4,000
                    feet

Horseshoe Trl.

Kabob
Hiking Club
monument

Old Rattling
Run tower site

Horseshoe Trl.–
Rattling Run Rd.

Appalachian Trl.

Dehart
Reservoir

Stony Creek Rail Trl.

Dehart
Dam

To
Tower City

325

Rattling Run Rd.

STATE GAME
LAND 211

Stony Mountain
Lookout Tower

food
plots

Appalachian Trl.

P

Lookout Tower
Trl.

Clark Creek

325

To Dauphin,
Harrisburg

2000

1800

1600

1400

1200

FEET 1000

800

600

400

2.87   5.75   8.62   11.50

MILES

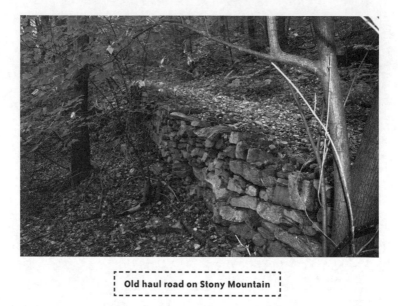

Old haul road on Stony Mountain

the creek, and tall hickory and oak trees stretching up the rocky and rugged hillside. The roadbed continues all the way to the crest of Stony Mountain, traversing the side of the mountain and providing nice views of the Clark Creek valley during the fall and winter. As you progress, the trail becomes a little steep, though never too bad. It does, however, get quite rocky after the first 0.5 miles or so.

At about 2 miles, the trail descends rather significantly for a short distance. In this area you'll notice remnants of old switchbacks and retaining walls of one of the old coal roads that used to climb the mountain. Just shy of 3 miles, the trail climbs for a short distance and then tops out on the ridge. At the ridge crest, two yellow blazes on a birch tree to your right indicate the beginning of the Horse-Shoe Trail. It extends for 141.4 miles to Valley Forge National Historic Park outside Philadelphia. Just ahead, the Horse-Shoe Trail and the A.T. part ways at a stone memorial dedicated to Cyril C. Sturgis Jr., an active member of the Horse-Shoe Trail Club during the 1960s. A yellow horseshoe is nailed to the tree next to it.

After a well-deserved break here, follow the Horse-Shoe Trail past a trail register, down the south side of the ridge contouring to the west. You are now entering a region known as St. Anthony's Wilderness, one of the largest open and wild areas in the state. The Horse-Shoe Trail descends rather steeply for the next half mile before leveling out by the old town site of Rattling Run. Rattling Run was the location of the Stony Valley's first coal shafts, named Reliance and Perseverance, which were mined from 1825 to 1850. Just left of the trail you can find the ruins of old buildings. One look at the terrain makes obvious the sorts of hardships people went through to mine coal. The forest floor is nothing but a huge talus field that the main creek, the Devils Race Course, flows beneath.

Just past the town site, the trail joins with the old Rattling Run Road. The Horse-Shoe Trail turns to the left here and descends into the Stony Creek valley.

This hike follows Rattling Run Road uphill and west along the Devils Race Course to the head of the drainage at the junction of the ridges that form Sharp Mountain (to your left as you are walking) and Stony Mountain (to the right). A large flat rock on the right provides a comfortable spot to rest about 100 feet up the road from the trail junction. Before heading uphill, however, be sure to walk downhill about a hundred yards to have a look at the monument commemorating the founding of the Kabob Hiking Club of Harrisburg and Vicinity.

From its junction with the Horse-Shoe Trail, Rattling Run Road climbs rather steeply at first, but it soon levels out and for the next several miles climbs at a gentle grade. The hiking here through a forest of birch and hickory trees is pleasant as the path is sandy and grassy. The occasional yellow blazes indicate that this was the old path of the Horse-Shoe Trail, now rerouted.

This hike follows Rattling Run Road for approximately 3.5 miles from the junction to the trail spur that leads to the Stony Mountain Lookout Tower. On the way, you'll pass a significant road cut on the right at 6.1 miles (the Henry Knavber Trail), and two large food plots numbered 5 and 6 (7.1 miles). These food plots provide food and shelter for wildlife on the game lands, and they are often planted with grasses or even with corn farther along the ridge.

Another 0.6 miles beyond the plots and you arrive at the junction with the spur to the lookout (7.75 miles). No sign marks the spur, though it is easily identifiable because it is a dead straight and flat dirt road with a swath of brush and brambles about 100 feet wide on each side of it. You'll undoubtedly feel a bit tuckered out when you reach the junction, but it is a flat, easy walk out to the lookout. An old fire tower, it's a large steel structure, 150 or so feet high, with a platform and small shelter on top.

Note: Climbing the tower is illegal, and a gate around the bottom is typically locked, but the clearing at the lookout's base is a nice place to rest and offers nice views to the north and east.

After the side trip to the lookout, you'll next head to the north extension of the Water Tank Trail. It can be a little difficult to locate. From the junction of Rattling Run Road and the road to the lookout tower, walk west along the road for 100 feet or so until you reach a small clearing to your right. Follow the road to the end of the clearing. On your left will be a tall oak with a blue blaze that marks the path of the Water Tank Trail as it enters the woods heading south. A small cairn is located on the right side of the road marking the path of the north extension, though the path is indistinct through the clearing. If you look into the woods, you should spot a blue blaze on a tree. Keep in mind that the Water Tank Trail crosses directly perpendicular to Rattling Run Road. If you don't spot the blaze, follow the edge of the clearing until you reach the woods. The trail is obvious when it enters the woods and is well marked with blue blazes all the way down the mountain. Significant deadfall obstructs the trail in several places and requires a little circumnavigation. Make sure that you get back on the trail and see the blazes before wandering too far.

After about 0.2 miles of walking through the woods along rather level terrain, the trail descends abruptly and drops left from a prominent cairn. Although steep, the trail surface is mostly dirt and offers good footing through a pretty forest of fir trees. After a while, the footing gets more rocky and rugged, demanding attention, but is manageable. At 8.9 miles, you'll reach a flat area on the hillside where you'll find a maple tree with a bunch of blazes. The trail bends to the right here.

The walking gets more significantly rocky for the next 0.8 miles from the bend, but is not as steep as above. In spots it is rather brushy and heavily eroded, appearing to be little more than a watercourse. But it is always well marked. At just about 10 miles into this hike, you emerge from the woods at a significant logging road. Turn right here (east) and follow the road for 1.5 miles to the end of the Water Tank Trail at its junction with the A.T. Along the way, you'll pass a large clearing (10.5 miles) to the south of the trail with some very tall trees. This is a great place to spot hawks.

At about 11.1 miles, the road enters an area that has been recently cleared of trees, with a new road cut heading into the woods to the east. The Water Tank Trail and the original roadbed make a left here, heading downhill toward the creek. A blue blaze marks the way on a tree just downhill from the clearing. At the time of this writing, the way was obvious, although I can imagine it getting less so if the area were to be cleared more extensively. The A.T. is 0.4 miles from this clearing and the parking area just a few minutes beyond.

You could, of course, reverse the route (though I think it walks better in a clockwise direction), or simply hike from the Clark Creek parking area up the Water Tank Trail to visit the lookout tower (a popular and much shorter hike of about 3.3 miles each way). If you choose that route, be certain to pick up the Water Tank Trail where it begins to climb at the right place (about 1.5 miles). Heading west, you'll pass three decent-sized meadows, all of which have an old logging road heading up the side of the mountain. The Water Tank Trail is obviously a footpath where it departs from the road, although there is no sign, just a few blue blazes on a tree to the left.

NEARBY ACTIVITIES

Clark Creek, which parallels PA 325, offers wonderful fishing for both bait and fly anglers.

STONY MOUNTAIN FROM THE SOUTH

19

IN BRIEF

This lovely hike begins by following the multi-use Horse-Shoe Trail (referred to variously on some maps and locally as the Stony Creek Trail or the Stony Valley Rail Trail) for 2 miles along the Stony Creek valley. At 2 miles, it picks up the Water Tank Trail and climbs steeply to the ridge of Stony Mountain, where it meets with Rattling Run Road. A short (1.2 miles round-trip) detour takes you to the Stony Mountain Lookout Tower. The descent follows Rattling Run Road down the south side of Third Mountain and back to Ellendale Road.

DESCRIPTION

Begin this hike at the Ellendale gate at the beginning of the Stony Valley Rail Trail, also the equestrian path of the Horse-Shoe Trail. This trail follows the path of the old Dauphin and Susquehanna Railroad, constructed in the early 1800s to support coal-mining operations in and around the Stony Creek valley. Now the railroad grade serves as a path for hikers, bikers, and horseback riders, and it extends for 24 miles to the Lebanon Reservoir in Schuylkill County. This hike follows the grade for the first 2 miles to the junction with the Water Tank Trail on the left.

Directions

From Harrisburg, follow US 322 West to Dauphin Boro/Stony Creek exit. Exit highway and drive over the creek. You are on Allegheny Street. Turn right on Schuylkill Street and then right on Erie Street (at stop sign). Signs point to Stony Creek. At end of Erie Street turn left on Stony Creek Road. Follow Stony Creek Road for approximately 5 miles where it turns to dirt and is called Ellendale Road. Follow for another 1.05 miles until the road ends at a gate with a large parking area.

KEY AT-A-GLANCE INFORMATION

LENGTH: 9.5 miles
CONFIGURATION: Loop
DIFFICULTY: Very strenuous
SCENERY: Stony Creek valley and ridge of Stony Mountain
EXPOSURE: About half sun and half shade
TRAIL TRAFFIC: Light
TRAIL SURFACE: Dirt and rock
HIKING TIME: 4.5–5.5 hours
DRIVING DISTANCE: About 9 miles from US 22/322 at the Dauphin Boro/Stony Creek exit west of Harrisburg
ACCESS: Open; on state game land
MAPS: USGS Enders; *Appalachian Trail in Pennsylvania, Sections 7 and 8: Susquehanna River to Swatara Gap;* the entire hike is on PA State Game Land 211, map 211a, which can be downloaded from www.pgc.state.pa.us/pgc/game/maps/default.asp?rgn=Southeast.
FACILITIES: None
WHEELCHAIR TRAVERSABLE: No

See additional comments at end of Description, page 98.

GPS Trailhead Coordinates

UTM Zone (WGS84) 18T
Easting 345729
Northing 4474455
Latitude N 40° 24′ 23.10″
Longitude W 76° 49′ 6.38

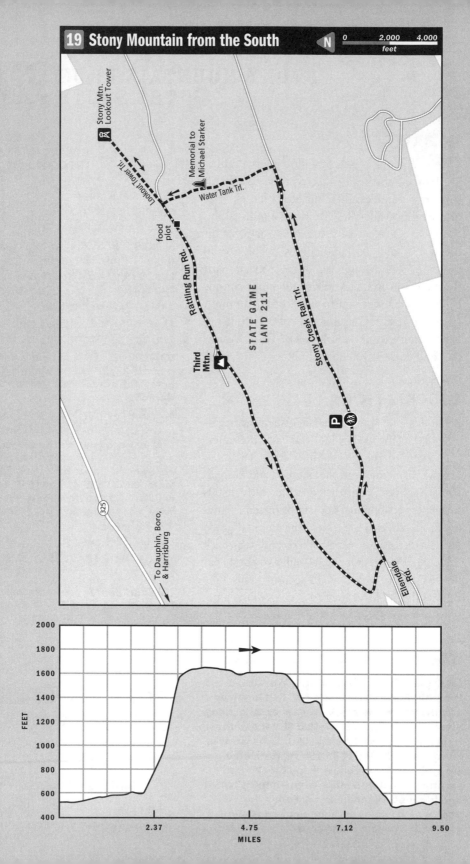

N

0   2,000   4,000
feet

Stony Mtn.
Lookout Tower

Memorial to
Michael Starker

Water Tank Trl.

Lookout Tower Trl.

food
plot

Rattling Run Rd.

Stony Creek Rail Trl.

STATE GAME
LAND 211

Third
Mtn.

P

325

To Dauphin, Boro,
& Harrisburg

Ellendale Rd.

2000
1800
1600
1400
1200
1000
800
600
400

FEET

2.37   4.75   7.12   9.50

MILES

Finding the junction with the Water Tank Trail can be difficult, as it is marked only by three blue blazes on a small maple tree on the left of the railroad grade. There is no sign. The trailhead is just beyond a spot where a small creek passes underneath the railroad grade creek via a stone aqueduct identified by two metal poles (one on each side of the trail) painted white on the bottom and red on the top (1.9 miles). The Water Tank Trail takes off left 0.1 mile farther on from a point about 100 feet before a tree on the right with a large blue-and-white sign with a disability symbol mounted just above a smaller green triangular sign with an equestrian symbol mounted just above a yellow blaze. The tree sits at the far end of what appears to be an old parking pull-out to the side of the trail under some hemlock trees. This was the site of Water Tank, where a wooden storage tank that provided water for the engines passing through the valley was located.

Once you gain the Water Tank Trail, the route-finding difficulties are finished, although the difficult hiking is just beginning. Over the next mile, the trail climbs just about 1,000 feet over very rough terrain. For the first 0.25 miles, the trail climbs moderately, and it is easy to follow through the woods with plenty of blue blazes. Then it joins what appears to be an old haul path for lumber and takes a direct route up the mountain. Soon you meet the course of a significant creek, and just beyond that point you pass a memorial marker for Michael Starker, a hiker who went missing in the area in the fall of 2000 (2.54 miles). From here the trail gets very wet, rugged, and steep, sometimes absurdly so, for about a half mile, as it passes by some rocky outcrops and a trail marked by orange blazes to the right. At times the path crosses back and forth through the creek. At times it goes straight up it.

If this sounds unpleasant enough to make you consider walking the loop in reverse, keep two things in mind: first, the climb is short and is over with soon enough; and second, the only thing more unpleasant than walking up this path would be walking down it, especially with 7 miles of hiking behind you. A mile from the railroad grade (3 miles), the trail levels out abruptly, curves decisively to the right and then back to the left, and after about 0.1 mile tops out on the ridge at the Rattling Run Road, a wide-open and generally flat road.

From here, turn right on the road and then left at the fork just ahead. The Stony Mountain Lookout Tower is 0.6 miles from the fork. Note that the tower is closed to the public, but from the clearing at its base, you can take in a decent view toward the Dehart Reservoir to the east and of the Clark Creek valley to the north.

After visiting the tower, return to the junction with the Water Tank Trail and continue hiking west along Third Mountain. After the mile-long hill climb, the flat ridge road could not be more pleasant. Thick brush and berry bushes line the road. Tall hickory, oak, maple, and pine trees make up the woods on either side. Occasionally, you pass by wildlife food plots. In the fall, the colors are beautiful. In late summer, you can find hundreds of butterflies, frogs, praying mantises, and snakes along the trail. I discovered a four-foot-long black rat snake in August sunning itself on the trail.

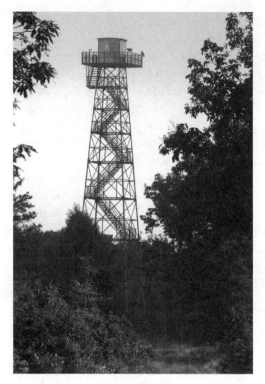

Stony Mountain Lookout Tower

The trail is mostly level for about 1.2 miles as it follows the ridge, and then it reaches a gate at a hairpin turn on the access road to the radio towers atop Third Mountain. I've never felt compelled to walk up the road to see the towers. With the exception of one just above the gate, they remain pleasantly hidden from view. This hike follows the road downhill for 2.5 miles back into the Stony Creek valley. You'll have wonderful views of the valley and Second Mountain along the way. The road is, however, south facing and is not especially shaded for a good bit of the walk, so it can be rather hot and dry in the summer time. At just about 8 miles into this hike, you'll reach Ellendale Road, where you turn left and walk another 1.25 miles back to the car at the trailhead.

Note: With the exception of the third mile of the hike, which ascends 1,000 feet along a rough and rocky path, all of the walking is on good roadbeds with easy or moderate grades. The Water Tank Trail is subject to flooding and may be impassable during and after heavy rains. Because this hike crosses state game land, care should be taken during hunting season. From November 15 through December 15, you must wear at least 250 square inches of blaze orange.

NEARBY ACTIVITIES

Stony Creek is a nice fishing creek, especially in the area of the trailhead and parking area. The Stoney Creek Restaurant and Lounge at the intersection of Erie Street and Stony Creek Road in Dauphin Boro is a nice place to grab a bite after the hike.

SWATARA STATE PARK RAIL TRAIL:
Waterville Bridge to Swopes Valley Road

20

IN BRIEF

This hike begins in Swatara Gap and follows the Appalachian Trail west over Swatara Creek via the Waterville Bridge (no automobiles). On the west side of the creek, it follows the Swatara State Park Rail Trail along the Swatara Creek for about 6 miles to the town of Suedberg. From Suedberg, the hike follows the shoulders of two roads for about 0.7 miles to a picnic area on Swopes Valley Road.

DESCRIPTION

Located in Lebanon County, Swatara State Park is a mostly undeveloped park that provides opportunities for a variety of activities, including hiking, biking, fishing, canoeing, and hunting. An 8-mile section of Swatara Creek flows the length of the park, exiting at its southern boundary in Swatara Gap, a large water gap through the flank of Blue Mountain. Interstate 81 passes through the gap directly above the creek, as does the A.T. directly below I-81. A significant tributary of the Susquehanna River, the Swatara Creek watershed encompasses a large area of the high country north and east of I-81. The creek through the park is part of the

KEY AT-A-GLANCE INFORMATION

LENGTH: About 12 miles or shorter if you walk only a portion (see the hike profile for options)

CONFIGURATION: Out-and-back

DIFFICULTY: Easy–moderate depending on length

SCENERY: Swatara Creek and Swatara Gap

EXPOSURE: About half sun and half shade

TRAIL TRAFFIC: Moderate

TRAIL SURFACE: Cinders; paved at the beginning of the hike

HIKING TIME: Depends on length; about 5.5 hours in full

DRIVING DISTANCE: 2.5 miles from Interstate 81 at Lickdale

ACCESS: Dawn–dusk

MAPS: USGS Indiantown Gap, Tower City, and Pine Grove; *Appalachian Trail in Pennsylvania, Sections 1 through 6: Delaware Water Gap to Swatara Gap*

FACILITIES: None

WHEELCHAIR TRAVERSABLE: The first mile or so from the parking area at the Waterville Bridge is paved and accessible.

SPECIAL COMMENTS: Several options exist for extending or shortening this hike.

Directions ⟶

Take the Lickdale exit off Interstate 81 and follow Monroe Valley Road east across PA 72. Veer left when it changes to Monroe Valley Drive. Turn left at the first T-intersection (Little Mountain Road goes right), left again at the second T-intersection, and then right on Old State Road. Pass beneath I-81, and you will begin to see white blazes for the Appalachian Trail. Just beyond the significant Waterville Bridge (over which the A.T. crosses Swatara Creek), you'll find a nice parking area on the left. Parking is also available along the road in the area of the bridge.

GPS Trailhead Coordinates

UTM Zone (WGS84) 18T

Easting 370575

Northing 4481986

Latitude N 40° 28′ 42.54″

Longitude W 76° 31′ 36.90″

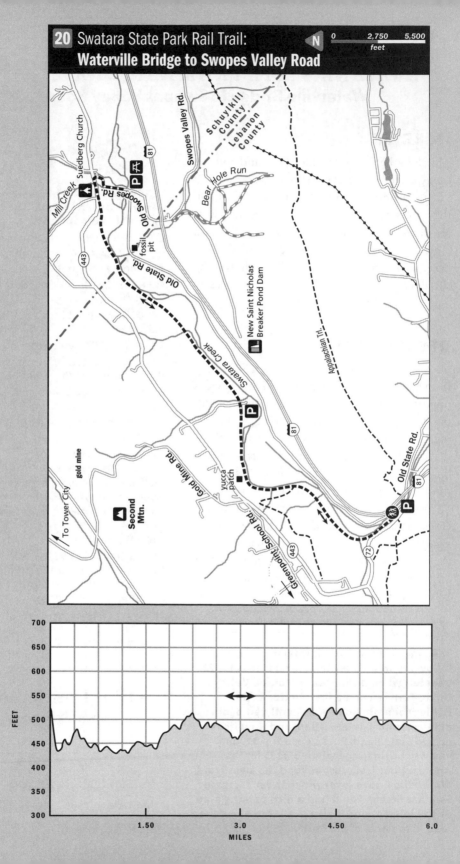

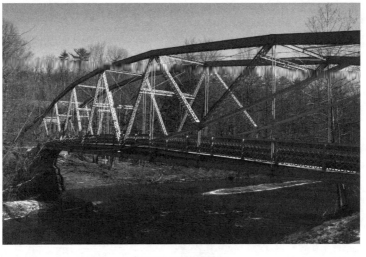

Waterville Bridge

Swatara Creek Water Trail, which extends from Pine Grove to the north to Middletown and the Susquehanna River to the southwest. A map of the water trail indicating all the points of interest is available at parking areas in the park.

Several options exist for hiking the rail-trail through Swatara State Park. The first, which this profile documents, is an out-and-back trip beginning from the Waterville Bridge. The rail-trail extends for approximately 6 miles through the park, leaving the park at PA 443 at the town of Suedberg, a good location to turn around. This makes a round-trip of about 12 miles. Or you can simply hike out for as long as you feel comfortable and turn back. A second option, if you have two cars, is to run a shuttle, leaving one car at the picnic and parking area on Swopes Valley Road just beyond Suedberg. Doing so allows you to make a pleasant hike of about 6.5 miles one-way.

A third option is to make a loop hike of about 12.3 miles hiking from the Waterville Bridge out the rail-trail to Swopes Valley Road and then returning south of the creek via the Old State Road back to the parking area at the bridge. I find this option the least appealing of all, though not because of the length, as you might suppose. If you choose to walk the Old State Road, you are likely to be sharing the path with automobiles and ATVs. Additionally, it passes close enough to Interstate 81 at times for the highway noise to be bothersome. Personally with a single car, I prefer the hike out to Suedberg and back. This description will provide directions for the rail-trail from the Waterville Bridge as far as the parking area at Swopes Valley Road.

Begin at the parking area in Swatara Gap and cross over the Waterville Bridge. The bridge was constructed in 1890 by the Berlin Bridge Company, of East Berlin, Connecticut. The bridge was originally located over Little Pine Creek in Lycoming County. It was moved to its current location in 1987. Turn right on

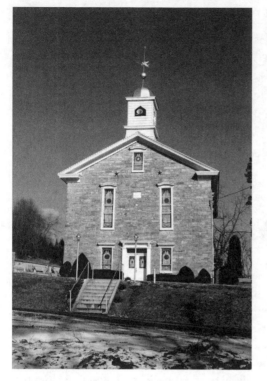

Suedberg Church of God

the paved rail-trail and follow it northeast along the creek. The trail begins a couple of miles to the south in Lickdale and runs for about 8.5 miles to the northern terminus of the park. With the exception of the first paved section, the trail surface is cinders and dirt.

After a short distance, a paved trail ascends to the left. Stay on the trail at the level of the creek where it becomes more of a road. After about 0.5 miles, the rail-trail departs from the paved road at a bend. The footpath follows the paved road for a long way and you can stick to the road if the trail is muddy or overgrown. After about a mile of walking, you should see the 3-mile trail marker (a brown post marked SW RT) just off of the road, and you pass a wonderful area of lots of thicket and grasses with scattered trees to the left of the road. This is a great place to look for wildlife, especially early in the morning. The red foxes seem to love this area.

Just shy of the 4-mile trail marker, the paved road ends and you are forced to walk along the old railroad grade. Here, the grade is carved through a shale outcrop and just beyond the cut, you'll come across a small patch of yucca growing along the right side of the trail. It is not what you would expect to see in central Pennsylvania, though according to one of my natural-history guides, small stands are not uncommon throughout the state. The plant is probably not native.

Continue along the rail-trail a fair distance above the creek. Soon you'll cross the 5-mile marker, and just beyond that a parking area. From the parking area, you can access the creek by following a footpath leading to the south. It meanders around the woods for a bit, by some old coal mining debris, and eventually comes to a nice spot on the creek among pines and hemlocks. The parking area at the trail can be accessed from PA 443 just east of Gold Mine Road. A park sign identifies the turn.

From the parking area, continue northeast along the rail-trail. The path follows the creek about 30 feet or so above its level, and at places offers nice views up and downstream. Between the 6-mile and 7-mile markers, some straggly trees stand on either side of the trail. I haven't yet been able to identify them. They have a distinctive appearance, however. Beyond the 7-mile marker, you'll reach a lovely large meadow on the right side of the trail. This is a great place for birding. Just past the meadow, you'll reach a gate on the trail at PA 443 (6 miles). The attractive Suedberg Church of God is across PA 443 to your left. If you are hiking out and back, this is a good place to turn around.

If you parked a car at the small picnic area on Swopes Valley Road or want a little more hiking, follow the trail for about 150 feet to a point where it dips down by a culvert. From this point, walk over to PA 443 and follow its shoulder east to Swopes Valley Road onto which you will turn right. At the corner, you'll find a scenic carcass of an old abandoned house. Follow Swopes Valley Road for about 0.6 miles to the bridge over Swatara Creek. The picnic area is on the left just beyond the bridge. If you feel compelled to make the loop hike, turn right onto Old State Road just past the bridge and follow it back to the car.

NEARBY ACTIVITIES

At the picnic area on Swopes Valley Road (just across from the end of Old State Road), you'll find a picnic table, a clearing, and a small pond surrounded by reeds and cattails. A fossil pit is located about 1 mile south and east from the picnic area along Old State Road. You are allowed to keep the fossils you find there.

21 TABLE ROCK AND PETERS MOUNTAIN HIKE

KEY AT-A-GLANCE INFORMATION

LENGTH: 2 miles to Table Rock; 3.1 miles to Peters Mountain Shelter; 4.15 miles to Victoria Furnace Trail. Double the distance for return.

CONFIGURATION: Out-and-back

DIFFICULTY: Easy–moderate

SCENERY: View of Clark Creek valley, Peters Mountain Shelter; very nice ridge walking

EXPOSURE: Mostly shaded

TRAIL TRAFFIC: Moderate–heavy on weekends

TRAIL SURFACE: Dirt

HIKING TIME: 2 hours for Table Rock, 3 hours for Peters Mountain Shelter; 4 hours for Victoria Furnace Trail

DRIVING DISTANCE: About 10 miles from intersection of Interstate 81 and US 22/322 outside of Harrisburg

ACCESS: Open

MAPS: USGS Halifax and Enders; *Appalachian Trail in Pennsylvania, Sections 7 and 8: Susquehanna River to Swatara Gap*

FACILITIES: Spring and privy at Peters Mountain Shelter

WHEELCHAIR TRAVERSABLE: No

SPECIAL COMMENTS: A pleasant hike year-round

GPS Trailhead Coordinates

UTM Zone (WGS84)   18T

Easting   336252

Northing   4475267

Latitude   N 40° 24′ 42.92″

Longitude   W 76° 55′ 47.68″

IN BRIEF

This hike heads east out of the parking area along the Appalachian Trail, along the Peters Mountain ridge to Table Rock, a wonderful sunny overlook. From there, you can follow the A.T. to the Peters Mountain Shelter, and from there to the Victoria Trail near the boundary of the Joseph E. Ibberson Conservation Area (see page 50).

DESCRIPTION

The first section of this hike, to Table Rock and back, is deservedly popular. The walking is easy, the distance is not too long, and the view from the rock is spectacular. Beyond Table Rock, the trail can still be busy, as a trip to the Peters Mountain Shelter and back makes for an easy overnight excursion. Beyond the shelter, you'll see fewer people, mostly folks exploring the A.T.

This hike offers pretty views along Peters Mountain, one of the significant long, level ridges that form the Valley and Ridge Physiographic Province of central Pennsylvania. Peters Mountain extends for nearly 30 miles from the Susquehanna River north of Harrisburg northeast to Tower City. Across the Susquehanna, which forms a large water gap in the ridge, it continues as Cove Mountain to the west.

Directions

Follow US 22/322 north from Harrisburg to PA 225 north toward Halifax. Follow PA 225 for about 4 miles to the crest of Peters Mountain. Immediately before the ridge and passing beneath the Appalachian Trail footbridge, a dirt road exits to the right at an Appalachian Trail sign. Drive up this dirt road and park in the large parking area atop. Note: Do not park by the house just north of the bridge on PA 225; that is private property.

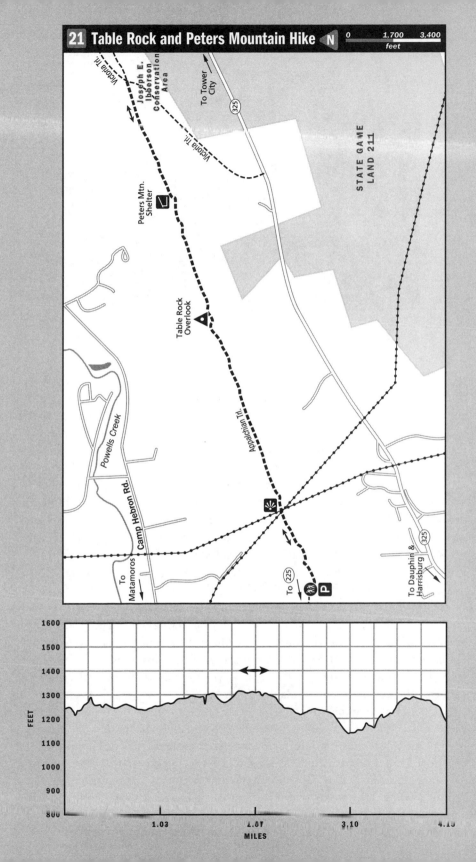

0   1,700   3,400
feet

Victoria Trl.

Joseph E.
Ibberson
Conservation
Area

To Tower
City

325

Victoria Trl.

STATE GAME
LAND 211

Peters Mtn.
Shelter

Table Rock
Overlook

Appalachian Trl.

Powells Creek

Camp Hebron Rd.

To
Matamoros

To 225

P

325

To Dauphin &
Harrisburg

1600
1500
1400
1300
1200
1100
1000
900
800

FEET

1.03   1.07   3.10   4.10

MILES

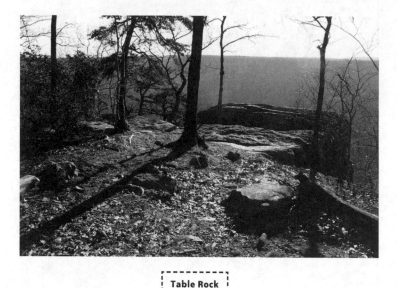

Table Rock

The top of Peters Mountain, like many of the other mountains in the Valley and Ridge Province, is formed of extremely hard, erosion-resistant sandstone. All across its crest you'll find large, blocky outcrops of rock. The ridge line is surprisingly narrow in places, though not so much on this hike. The top of the mountain varies very little in elevation, and because this hike begins at the top of the ridge, you'll have very little climbing. It is mostly flat walking on a good trail.

From the parking area above PA 225, head east along the Appalachian Trail. You may get slightly confused as you leave the parking area because an inviting dirt road leads directly up the ridge. The A.T. actually heads over to the south side of the mountain right away to bypass the radio towers to which the road leads. Look for the white blazes and a trail sign for Table Rock (2 miles) and Peters Mountain Shelter (3 miles) pointing the way over some rocks.

After passing below the radio towers, the trail climbs back to the ridge, crosses over the top and joins an old roadbed. The walking here is extremely pleasant. You'll begin to see some of the outcrops along the ridgetop here and if you are feeling ambitious you might scramble to the top of one or two for a view. Soon, however, the trail passes beneath a power line dropping off to the north from a large outcrop. You'll get a great view of the Susquehanna River and the valley to the north up toward Halifax from here.

Continue along the trail, which quickly becomes more of a footpath through the woods. At 2 miles, you'll reach Table Rock. Although there is no sign, it is hard to miss. It is a large sandstone outcrop that forms a cliff on the south side of the ridge, offering an incredible view of Clark Creek and the ridge of Stony Mountain. Surrounded by Table Mountain pine trees that add to the beauty of the setting, I would have to say that this is one of the prettiest views along the ridges east of the Susquehanna River. If you look to the east across the valley, you should be able spot the Stony Mountain lookout tower 4 or 5 miles distant.

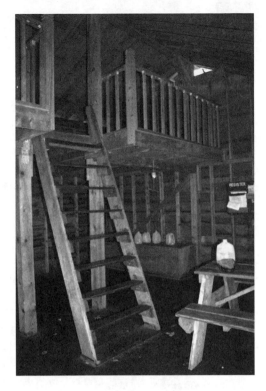

After you've had your fill of the view, continue east along the A.T. Just past Table Rock, you'll pass a junction with an orange-blazed trail dropping off the north side of the ridge. That is a private path, according to my A.T. map. Continue along the ridge for another mile to the Peters Mountain Shelter, constructed in 1994 by the Susquehanna Appalachian Trail Club. You'll find a privy here and a spring on the north side of the mountain (follow the sign from the shelter), though the water should be treated.

From the shelter, continue east through more oak trees along the ridge, and descend into a saddle via some rock steps at 4.15 miles. At the saddle, the A.T. continues along the ridge, crossing a dirt road rising from the south and descending to the northeast. This is the Victoria Trail, an old road used for hauling lumber to the Victoria Furnace in the Clark Creek valley from the Powell Creek valley to the north. Below the ridge to the north is the Joseph E. Ibberson Conservation Area. This is a nice place to rest before completing the trip by retracing your steps.

A suggestion for an alternate hike: if you have two cars, you can run a shuttle leaving one car at the parking area at the conservation area lot and the other at the A.T. lot at PA 225 on Peters Mountain. If you do that, you can follow this hike across Peters Mountain and then take the Victoria Trail down to the parking area at the conservation area (see page 50). Doing so will give you a one-way hike of about 6 miles.

22 WILDWOOD LAKE LOOP

KEY AT-A-GLANCE INFORMATION

LENGTH: 4.4 miles

CONFIGURATION: Loop

DIFFICULTY: Easy

SCENERY: Wildwood Lake Sanctuary and environs; great bird-watching

EXPOSURE: Mix of sun and shade

TRAIL TRAFFIC: Moderately heavy

TRAIL SURFACE: Varies among paved, dirt, boardwalk, and gravel

HIKING TIME: 1.5–2 hours

DRIVING DISTANCE: About 4.5 miles from downtown Harrisburg

ACCESS: Dawn–dusk

MAPS: USGS Harrisburg West; the nature center also provides a trail map, also available online at www .wildwoodlake.org/lake-sanctuary/ map.aspx.

FACILITIES: Water and restrooms available at the nature center; portable toilets en route

WHEELCHAIR TRAVERSABLE: Wildwood Way and the boardwalks on the east side of the lake are traversable as far as the Towpath Trail, 0.1 mile beyond the Susquehanna Spillway.

SPECIAL COMMENTS: Although subject to considerable road traffic noise, the sanctuary is visited year-round by many species of birds.

IN BRIEF

This 4.4-mile loop hike follows boardwalks and some of the lesser-used paths around the perimeter of Wildwood Lake.

DESCRIPTION

Formerly known as Wetzel's Swamp, the Wildwood Lake Sanctuary was constructed in 1907 as part of a movement to enhance recreational opportunities in urban areas and in order to control flood runoff from Paxton Creek, its main watershed. Located in northern Harrisburg, the sanctuary has a distinctly urban character. Industrial Road, which parallels the lake to the west, is lined with warehouses and distribution centers and sees plenty of truck traffic. To the south, the sanctuary is bordered by Interstate 81. US 322 forms its eastern and northern boundaries. The drone of traffic is a pervasive element of a hike around the lake.

Nonetheless, the lake and its environs are looked upon quite favorably by an abundance of wildlife that make it their permanent home or that use it as a layover on their migratory routes. Every time I visit the lake, I am amazed by the variety of wildlife I see. On a single trip in August, my sons and I saw osprey, herons, egrets, several varieties of turtles and

GPS Trailhead Coordinates

UTM Zone (WGS84) 18T

Easting   339931

Northing 4463503

Latitude   N 40° 18′ 24.63″

Longitude W 76° 53′ 1.22″

Directions

From Interstate 81, take the Front Street exit #66. Head north on Front Street to the first traffic light and turn right onto PA 39 (Lingles-town Road). Turn right at the next traffic light onto Industrial Road. Follow Industrial Road for about a mile. Turn left onto Wild-wood Way at a sign that says NATURE CENTER. If you go underneath I-81, you have gone too far. Follow the paved road to the parking lot.

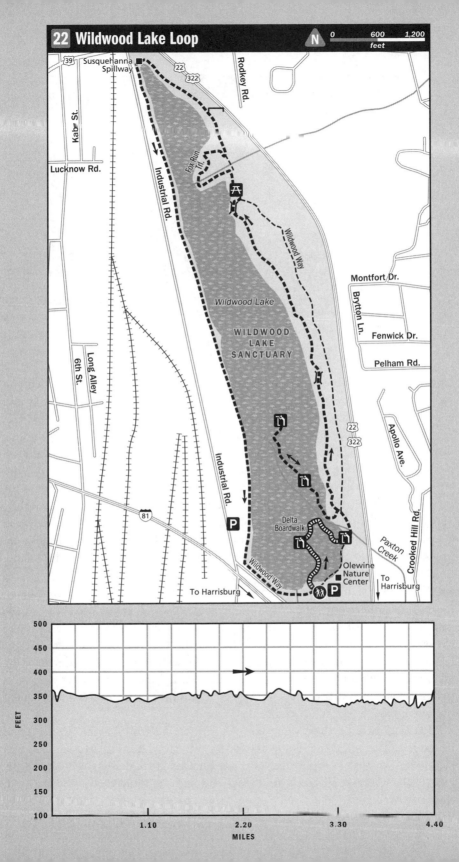

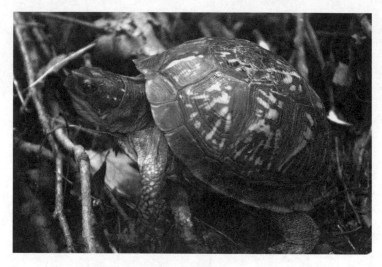

Painted turtle

frogs, a snake, and a woodchuck, whose sudden appearance on the trail made us all jump. The variety of flora is impressive, particularly the abundance of American lotus plants, which cover the surface of the lake by late summer.

A 3.1-mile loop following the main lakeside trails (Wildwood Way and the Towpath Trail) around the lake is popular with local walkers, joggers, and bicyclers, and the section from the nature center parking lot to the north on Wildwood Way is wheelchair accessible. At 4.4 miles, however, our hike follows the boardwalks along the east shore, providing nice side excursions to wildlife-viewing stations out in the center of the lake, before joining with Wildwood Way and the Towpath Trail for the remaining 1.2 miles. Sections of this hike are accessible to wheelchairs, and the boardwalks are closed to bicycles, skateboards, and inline skates.

This hike begins at the entrance to the Benjamin Olewine III Nature Center, located at parking area at the south end of Wildwood Lake. Walk toward the southeast corner of the lake along a paved path through wildflowers. Just beyond the wildflowers, turn right onto the Delta Boardwalk. It begins 360 feet from the nature center. The boardwalk passes through the wetlands area on the edge of the lake, and you'll find benches for resting and wildlife watching frequently along its length. This is a good area for spotting egrets and herons, both of which frequent the open water at the south end of the lake.

At 0.25 miles, a short spur takes you to viewing scopes about 50 feet or so to the left. The boardwalk is surrounded by waterfowl nesting areas. In addition to looking for birds, keep your eyes trained on the ground along the edge of the boardwalk where you'll likely find frogs and perhaps a turtle. Beyond the spur, the boardwalk meanders along Paxton Creek, passing another short spur to the left at 0.45 miles, just before it ends at the junction with Wildwood Way.

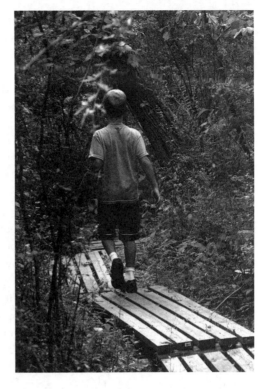

Jackson Willen explores the Fox Run Trail

Turn left on Wildwood Way and cross over Paxton Creek via a large footbridge. After you cross the bridge, the trail will come to a T-intersection. To the right, it goes under US 322, exiting the natural area. Turn left and continue along Wildwood Way for 100 feet or so to the intersection with the North Boardwalk on the left (0.55 miles). Turn left onto the dirt path and left again onto the boardwalk. The trek along the North Boardwalk is 0.7 miles long (out-and-back) through wetlands to a viewing area situated among the lotuses in the middle of the lake. It is worth the walk just to see the lotuses.

Along the way, you'll encounter plenty of swamp rose mallow (purple flowers), cattails, and common arrowhead (yellow flowers) among other flowering plants. About 0.15 miles along, a short spur leads to a bird-watching station on the right. A bird-identification guide is located on the trail at the spur. Just beyond the spur, another spotting scope is located on the right. At the end of the boardwalk, you'll find another bird-watching station situated amid a landscape of lotus plants, which are not especially common in Pennsylvania. I've seen herons out in this area, though patience is necessary since they can be tough to spot among the foliage.

After a break at the end of the boardwalk, return to its beginning. Rather than going back to Wildwood Way, turn left at the end of the boardwalk onto the dirt path that follows the shore of the lake through the forest of oak, sycamore, tulip poplar, and hickory trees. This is the East Shore Trail, and you'll follow it for 0.9 miles back to Wildwood Way. Although the path can be a little damp in places, its proximity to the shore of the lake and its distance from the main path make it ideal for spotting wildlife. Along the way, it crosses a couple of short boardwalks through especially marshy areas and crosses two footbridges before joining with the main trail.

Turn left at the junction with Wildwood Way, which is wide and paved in this area. A picnic table sits aside the path just after you join it. From the junction, continue north for about 0.15 miles to the junction with the Fox Run Trail on the left. This 0.25-mile loop through wooded wetlands is another good place to spot wildlife, as it is also off the main path. It is the location of our famed woodchuck encounter. If you'd prefer to stick to the paved path, the Fox Run Trail joins Wildwood Way again about 50 feet from where it departs.

Upon completing the Fox Run loop, turn left on Wildwood Way and follow it over a hill and down to the north end of the lake at the Susquehanna Spillway, just below Linglestown Road. This is a rather noisy section of trail. After another 0.1 mile, Wildwood Way ends at the Egret parking lot off Industrial Road, where you'll find a picnic pavilion and portable restrooms.

From the lot, you'll want to pick up the Towpath Trail and follow it along the west shore of the lake for a mile or so to its southern edge, passing another small parking area at 0.3 miles (the Turtle lot) with no facilities. The Towpath Trail is wide, surfaced with mulch and dirt, and not wheelchair accessible. Watch the lake through the trees as you walk this path, and you may see herons or egrets or other waterfowl in the small areas of open water. To the right of the trail are the remains of the old Pennsylvania Canal, which ceased operations in 1854. It is a good place to watch for turtles and waterfowl.

At the end of the Towpath Trail, turn left onto the paved road at the southern end of the lake and walk back toward the parking area and nature center. Near the end of the hike, you'll see the Morning Glory Spillway, so named because its funnel-shaped overflow channel resembles a morning-glory flower. It was constructed by the Harrisburg Department of Public Works in 1908 to regulate the height of the water in the lake.

NEARBY ACTIVITIES:

The Benjamin Olewine III Nature Center provides interpretive information about the flora and fauna of the lake and surrounding wetlands. It is open daily from 10 a.m. to 4 p.m. except on Thanksgiving, Christmas, and New Year's days. The State Museum of Pennsylvania, located next to the state capitol in downtown Harrisburg, is definitely worth a visit. Its address is 300 North Street in Harrisburg. Call (717) 787-4980 for hours and information.

YELLOW SPRINGS LOOP HIKE

IN BRIEF

Cross Clark Creek just out of the parking area. Follow the Stone Tower Trail a short distance to an old roadbed and connector trail. Turn left and follow the road for a mile to the Sand Spring Trail. Head south, cross over Stony Mountain, and descend into upper Rausch Creek. A short side trip takes you to the site of "The General," an iron excavator used for digging gravel in the late 19th century. From Rausch Creek, follow the Appalachian Trail west to the Yellow Springs Trail. Head north to the Stone Tower ruins on Stony Mountain. Follow the Stone Tower Trail back to the parking area.

DESCRIPTION

This hike traverses the rugged and remote upper reaches of Rausch Creek in the St. Anthony's Wilderness. The terrain is prime habitat for white-tailed deer and black bear. A variety of birdlife, including flycatchers, warblers, thrushes, bluebirds, and tanagers, inhabits the area during the spring, summer, and fall. The riparian habitat along Rausch Creek is home to frogs, salamanders, and snakes, as well

Directions ———————▶

Exit US 22/322 west from Harrisburg on PA 225 north toward Halifax. Follow PA 225 for about 1.8 miles, and then turn right (east) on PA 325. Follow PA 325 for 16.4 miles. A small parking area is located on the right just beyond the end of the Dehart Reservoir. It is identified by two large red blazes on a tree above a large area of fluorescent pink spray paint on the same tree. Space is available for 6 or 7 cars. Parking for an additional 2 or 3 cars is located a mile up the road on the right. You can cross the creek and pick up the Sand Spring Trail there.

KEY AT-A-GLANCE INFORMATION

LENGTH: 8 miles

CONFIGURATION: Loop

DIFFICULTY: Moderately strenuous

SCENERY: Upper Rausch Creek; "The General" (an abandoned excavator); ghost town of Yellow Springs; and the Stone Tower ruins, an old mine ventilation shaft.

EXPOSURE: Shade

TRAIL TRAFFIC: Light

TRAIL SURFACE: Mostly dirt and rather rocky on the ascent and descent

HIKING TIME: About 5 hours

DRIVING DISTANCE: About 19.2 miles from the PA 225 exit off of US 22/322 west of Harrisburg

ACCESS: Open; on state game land

MAPS: USGS Grantville and Lykens; *Appalachian Trail in Pennsylvania, Sections 7 and 8: Susquehanna River to Swatara Gap*; the entire hike is on PA State Game Land 211, map 211b, which can be downloaded from www.pgc.state.pa.us/pgc/game/maps/default.asp?rgn=Southeast.

FACILITIES: None

WHEELCHAIR TRAVERSABLE: No

SPECIAL COMMENTS: Take care descending the Stone Tower Trail, which is rocky and has a very steep section.

GPS Trailhead Coordinates

UTM Zone (WGS84) 18T

Easting 358658

Northing 4484149

Latitude N 40° 29′ 45.65″

Longitude W 76° 40′ 4.58″

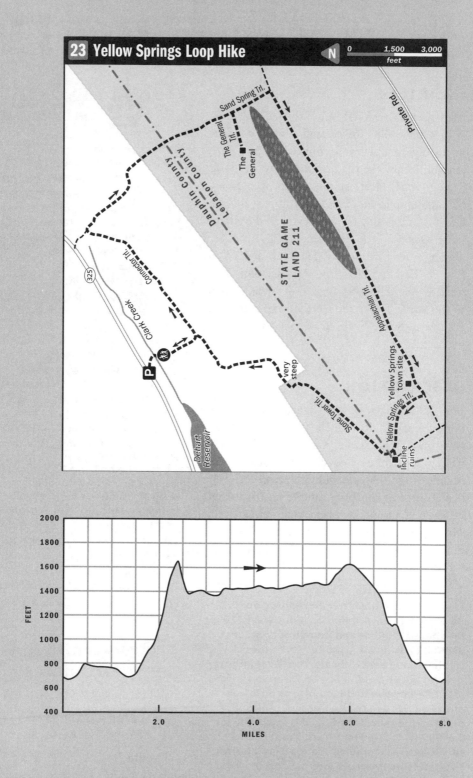

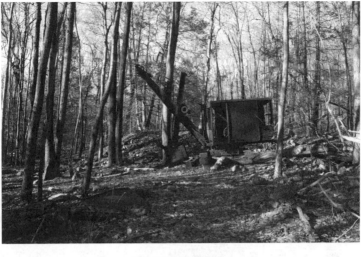

"The General"

as a variety of ferns and mosses. I highly recommend getting an early start on this hike, not because of its length but because the quality of morning light on the Stony Mountain ridge is quite stunning.

Begin the hike by following red blazes directly south out of the parking area. You'll come to the crossing at Clark Creek in no time. Consisting of a thin log with flat boards nailed to it and a steel cable for your hands, the crossing can be tricky if wet or covered in frost. Once over the creek, you'll see a sign pointing to the Stone Tower Trail. Veer right and follow red blazes through the mountain laurel, across a couple of small streams, and uphill for about 0.6 miles to a road-bed. The Stone Tower Trail continues to the right, and a pink-blazed connector trail to the Sand Spring Trail follows the roadbed to the left. Turn left here and walk east for 1 mile to the Sand Spring Trail, marked by two prominent blue blazes on a tree.

Turn right onto the footpath and begin the ascent of Stony Mountain through a forest of hemlock and mountain laurel. Given that this trail, like many others in the area, was originally developed to move coal and lumber down the hillside, its direct route up the mountain is not surprising. Gravity was a big help moving the loads. Except for a steep and rocky section beginning at about 0.6 miles along the trail, though, the climb is neither too rugged nor too steep. Just beyond the steep section, you'll come to the flat ridge of Stony Mountain.

Cross over the ridge and begin the descent into Rausch Creek down a short, steep, and slippery section. At the end of this section, you'll come to a pair of blazes where the trail bends right near a large boulder. The A.T. map indicates that a yellow-blazed trail traverses east from this area to a lookout below the ridge, though I've not been able to locate it. Continue into the drainage to a pair of blazes on a birch tree next to a hemlock. Here a side trail, marked by a sign that reads

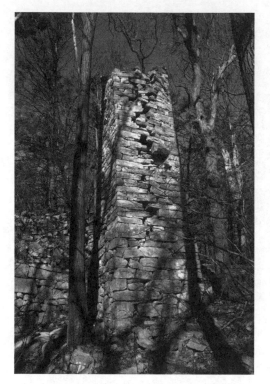

The Stone Tower

THE GENERAL, heads off to the right. Turn right and follow it for about 0.25 miles. At the end of the trail, you'll find "The General," a large steel excavator dating to the early 1900s. It was likely used for removing gravel from the pit on the hillside behind it. Considering the remote location, the presence of this piece of heavy machinery is rather remarkable, and it causes you to realize the extent of change this area has undergone since the heyday of mining operations more than a hundred years ago.

From "The General," return to the main trail, turn right, and walk over to Rausch Creek. The easiest crossing is just right of where the trail meets the creek. The area surrounding the creek is a serene wetlands, populated by hemlocks, mountain laurel, and carpets of moss and fern. A couple of hundred yards beyond the creek, the Sand Spring Trail ends at the A.T. Turn right and walk west through oak and hickory forest for about 2 miles to the Yellow Springs town site and the Yellow Springs Trail. The trail junction is identified by a white mailbox containing a trail register and by a campsite used by A.T. hikers. This hike turns right onto the Yellow Springs Trail and follows it back up to the crest of Stony Mountain.

Like the nearby settlements of Rausch Gap and Rattling Run, Yellow Springs was a coal mining town that was in operation during the 1800s. Along the Yellow Springs Trail, you'll find the stone foundations of many of the original buildings. Most of the ruins are visible from the trail, though if you wander around a little bit you'll notice that this was really an extensive community. The most interesting ruin is the Stone Tower near the crest of Stony Mountain about 0.7 miles along the Yellow Springs Trail. Standing about 30 feet high, the tower is located at the head of several old coal shafts extending into Stony Mountain. When in use, it served to ventilate the deep mines by channeling air out of the shafts via a cast iron pipeline, the remains of which can be seen near the opening of the shaft. Please use caution in this area, as people die each year in Pennsylvania from accidents in abandoned mines. Beyond the tower lies the junction of the blue-blazed Yellow Springs and red-blazed Stone Tower trails. If you follow blue blazes into the woods a short distance, you'll soon come to the remains of an old incline used for moving coal down the mountain to the Dauphin and Susquehanna Railroad in the Stony Valley.

From the ridge crest above the tower, follow the red blazed Stone Tower Trail to the north and then to the east as it descends from the ridge. At first the walking is rocky, but not too steep because the trail traverses the hillside. About 0.8 miles from the trail junction, however, the trail takes a rather illogical path straight down a steep, but short, section of hillside over large boulders. Use extra caution in this area; it is as good a place to break an ankle as any place I have been. Just before reaching the bottom of the hill, red blazes lead off to the east over the rocks. Soon the path joins an old roadbed and turns right. Follow the roadbed for about 0.3 miles, keeping your eyes open for the point where the Stone Tower Trail drops down to the crossing at Clark Creek and the road turns into the pink-blazed connector trail. The junction is easy to miss, even though you passed by it a few hours earlier. Follow the trail back to the creek crossing and to the car.

NEARBY ACTIVITIES

Because the Dehart Reservoir is a watershed, the area immediately around it is closed to all public use. However, above and below the reservoir, Clark Creek on public land provides some wonderful fishing.

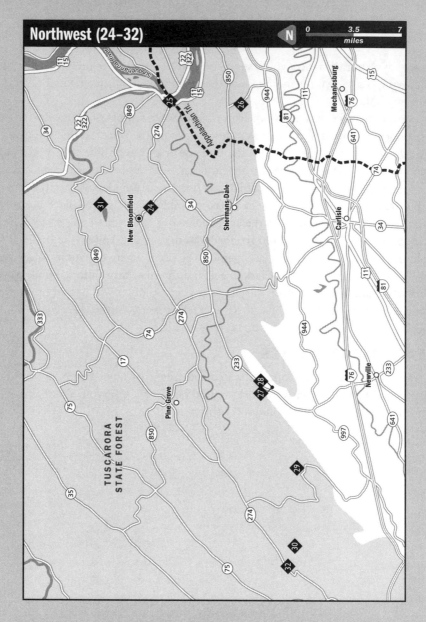

N

0   3.5   7
miles

NORTHWEST

24 BOX HUCKLEBERRY NATURAL AREA

KEY AT-A-GLANCE INFORMATION

LENGTH: About 0.5 miles

CONFIGURATION: Loop

DIFFICULTY: Easy

SCENERY: Box-huckleberry bushes and pretty forest

EXPOSURE: Shade

TRAIL TRAFFIC: Light

TRAIL SURFACE: Dirt

HIKING TIME: About 30 minutes

DRIVING DISTANCE: 1.5 miles from PA 274 in New Bloomfield; about 10 miles from US 11 in Duncannon

ACCESS: Dawn–dusk

MAPS: USGS Newport; a trail guide might be available in the information box near the trailhead.

FACILITIES: None

WHEELCHAIR TRAVERSABLE: No

SPECIAL COMMENTS: Although a short hike, you can spend several hours at the natural area admiring the flora. A great place for the kids.

GPS Trailhead Coordinates

UTM Zone (WGS84) 18T

Easting 315456

Northing 4474847

Latitude N 40° 24′ 13.68″

Longitude W 77° 10′ 29.07″

IN BRIEF

From the parking area, follow the steps up the hillside to the beginning of the short loop. Follow the loop counterclockwise.

DESCRIPTION

Although a very short hike, this excursion around the Box Huckleberry Natural Area in Perry County is well worth a visit. The area is home to the rare box-huckleberry plant, which is estimated to be about 1,300 years old. Perhaps equally as remarkable as its age is that the huckleberry found there, which covers much of the natural area's ten acres, consists of a single colony. In the spring, the plant has pretty pink and white flowers. In the fall, it turns bright red. When the huckleberry is in bloom, you are likely to spot the beautiful pink lady's slipper, as well as flowering dogwood, mountain laurel, and azalea.

According to a Pennsylvania Bureau of Forestry brochure on the area, the plant colony was discovered in 1845 by a professor from Dickinson College. Apparently, this was neither the oldest nor the largest colony of huckleberry to be discovered in the area: another one was discovered along the Juniata River not far away. That colony covered almost

Directions

From Duncannon, follow PA 274 west for 7 miles. Bear right onto PA 34 north and follow that for about 2.3 miles to Seiders Road, identified by a sign for Perry County Archers on PA 34 at the intersection. Turn left and left again onto Huckleberry Road. The entrance to the natural area is about 0.2 miles farther on the left, just before Arbutus Lane. Limited parking is available on either side of the road. Please do not block the private drive.

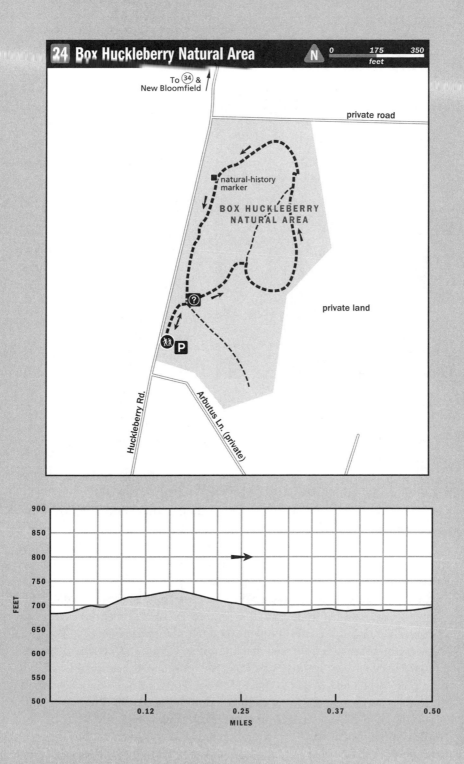

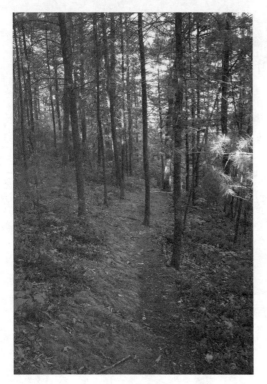

The path among the huckleberries

100 acres and was estimated to be about 13,000 years old. Unfortunately, much of it was destroyed by the construction of US 22/322.

The natural area is home to a wide variety of plant life in addition to the huckleberry. You'll also find witch hazel, hemlock, sassafras, pines, cherry, and oak trees, among many others. Aside from the flora, the natural area has been designated as an important birding area by Audubon Pennsylvania. If you arrive early in the morning, you are likely to encounter deer and perhaps a fox or two in the area.

This hike follows the Nature Trail through the natural area. Begin at the parking area just north of Arbutus Lane. You may have to look around to find the trailhead; the sign is posted above the level of the road. When you find it, walk along the trail above the road for about 100 feet to an information box that contains a trail guide and information on the area's natural history.

From the information box, look uphill and you'll see a fork in the trail. The main Nature Trail heads left at the fork (there is a sign). Walk up a gentle hill for a hundred yards or so to a T-intersection with another trail. Turn right to follow the entire Nature Trail. If you turn left, you will make the short hike even shorter as it soon leads to the halfway point. Follow the Nature Trail to the right back to private property, at which point it heads to the left and loops back down eventually passing above a small but steep-sided hollow to your right.

Soon you'll reach the halfway point, identified by a sign. Stay to the right and follow the trail as it bends down and around to the south. The trail is very beautiful in this section as it passes through some tall pine trees. Next you'll descend a couple of steps to a monument that indicates the natural area is a Registered National Landmark and explains that the "site possesses exceptional value in illustrating the natural history of the United States." Continue following the path to the south as it traverses a hillside above the road, through pine and mountain laurel.

Soon enough you'll reach the end of the trail. I typically walk the loop a couple of times when I visit the natural area, as I always seem to notice something that I missed the first time.

COVE MOUNTAIN–HAWK ROCK LOOP

IN BRIEF

This hike ascends Cove Mountain to the Hawk Rock Overlook via the Appalachian Trail. From the overlook, it traverses Cove Mountain, makes a brief side trip to the Cove Mountain Shelter, and picks up a side trail that descends to the north. At the bottom of the trail, this hike heads east on a dirt road along a tributary of Sherman Creek and joins Sherman Creek proper about a mile from the end.

DESCRIPTION

Although the first mile of this hike up to Hawk Rock is a popular outing, the rest of it sees relatively little traffic. I pieced the loop together after studying a couple of maps and thought it would make for a pleasant trip. You'll get a great view from Hawk Rock, some wonderful ridge walking through the woods along Cove Mountain, and then a walk along a wildlife-management road through more of a wetlands terrain on the return.

Directions ⟶

From Harrisburg, follow US 22/322 west. Cross the Susquehanna River over the Clark Ferry Bridge and take the first exit (on the left) for PA 849/Duncannon. Follow PA 849 over the Juniata River and when it bears to the right, make a left onto Market Street. Follow Market Street through Duncannon and follow signs for US 11/15 south. Once through town, pass beneath US 11/15 and make the first left onto Main Street. Go past the on-ramp for US 11/15 south (don't get on the highway!), and continue straight until the road crosses Sherman Creek. Turn right onto Little Boston Road and make the first right onto Waterworks Road. Follow the signs to the recycling center and park on the left.

KEY AT-A-GLANCE INFORMATION

LENGTH: 8.1 miles

CONFIGURATION: Loop

DIFFICULTY: Moderately strenuous

SCENERY: Beautiful view of Susquehanna River from Hawk Rock; Cove Mountain ridge

EXPOSURE: Shade

TRAIL TRAFFIC: Moderate

TRAIL SURFACE: Dirt and rather rocky at times

HIKING TIME: 4–5 hours

DRIVING DISTANCE: About 2.2 miles from US 22/322 and PA 849 north of Harrisburg

ACCESS: Open

MAPS: USGS Wertzville and Duncannon; *Appalachian Trail, Susquehanna River to PA Route 94* (Sections 9, 10, and 11)

FACILITIES: None

WHEELCHAIR TRAVERSABLE: No

SPECIAL COMMENTS: The first mile of the hike to Hawk Rock is very popular and also very steep. The walk across Cove Mountain is quite secluded.

GPS Trailhead Coordinates

UTM Zone (WGS84)   18T

Easting   327395

Northing   4472243

Latitude   N 40° 22′ 58.48″

Longitude   W 77° 2′ 0.34

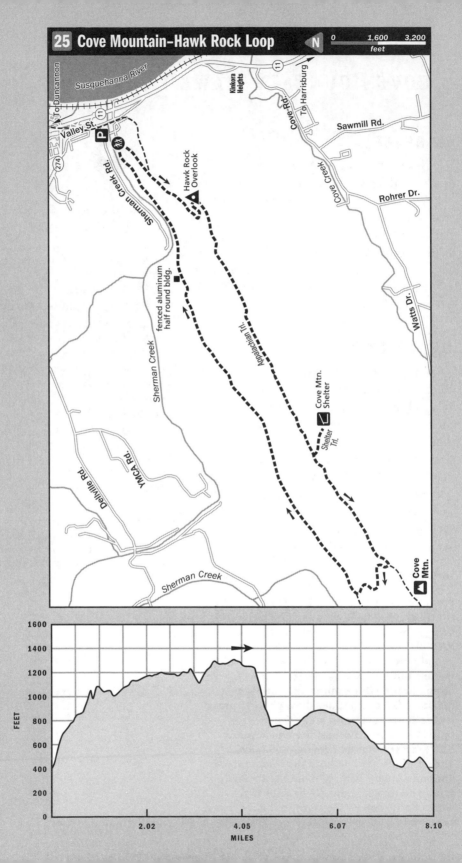

N

0   1,600   3,200
feet

Susquehanna River

To Duncannon

Valley St.

Kinkora Heights

To Harrisburg

Cove Rd.

Sawmill Rd.

Cove Creek

Rohrer Dr.

Watts Dr.

Hawk Rock Overlook

Sherman Creek Rd.

fenced aluminum half round bldg.

Appalachian Trl.

Cove Mtn. Shelter

Shelter Trl.

YMCA Rd.

Dellville Rd.

Sherman Creek

Sherman Creek

Cove Mtn.

FEET

1600
1400
1200
1000
800
600
400
200
0

2.02   4.05   6.07   8.10

MILES

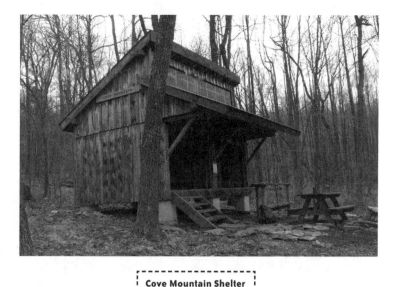

Cove Mountain Shelter

From the parking area at the recycling center in Duncannon, begin hiking uphill on an obvious (though unmarked) path heading to the west. It looks to be an old logging road of sorts and is easy to locate as it leaves right from the small parking area. After about 0.2 miles, the Appalachian Trail (A.T.) enters from the left and the old road is marked with white blazes. Follow it uphill for about a mile (at times rather steep) and just beyond a switchback the trail comes out to Hawk Rock, a small sandstone outcrop among the pines. From this location, you'll get an excellent view of Sherman Creek about 600 feet directly beneath you, the Susquehanna River upstream from Duncannon to the east, and the mountains off to the north. It is a great place on a nice clear day. Unfortunately, the ease of access to this spot has also led to it being repeatedly covered in graffiti.

After you've had your fill of the view, pick up your pack and hike up the A.T. to the ridge just above you. Now begins a long ridge walk to the west along Cove Mountain. The mountain—which is, in effect, the continuation of Peters Mountain on the east side of the river—is so named because it is a long ridge of about 12 miles that extends west from the river for 5 miles before making a complete **U**-turn and heading back to the river. The valley that remains within the **U** has the appearance of a large isolated cove just west of the river.

After about 2 miles of walking along a beautiful, wide, oak-covered ridge with many mountain laurels (very pretty in late May), you'll reach the junction with the trail to the Cove Mountain Shelter. This is the site of the old Thelma Marks Shelter. As is the case with most of the A.T. shelters, you'll find a picnic table, access to a spring, and a privy there. It is also a haunt for a mischievous porcupine. Bear in mind that the 0.25-mile walk to the shelter is all down a rather steep hill. If you don't want to walk back up, stay on the ridge.

Just about a mile beyond the shelter trail, the A.T. veers to the left and over the crest of the ridge at the head of an obvious north-tending hollow. Just after you pass the hollow, an unnamed, but well-marked, blue-blazed trail heads off to the north. Turn right and follow this trail into the valley below. The descent is rather steep at times, though for the most part the footing is good. Soon it levels out in the bottom of a small valley where it ends at a dirt road onto which you will turn right (east).

If you look at a map, you'll notice that this is an interesting valley, topographically speaking. Even though you've descended a good bit, the valley is still about 300 feet in elevation above Sherman Creek, which flows on the other side of the low ridge (Pine Ridge) to your north. The creek flowing through the woods to your left will actually exit the valley through a small water gap in Pine Ridge just east of the junction. You can see this gap if you keep your eyes on the ridge as you head east.

Follow the road for about 3.5 miles back to your car. It climbs to a small saddle first and then begins the descent to Sherman Creek, which will appear from the north after about 2.7 miles. To gauge your progress, at 2.3 miles you will pass a large, half-round aluminum building surrounded by a chain-link fence. When Sherman Creek is in view, you'll pass another road that follows it to the north. Stay to the right here.

If you are hiking during April, keep your eyes open on the forest floor for Dutchman's-breeches, a cluster of small yellow and white flowers that appear early in the spring. They are a pretty, if not unusually shaped, flower that grows in abundance along the side of the road above the creek.

NEARBY ACTIVITIES

Duncannon is a prominent layover for thru-hikers on the A.T. The town has restaurants, pubs, and hotels, all of which are quite accommodating to hikers. The Doyle Hotel is a common haunt for hikers. Just outside of town at the end of Main Street and Inn Road, about 0.2 miles south of Little Boston Road, is Tubby's Night Club on the left. The food is good and the proprietors very friendly. Tubby's is nearly across the street from where the A.T. proper meets the road, and you can use the parking area across from Tubby's as an alternate beginning for the hike. The owner, however, asks that you please don't leave cars parked overnight and don't make a mess.

DARLINGTON TRAIL LOOP 26

IN BRIEF

From the parking area, follow Idle Road to the Darlington Trail at Lambs Gap. Walk the ridge west along the Darlington Trail to Millers Gap Road. The hike follows Millers Gap Road downhill to the north where it picks up a game lands road and footpath that leads back to the car.

DESCRIPTION

I discovered this hike on the "Our Favorite Hikes" page of the Susquehanna Appalachian Trail Club Web site (www.satc-hike.org). Over the years, it has become one of my favorite excursions in the area, especially during the fall, when the trees are quite colorful, and during the spring before the leaves have sprouted, when you can get some nice views. The hike makes a loop between Lambs Gap and Millers Gap on Blue Mountain west of Harrisburg. It uses the Darlington Trail across the ridgetop and a game-land trail below. Two sections of dirt road connect the two. You can park at any one of four parking areas that the route passes by, but my experience suggests that the hike walks best in a clockwise direction beginning from the parking area on Idle Road below Lambs Gap.

Beginning at the parking area, follow Idle Road downhill to the south into Trout

KEY AT-A-GLANCE INFORMATION

LENGTH: 7.3 miles
CONFIGURATION: Loop
DIFFICULTY: Moderate
SCENERY: Beautiful wooded ridge walk, remote game lands
EXPOSURE: More shade than sun
TRAIL TRAFFIC: Light
TRAIL SURFACE: Dirt, short sections of dirt road
HIKING TIME: 4 hours
DRIVING DISTANCE: 3.75 miles from Interstate 81 and PA 944
ACCESS: Dawn–dusk
MAPS: USGS Wertzville
FACILITIES: None
WHEELCHAIR TRAVERSABLE: No
SPECIAL COMMENTS: One of my favorite hikes in the area

Directions

From Interstate 81, south of the Susquehanna River, take exit 61, PA 944. Follow PA 944 west for about a mile to Lambs Gap Road. Turn right on Lambs Gap Road and follow it over the top of the mountain. Just beyond the parking area at the top, turn left onto Idle Road. The trailhead is at a large parking area 1.25 miles along on the left, where the road bends right after climbing out of Trout Run.

GPS Trailhead Coordinates

UTM Zone (WGS84) 18T
Easting 327216
Northing 4464640
Latitude N 40° 18′ 51.93″
Longitude W 77° 2′ 0.51″

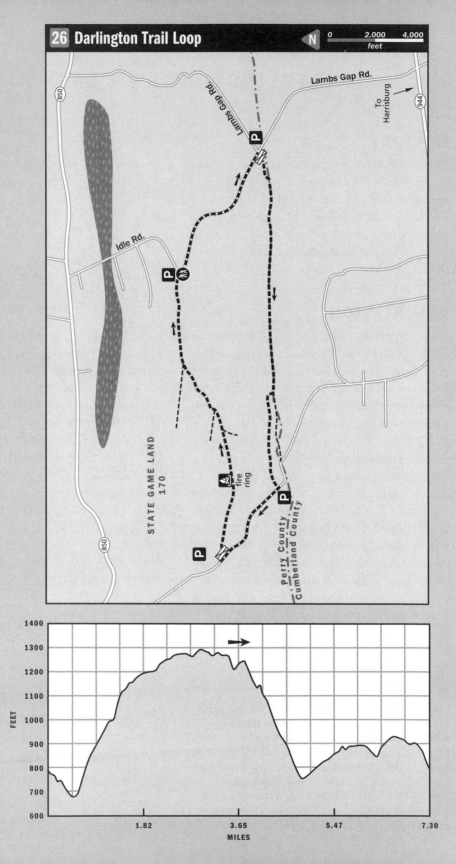

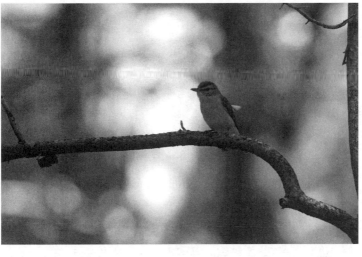

Yellow-eyed vireo

Run and then uphill to Lambs Gap Road. While not unpleasant or heavily traveled, the climb from Trout Run up to Lambs Gap is about 0.75 miles long. My preference is to get this out of the way first, and then the rest of the hike has only short moderate climbs. When you reach the stop sign at Lambs Gap Road, turn right and then make an immediate right turn onto the Darlington Trail, identified by a game lands gate and orange blazes. The Darlington Trail is one of the older hiking trails in this part of the state, having been established by the Alpine Club of Pennsylvania in the early 1900s. An organization of conservation-minded outdoorsmen, the club established routes up many of the mountains and through much of the backcountry all around the state. Several libraries, including the Pennsylvania State University Library, have copies of the club's journals, which are entertaining to read at least for antiquarian interest.

The original Darlington Trail extended along Blue Mountain east and west of the Susquehanna River, although now much of that path belongs to the Appalachian Trail corridor. According to the SATC Web site, the Darlington Trail today stretches for 7.75 miles along Blue Mountain west of Harrisburg, much of which is along a footpath constructed by the club in the past ten years.

From Lambs Gap Road, pass the gate and climb up a short hill until the trail levels out and traverses the ridge though a pretty forest of birch and hickory trees. The wildflowers are abundant here during the spring, and the area is prime habitat for white-tailed deer. Follow the pleasant trail along the ridge for about 2 miles until you encounter a pair of double blazes indicating a change of direction. The trail forks here with the main path continuing straight along the ridge eventually into private property. Take the right fork, which heads over to the north side of the ridge through a more densely wooded section of forest.

In about 0.3 miles, the trail begins a long, level traverse along a very steep hillside about 50 or 60 feet below the crest of the ridge on what appears to be an

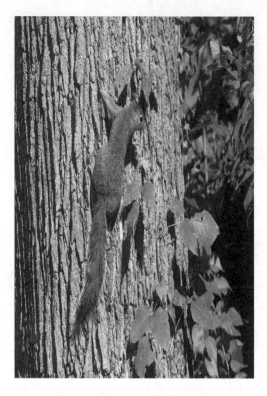

Gray squirrel along Trout Run

old stone road grade. At 2.7 miles from Lambs Gap Road, you'll reach Millers Gap Road. Turn right and follow Millers Gap Road downhill for 0.75 miles to a trailhead with a gate across a state-game-lands track. A sign indicates that this is State Game Land 170, encompassing 9,092 acres. There is a triangular sign on the gate indicating that this is a bicycle and horse path.

Follow the grassy track east for about a mile, past a small meadow and over a culvert, to a small clearing with a fire ring. The trail enters the woods on the other side of the camp and becomes more of a footpath than a road. Keep your eyes open for occasional blazes consisting of black with a white bulls-eye wherever the path joins with others. At about 1.5 miles from Millers Gap Road, you'll reach a swampy area—the headwater of Trout Run—and pass a trail entering from the right and not long afterward a trail entering from the left.

Climb out of the swampy section along a hillside to a junction with a significant trail entering from the left. Stay to the right and follow this old roadbed through a long section of beautiful and fairly open pine and hardwoods back to the parking area at Idle Road.

FLAT ROCK OVERLOOK 27

IN BRIEF

Departing from the environmental education center at Colonel Denning State Park, follow the Flat Rock Trail uphill for 1 mile to the Wagon Wheel, a junction of five trails. From here, the Flat Rock Trail follows the path of the Tuscarora Trail for another mile out to the Flat Rock Overlook. Retrace the route back to the state park or continue following the Flat Rock and Warner Loop through Wildcat Hollow (see page 135).

DESCRIPTION

The first thing you will encounter when you do this hike is a sign that says YOU MAY ENCOUNTER RATTLESNAKES ALONG THIS TRAIL. Then the trail climbs moderately for a half mile before it gets really steep for another half mile. You should not, however, allow these two facts to dissuade you from doing this hike. The rattlesnakes are not hanging from trees and hiding beneath every rock (though you do need to be aware that this is timber rattler country and exercise appropriate caution), and the hill climb is rather short-lived. The reward for completing the hike is one of the best views in central Pennsylvania. I've made this hike on

KEY AT-A-GLANCE INFORMATION

LENGTH: 4 miles

CONFIGURATION: Out-and-back

DIFFICULTY: Strenuous hill climb for 0.5 miles and the rest is moderate walking.

SCENERY: Outstanding view of the Cumberland Valley

EXPOSURE: Shade

TRAIL TRAFFIC: Moderate— somewhat busy on weekends

TRAIL SURFACE: Dirt and rock

HIKING TIME: About 1 hour each way

DRIVING DISTANCE: About 25 miles from the junction of Interstate 81 south and PA 114 south of Harrisburg

ACCESS: Dawn–dusk

MAPS: USGS Andersonburg; Colonel Denning State Park map has part of the route; *Tuscarora Trail, Map J: Appalachian Trail, PA, to PA Route 641*

FACILITIES: Water and restrooms near trailhead

WHEELCHAIR TRAVERSABLE: No

SPECIAL COMMENTS: The second half mile of the hike is a real grind; afterward it is much more pleasant. The area is home to timber rattlesnakes.

Directions

Follow Interstate 81 south from outside of Harrisburg. Take exit 57 and turn right on PA 114 for about a mile. Turn left on PA 944 and follow it for 4.5 miles to PA 34. Turn right on PA 34 and follow it for another 5 miles to PA 850. Turn left and follow 850 into Landisburg. At Landisburg, proceed straight on PA 233. Follow that over the mountain. Colonel Denning State Park is 7.7 miles from Landisburg on the left. Park near the environmental center along the creek.

GPS Trailhead Coordinates

UTM Zone (WGS84)   18T

Easting   294401

Northing   4461634

Latitude   N 40° 16′ 47.76″

Longitude   W 77° 25′ 0.24″

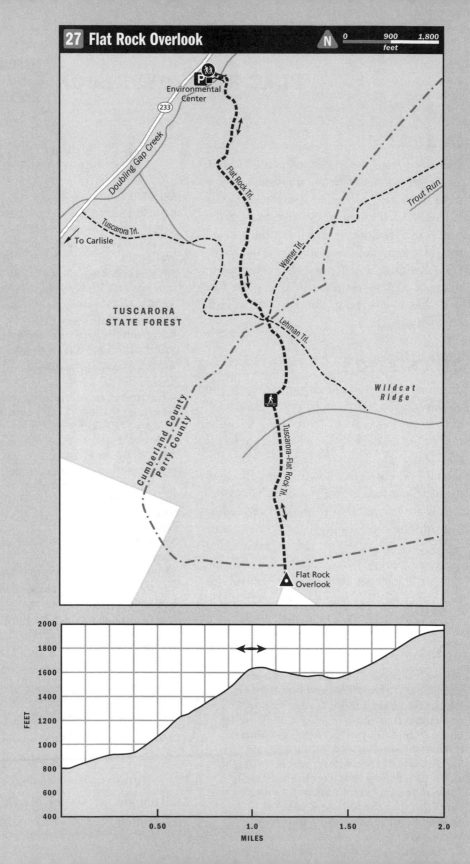

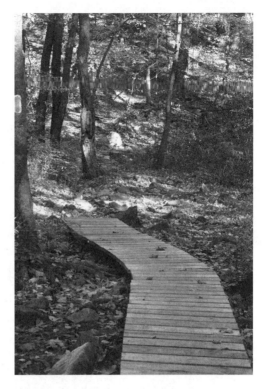

Boardwalk in upper Wildcat Hollow

several occasions, in a variety of weather conditions, and degrees of good and bad moods, and have never regretted doing so.

You begin this hike from the nature center parking area in Colonel Denning State Park. Walk south past the picnic shelter, keeping the amphitheater to your right and cross the creek at a bridge, where you will see the rattlesnake sign. From the bridge, the trail ascends Blue Mountain by way of a series of wooden steps constructed into the hillside. Blue Mountain in this area makes a Z-shape, formed by the uplifting of the Valley and Ridge Province during the Allegheny Orogeny, the formation of these mountains millions of years ago. In effect, this hike begins in the southwestward-tending valley formed by the Z, climbs over the center ridge and across the head of the northeastward-tending valley (Wildcat Hollow) to the Flat Rock Overlook, which is situated at the very bottom of the Z.

From the steps, continue past the tent-camping area on the left along a gradual incline through a beautiful forest of oak and hickory trees. If you are a fan of oranges and yellows, this place cannot be beat in the fall. I have spotted quite a few deer here early in the morning, and judging by the amount of mast on the ground here during the fall, I wouldn't be surprised if black bears frequent the area.

After 0.25 miles, the trail reaches a prominent dirt road. Turn left on this road and follow it up a steeper incline for another 0.25 miles to the remains of an old spring house. Here, the road ends and the trail begins to climb steeply to the right of a watercourse for the next half mile. Just when your hamstrings are beginning to feel like piano strings, it abruptly levels out at the Wagon Wheel, the meeting place of five trails on the Blue Mountain ridge. Here, the Flat Rock Trail joins the blue-blazed Tuscarora Trail, a 252-mile-long path that extends from the crest of the Blue Ridge Mountains in Shenandoah National Park, Virginia, to just shy of the Susquehanna River near Harrisburg. Follow the Tuscarora–Flat Rock Trail south from the Wagon Wheel down into the head of Wildcat Hollow, passing by a trail shelter and outhouse on the left after 0.2 miles.

Soon the trail levels out in a swampy area and crosses several wooden boardwalks and a couple of areas where stones have been positioned as treads. The hickory trees here are tall and provide habitat for many birds. When I last passed through this area, I spotted an owl in the early morning flying silently just above the forest floor. After passing the swampy section, the trail begins to climb again to the ridge of Blue Mountain, only much more gently this time. The 0.6-mile ascent is rather remarkable as the trail—and indeed the entire forest floor—consists of large plates and boulders of sedimentary rock. The trail levels out gradually as it reaches the ridge, and the overlook is actually beyond the ridge, downhill from its crest about 75 vertical feet or so. The overlook is, as its name implies, a large flat rock wedged into the mountainside and clear of trees to the south and east. The view of the Cumberland Valley is the stuff of calendars and postcards. Remarkable. Beneath you, Blue Mountain drops steeply away into a large open talus field, giving the whole experience a vertiginous feel. Bear in mind that the Cumberland Valley is only part of the Great Valley, a geological formation that extends from New York to Georgia.

As you cross the ridge and approach the overlook, try to be as quiet as possible. The entire ridge line is a wonderful roost for birds of prey and other large birds, and you'll have a better chance of seeing some if you approach the overlook silently. In addition to the abundant turkey vultures that can often be found soaring on the wind currents along the ridge, I have seen peregrine falcons from the overlook and several species of hawks.

From the overlook, you can continue along the Tuscarora Trail to the east and make a loop back to the Wagon Wheel via the Lehman Trail or the Warner Trail (see next hike profile), both of which are significant undertakings as the terrain gets very rugged to the east. Or you can simply retrace your steps, the common excursion. Be sure to watch your footing when descending from the Wagon Wheel to the spring house.

NEARBY ACTIVITIES

Colonel Denning State Park has plenty of things to do. The park has a very nice tent-camping area. It also has a lake with a swimming beach and a seasonal concession area. Environmental programs are often scheduled at the nature center. And plenty of space is available for picnicking.

FLAT ROCK OVERLOOK AND WARNER TRAIL LOOP 28

IN BRIEF

Beginning at the Flat Rock Overlook (see previous hike profile), this hike follows The Tuscarora Trail east through Wildcat Hollow. After several miles, it joins the Warner Trail and follows Trout Run to the Wagon Wheel trail junction a mile above the parking area at Colonel Denning State Park.

DESCRIPTION

For the first 2 miles of this hike, follow the directions to the Flat Rock Overlook, provided in the previous profile. After enjoying the view, it's time to grab your pack and take to the Tuscarora Trail. From the overlook, head back uphill a short distance and keep your eyes open for the not-so-obvious blue-blazed trail heading off to the east. If you backtrack as far as the ridge crest, you've passed it. For the first 0.25 miles or so from the overlook, the route passes over talus in the woods. Nothing suggests a trail except the blazes (which are prolific), although the path generally follows the ridge of Blue Mountain until it begins to descend into Wildcat Hollow. Although not steep, the descent is rather rocky with uncertain footing in places and would be

Directions

Follow Interstate 81 south from outside of Harrisburg. Take exit 57 and turn right on PA 114 for about a mile. Turn left on PA 944 and follow it for 4.5 miles to PA 34. Turn right on PA 34 and follow it for another 5 miles to PA 850. Turn left and follow 850 into Landisburg. At Landisburg, proceed straight on PA 233. Follow that over the mountain. Colonel Denning State Park is 7.7 miles from Landisburg on the left. Park near the environmental center along the creek.

KEY AT-A-GLANCE INFORMATION

LENGTH: 8.5 miles including the hike to Flat Rock Overlook

CONFIGURATION: Balloon

DIFFICULTY: Quite strenuous

SCENERY: Outstanding view of the Cumberland Valley; the dark and remote Wildcat Hollow

EXPOSURE: Shade

TRAIL TRAFFIC: Light

TRAIL SURFACE: Dirt; sections are very rugged and rocky.

HIKING TIME: 5–6 hours

DRIVING DISTANCE: About 25 miles from the junction of Interstate 81 south and PA 114 west of Harrisburg

ACCESS: Dawn–dusk

MAPS: USGS Andersonburg; Colonel Denning State Park map has part of the route; *Tuscarora Trail, Map J: Appalachian Trail, PA, to PA Route 641*

FACILITIES: Water and restrooms near Flat Rock Trail trailhead

WHEELCHAIR TRAVERSABLE: No

SPECIAL COMMENTS: This is a strenuous hike through a remote section of the Tuscarora State Forest. In spots the trail is very rugged. Use caution and common sense on this route, and allow plenty of time.

GPS Trailhead Coordinates

UTM Zone (WGS84) 18T

Easting 294401

Northing 4461634

Latitude N 40° 16′ 47.76″

Longitude W 77° 25′ 6.24″

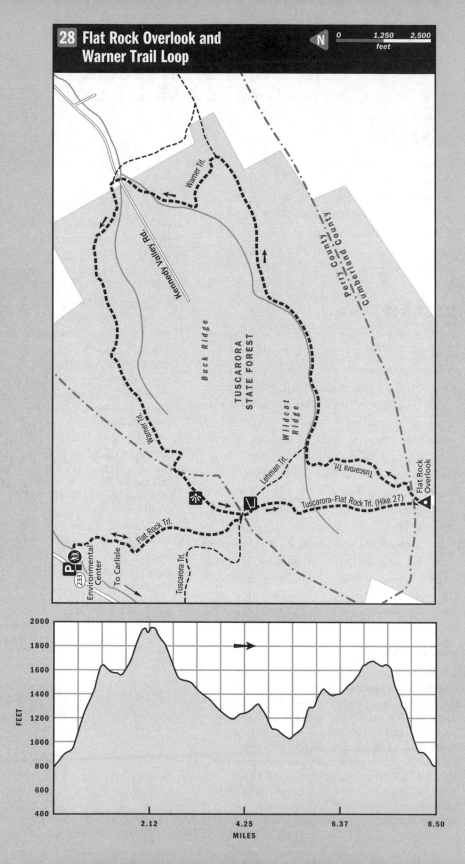

N

0   1,250   2,500
feet

Warner Trl.

Kennedy Valley Rd.

Perry County
Cumberland County

Buck Ridge

**TUSCARORA
STATE FOREST**

*Wildcat
Ridge*

Warner Trl.

Lehman Trl.

Tuscarora Trl.

Flat Rock
Overlook

Tuscarora–Flat Rock Trl. (Hike 27)

Flat Rock Trl.

To Carlisle

Tuscarora Trl.

P

233

Environmental
Center

FEET

2000
1800
1600
1400
1200
1000
800
600
400

2.12   4.25   6.37   8.50

MILES

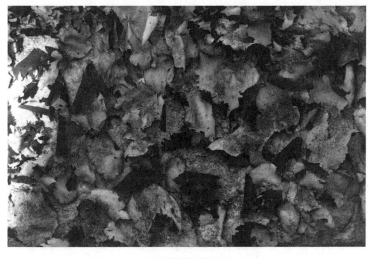

Giant rock tripe

unpleasant in the rain. If you pay attention, you'll find some wonderful patches of giant rock tripe, a leathery brown-and-green lichen growing on the rocks in the woods. This distinctive lichen grows in large flakes over many years.

As the trail descends into Wildcat Hollow, it gets a little steeper, though a little less rocky. After a rather long 0.85 miles, the terrain levels out and the trail joins an old logging road at the junction with the Lehman Trail. Have a look down the Tuscarora Trail, which follows the logging road next to the creek. Rugged, dark, and rocky, with several fallen trees across it, the trail appears rather forbidding. If the passage looks undesirable, turn left on the Lehman Trail and follow that for about a half mile uphill to the Wagon Wheel. If you decide to continue, you'll traverse some wild and remote terrain. As it descends farther along the creek, the Tuscarora Trail passes through dark stands of hemlock trees. If you are lucky, you may spot signs of the wildlife for which the hollow is named. On my most recent excursion into the hollow, I came across a tree on the trail that was obviously used as a scratching post by a bobcat. Its bark was streaked with long thin claw marks, too narrow to be those of a bear, which also will mark trees with its claws.

The farther you travel into the hollow, the better the trail gets. Around a mile from the junction with the Lehman Trail, the Tuscarora Trail begins to climb away from the creek, which makes a bend to the north around the end of Wildcat Ridge toward Buck Ridge. The forest in this area is populated by some mature maple and oak trees towering above. The forest floor is matted with ferns and filled with carcasses of large trees in various stages of decay. At about 2.1 miles from the Flat Rock Overlook, the trail passes onto private property identified by two prominent NO TRESPASSING signs nailed to trees astride the path. Just about 0.1 mile beyond those signs, you'll reach the junction with the red-blazed

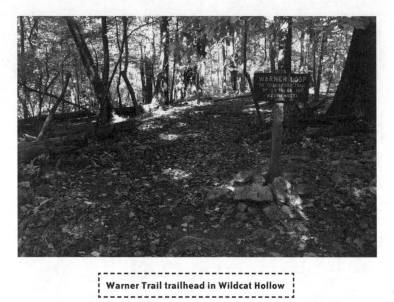

Warner Trail trailhead in Wildcat Hollow

Warner Trail marked by a sign. Turn left on to the Warner Trail, an old roadbed, and follow that through more tall oak and hickory trees back to the creek in Wildcat Hollow. You may notice a significant change in geology in this area. Whereas this hike passed over large boulders of coarse gray sandstone along top of Blue Mountain, now it passes through an area characterized by plates of dark-maroon Tuscarora sandstone. Soon the forest becomes more populated with hemlock trees, and the creek below is surrounded by large areas of willows.

At 0.7 miles from the Tuscarora Trail, the Warner Trail crosses the creek and immediately heads to the right through the willows (if you continue straight uphill along an obvious path from the creek, you'll soon reach a cabin and private property). Continue along the trail for a short distance and cross the Kennedy Valley Road, accessible in this area only by four-wheel-drive vehicle. You should spot a sign for the Warner Trail at the road. If you don't, look uphill as the trail gets braided in the willows and several paths come out to the road a little farther downhill. Cross the road and begin the 2-mile climb up Trout Run back to the Wagon Wheel.

After a half mile, you'll reach a woven wire fence surrounding a forest-management area, which you will enter by a hanging gate constructed of rebar. You'll eventually leave the area by the same type of gate. These gates can only be lifted outward from the forest-management area and are designed to allow wild-life, deer in particular, to escape but not enter the area. Within the fence are many oak and hickory saplings and young growth trees, the bark of which is a favorite for deer to browse on. The fence and gates keep the deer away, and hunting is encouraged within these fenced areas.

After exiting the management area, the trail soon joins a very old roadbed, and comes out to a significant logging road about 1.7 miles from the creek crossing below. Follow the logging road uphill for a short distance and around a bend to the right. Before it bends back to the left, look for a sign for the Warner Trail on the right conveniently hidden behind a tree. The Warner Trail departs from the road and traverses beneath the crest of Blue Mountain on an old coach road above Colonel Denning State Park. In the fall and winter, this section of trail offers great views across the valley toward Doubling Gap to the north. Soon you reach the Wagon Wheel, completing the 6.5-mile loop, very little of which was on flat ground. Take a well-deserved break and then follow the Flat Rock Trail back to the car.

NEARBY ACTIVITIES

Colonel Denning State Park has plenty of things to do. The park has a nice tent-camping area. It also has a lake with a swimming beach and a seasonal concession area. Environmental programs are often scheduled at the nature center. And plenty of space is available for picnicking.

29 FRANK E. MASLAND JR. NATURAL AREA TREK

KEY AT-A-GLANCE INFORMATION

LENGTH: 5 miles

CONFIGURATION: Balloon

DIFFICULTY: Moderate

SCENERY: Pretty hollow of Laurel Run; open forest along the ridges

EXPOSURE: Half sun, half shade

TRAIL TRAFFIC: Light

TRAIL SURFACE: Dirt

HIKING TIME: 2.5–3 hours

DRIVING DISTANCE: About 15 miles from intersection of PA 233 and PA 850 in Landisburg

ACCESS: Dawn to Dusk

MAPS: USGS Blain and Newburg; Frank E. Masland Jr. Natural Area pamphlet provided by the Pennsylvania Bureau of Forestry has a good map, as does the Tuscarora State Forest public-use map available at the forest headquarters in Blain.

FACILITIES: None

WHEELCHAIR TRAVERSABLE: No

SPECIAL COMMENTS: You might do well to bring your fishing rod for Laurel Run.

IN BRIEF

This hike begins with a pretty walk along the North Branch Trail through the Laurel Run hollow, then climbs a hollow to the south of the creek on the Deer Hollow Trail out to Laurel Road. After a short walk along the road, it descends back to Laurel Run via the Turbett Trail, goes west and retraces the first mile to the parking area.

DESCRIPTION

Located in the Tuscarora State Forest in western Perry County, the Frank E. Masland Jr. Natural Area is a 1,270-acre tract of land that encompasses a hemlock-filled section of the north branch of the Laurel Run valley and a ridge covered with oak and mountain laurel rising to its south.

According to a Bureau of Forestry pamphlet, Frank E. Masland Jr. owned a carpet-manufacturing business in nearby Carlisle during the early 1900s. The naming of this tract of land, however, was a result of his commitment to natural-resources conservation around the state and the nation. As the sign at the beginning of the Turbett Trail on Laurel Road explains, Masland "dedicated a lifetime to the enrichment of human lives through the conservation of our natural resources." Among the lasting effects

GPS Trailhead Coordinates

UTM Zone (WGS84) 18T

Easting 284860

Northing 4458692

Latitude N 40° 15′ 3.80″

Longitude W 77° 31′ 46.35″

Directions

From Landisburg, follow PA 233 west for 3.75 miles to Laurel Run Road on your right. Turn right on Laurel Run Road and follow it for another 11 miles to a bridge over Laurel Run in a hemlock-filled hollow. Parking is available on the right at the trailhead before crossing the creek.

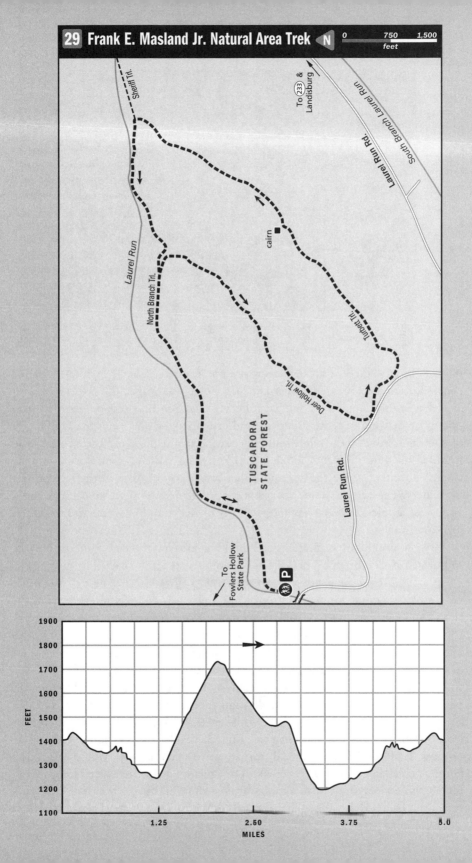

Sheriff Trl.

To 233 & Landisburg

South Branch Laurel Run Run

Laurel Run Rd.

cairn

Laurel Run

North Branch Trl.

Turbett Trl.

Deer Hollow Trl.

Laurel Run Rd.

TUSCARORA STATE FOREST

To Fowlers Hollow State Park

P

1900
1800
1700
1600
1500
1400
1300
1200
1100

FEET

1.25   2.50   3.75   5.0

MILES

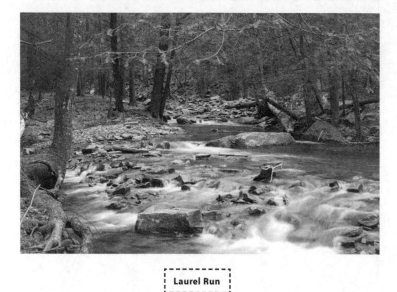

Laurel Run

that can be attributed to his dedication are the Box Huckleberry Natural Area (see page 120) and the Kings Gap Environmental Center (see page 50).

The natural area was founded for the protection of a second-growth stand of timber that may be the oldest second-growth stand in the state. The largest trees—the hemlocks, the white and red oak, the red maples, and the poplars—are found in the beautiful valley along Laurel Run. The oaks and pines located on the ridges above tend to be shorter and rather brushy, offering an attractive contrast in scenery. The area is home to a diverse population of woodland birds and a variety of reptiles, and is a habitat for many of the common woodland mammals of Pennsylvania.

Begin this hike from the small parking area on Laurel Run, where the red-blazed North Branch Trail begins. Follow the trail downstream through the valley not far from the south bank of the creek. Laurel Run has many large pools that provide habitat for native brook trout. The fish are often visible from the shore, and you may wish to bring some tackle along with you to test the waters.

At 0.6 miles, the trail climbs above the creek a couple of hundred feet to bypass a cliff along its south bank. Initially the climb is quite steep, but it eases off quickly. The trail walking is pleasant with good footing, but the hillside that the trail traverses is quite steep and probably not a good place for children. After passing through the high section, descend into a marshy area where the path becomes less distinct. Follow the red blazes through it, and shortly thereafter (1.2 miles), you'll cross a small creek. Just beyond it is the sign for the Deer Hollow Trail onto which you will turn right to make a loop over the ridgetop before descending back to the creek. The junction with the Deer Hollow Trail marks the end of the North Branch Trail proper, although the trail continues down the Laurel Run valley. The name of it changes here to the Sheriff Trail, and you'll pick that up in a couple of miles at the end of the loop and use it to return to this spot.

From the junction, follow the Deer Hollow Trail uphill along the bed of an intermittent creek. The trail gets a bit indistinct in places and the red blazes are not as prolific as they are in the valley. If you stick to the creek bed at places of uncertainty you should have no problems. The creek passes through pretty upland populated by small oak, pine, and much mountain laurel—great habitat for deer and very pleasant in late May and June when the mountain laurel is in bloom.

After 0.75 miles, the trail ends at Laurel Road (2 miles), which forms the boundary of the natural area. Turn left on the road and follow it south for about 0.15 miles to the trailhead for the Turbett Trail. The trailhead is obviously marked with a large sign and there is some room for parking. Turn left onto the Turbett Trail and follow it across a ridge in an ecosystem similar in character to that encountered along Deer Hollow.

At about 2.5 miles, you'll pass an enormous, well-constructed cairn in the middle of the Turbett Trail. Continue down the obvious path along rather flat terrain for what feels like a long way, and then begin the descent back to Laurel Run. The descent gets rather steep before reaching the level of creek. If you are thinking about doing the Deer Hollow–Turbett loop in the opposite direction, take the topography into consideration. The loop walks better counterclockwise.

At 3.3 miles, you'll reach the end of the Turbett Trail at the Sheriff Trail by the creek. A large log is located at the junction, and it makes a fine place to rest your feet after the descent. Turn left onto the Sheriff Trail and follow it west. After about 0.7 miles, you'll cross a significant wooden footbridge and just beyond that is the junction with the Deer Hollow and North Branch Trails. Follow the North Branch Trail back to the car.

NEARBY ACTIVITIES

The natural area has a certain middle-of-nowhere quality to it. However, Laurel Run and South Branch Laurel Run (accessible from Laurel Road) are both excellent fishing streams. Fowlers Hollow State Park is not far to the north and it has picnic facilities. Colonel Denning State Park is not far to the east on PA 233, and that park has picnic and recreational facilities.

30 HEMLOCKS NATURAL AREA LOOP HIKE

KEY AT-A-GLANCE INFORMATION

LENGTH: 3.1 miles

CONFIGURATION: Balloon

DIFFICULTY: Easy with some rocky sections

SCENERY: Old-growth-hemlock forest

EXPOSURE: Shaded

TRAIL TRAFFIC: Light

TRAIL SURFACE: Mostly dirt

HIKING TIME: 1.5–2 hours

DRIVING DISTANCE: About 31.5 miles from intersection of PA 34 and PA 274 in New Bloomfield

ACCESS: Dawn–dusk

MAPS: USGS Doylesburg; map of natural area is available at the Tuscarora State Forest office on PA 274 in Blain

FACILITIES: Pit toilet near south trailhead, seasonal water and restrooms at nearby Big Spring State Park

WHEELCHAIR TRAVERSABLE: No

SPECIAL COMMENTS: Although it's a long drive from Harrisburg for a short hike, the scenery here is outstanding. The outing can easily be combined with a hike on the nearby Tunnel Trail (see page 153) and a picnic at Big Spring State Park for a wonderful day, rich in natural and cultural history.

IN BRIEF

From the north trailhead for the Hemlocks Natural Area, this hike follows the Patterson Run and Rim trails along the east side of the Patterson Run. About halfway through the natural area, the hike crosses the creek and follows the Hemlock Trail along the west side of the ravine to the south end of the natural area. From there, the hike returns via the Rim and Patterson Run trails along the east of the ravine.

DESCRIPTION

Located in western Perry County, the Hemlocks Natural Area is a 120-acre tract of land that is home to a stand of virgin eastern hemlock trees. The extent of the natural area is located in the steep-sided ravine through which Patterson Run flows, and in all likelihood this stand of trees was saved from the bite of the saw by the topography. According to the information brochure provided by the Tuscarora State Forest, the oldest trees date back 280 years. Many of them measure more than 2 feet in diameter and more than 100 feet tall. Some of the trees are absolutely huge, and few places exist in the east where you can see trees with the stature of these hemlocks.

GPS Trailhead Coordinates

UTM Zone (WGS84)   18T

Easting   275995

Northing   4459458

Latitude   N 40° 15′ 20.24″

Longitude   W 77° 38′ 2.18″

Directions

From PA 34 in New Bloomfield, follow PA 274 west for approximately 29 miles to Big Spring State Park. Turn left onto Hemlock Road at the park sign. The trailhead and parking are 2.5 miles along on the left at a sign.

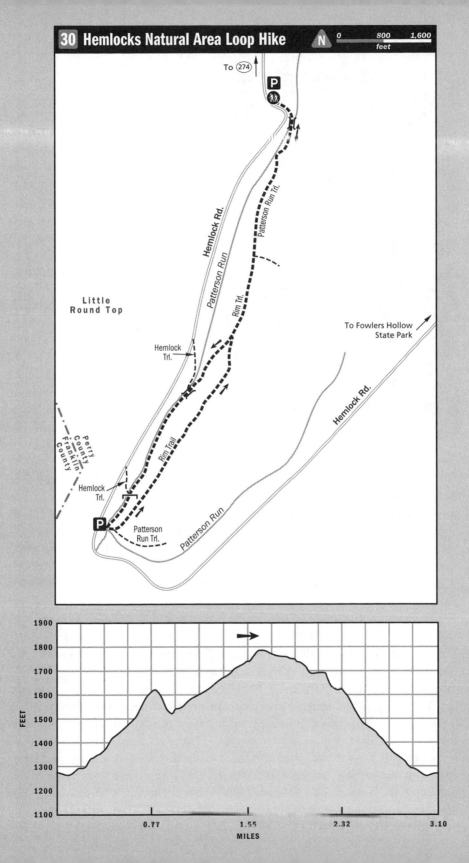

N

0   800   1,600
feet

To (274)

P

Hemlock Rd.

Patterson Run

Patterson Run Trl.

Rim Trl.

Little
Round Top

Hemlock
Trl.

To Fowlers Hollow
State Park

Hemlock Rd.

Rim Trail

Perry
County
Franklin
County

Hemlock
Trl.

P

Patterson
Run Trl.

Patterson Run

1900
1800
1700
1600
1500
1400
1300
1200
1100

FEET

0.77   1.55   2.32   3.10
MILES

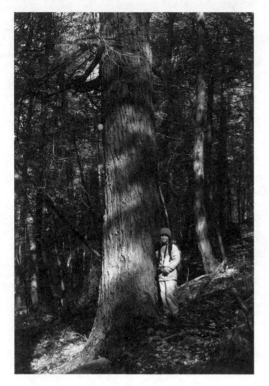

Jackson Willen dwarfed by a hemlock

The Pennsylvania state tree, the eastern hemlock, was all but eradicated during the lumber boom in the 19th century. Interestingly, the timber provided by the tree is not considered especially valuable for lumber purposes. It was cut instead for its bark to use for tanning leather. In 1973, the natural area was designated as a National Natural Landmark by the National Park Service. In addition to the hemlock, you will also find here white pine, several varieties of birch, maple, and oak trees, and a healthy understory of mountain laurel, Pennsylvania's state flower. Visiting the natural area in late May and early June will give you the opportunity to see the mountain laurel in bloom.

From the north parking area, follow the orange-blazed Patterson Run Trail down to the creek and cross a small footbridge. After crossing the bridge, be sure to veer left on the Patterson Run Trail heading uphill away from the creek. After about 0.3 miles, you'll reach the junction of the Patterson Run Trail and the yellow-blazed Rim Trail. The prior turns left, heading uphill, while the latter continues straight traversing the hillside. Continue straight on the Rim Trail. As you begin this trail, you'll notice the hemlocks getting large, and some of them have a very rough alligator-like bark.

Follow the Rim Trail to a fork in the trail at 0.8 miles. At the fork, turn right and drop down to a footbridge over Patterson Run. On the west side of the creek, you are following the red-blazed Hemlock Trail. From the bridge a spur of that trail heads uphill to the right to Hemlock Road. Turn left and follow the Hemlock Trail to the south along Patterson Run. The terrain is rather rocky for the next half mile, and in the summer the trail can be a bit overgrown. But from the bottom of the ravine you'll have an excellent view of some of the tallest trees on the steep east slope. Although Patterson Run is not very large, the pools all along it are home to small native brook trout that are easy to spot from the trail. During spawning season they have beautiful colors, speckled on top and bright red or orange on the bottom. They are small, only about six inches or so, but every large pool seems to sport one or two.

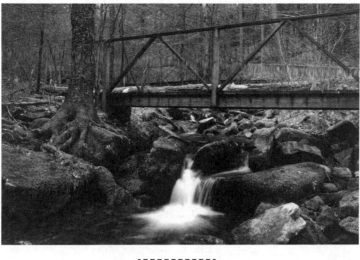

Patterson Run

At 1.4 miles, the trail passes a bench beside the creek and another spur of the Hemlock Trail heads up to the road. The spur is marked by a sign. From the bench, continue following the trail along the creek and in a few moments you'll reach a pair of footbridges over the creek and a small tributary. Cross the two bridges and you'll see some yellow blazes and a sign indicating the path of the Rim Trail traversing the east slope of the ravine back down the valley. As you follow the Rim Trail above the creek, you'll pass by some of the largest trees in the area, giving you a sense of what Pennsylvania might have been like when it was first settled. In about a half mile, the trail begins to descend and shortly thereafter meets the fork above the Hemlock Trail and footbridge you passed earlier. Continue straight and follow the Rim Trail and then the Patterson Run Trail back to the car.

NEARBY ACTIVITIES

Camping and picnicking facilities are located at Fowlers Hollow State Park, 7 miles to the southeast just beyond the end of Hemlock Road. Picnic facilities are located at Big Spring State Park. The Tuscarora State Forest has many unpaved forest roads that make for good bike riding. The forest headquarters, located on PA 274 in Blain, has maps and information on historical and natural landmarks.

31 LITTLE BUFFALO STATE PARK

KEY AT-A-GLANCE INFORMATION

LENGTH: 5.6 miles

CONFIGURATION: Loop

DIFFICULTY: Moderately strenuous

SCENERY: Nice views of Little Buffalo State Park environs and Little Buffalo Creek

EXPOSURE: More shade than sun

TRAIL TRAFFIC: Light

TRAIL SURFACE: Dirt, with short sections of grass and pavement

HIKING TIME: 3–4 hours

DRIVING DISTANCE: 5.75 miles from US 22/322 and PA 34 near Newport, west of Harrisburg

ACCESS: Dawn–dusk

MAPS: USGS Newport; Little Buffalo State Park map

FACILITIES: Restrooms and water at visitor center; a seasonal concession area

WHEELCHAIR TRAVERSABLE: No

SPECIAL COMMENTS: This hike generally follows the 6.2-mile Volksmarch route through the park, though it is a little shorter and stays more to trails than roads.

IN BRIEF

Beginning at the visitor center, this hike makes a circuit of Holman Lake by following trails on ridges to the north and south of the lake.

DESCRIPTION

Little Buffalo State Park is rich with natural and cultural history. The land in the valley along Little Buffalo Creek was purchased from the Iroquois League of Nations around the time of the Revolutionary War, and farming settlements began to be established in the early years of the 1800s. During the 19th century, the land around the present day park was the site of a large charcoal furnace, a forge (the Juniata Iron Works), a gristmill (Shoaff's Mill), and the Newport and Sherman's Valley Railroad. These businesses contributed to the development of the valley, as well as to the clearing of its forest. As the timber industry declined, the industries and railroad closed down, leaving farming as the area's primary industry. The park was opened in 1972, and in addition to recreational opportunities it has served to preserve some of the cultural history. This hike, which makes a circuit of the park around its 88-acre Holman Lake, passes by several of the historic sites and provides access to some of the park's charming backcountry.

GPS Trailhead Coordinates

UTM Zone (WGS84) 18T

Easting 316137

Northing 4480921

Latitude N 40° 27′ 31.08″

Longitude W 77° 10′ 6.52″

Directions

From US 22/322 at Newport, follow PA 34 south for about 4 miles to Little Buffalo Road (SR 4010). Turn right and follow the road for 1.75 miles to New Bloomfield Road. Turn left and the Little Buffalo State Park visitor center is on the left.

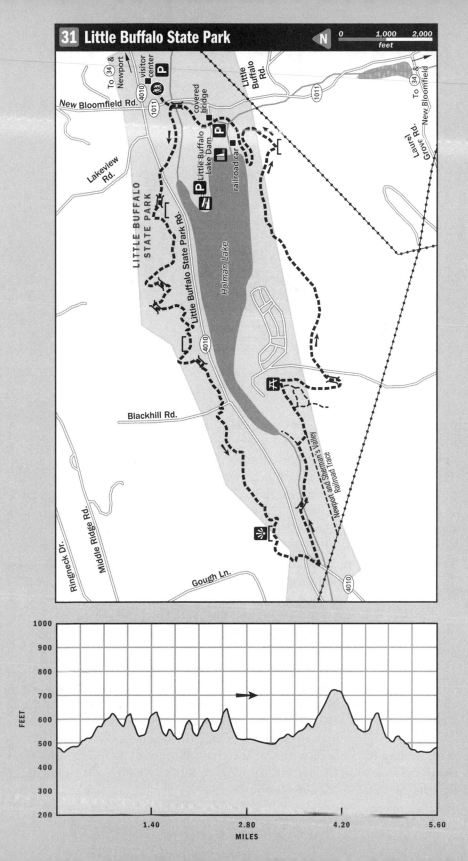

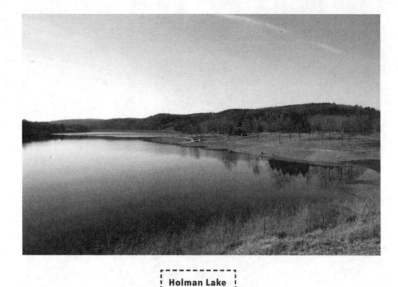

Holman Lake

Beginning from the visitor center, walk west across the park road toward the Blue Ball Tavern. Originally opened in 1811 by John Koch, a farmer, the tavern served as a resting place for messengers traveling between Carlisle and Sunbury during the War of 1812. A farmhouse built in 1865 now stands on the site. Pass the farmhouse (now a museum) and a bridge over the creek (don't cross the bridge!) and hike west along the Exercise Trail, keeping the creek to your left. This grassy, mown path passes through a pretty meadow with many nesting boxes for eastern bluebirds, a common resident of the park. As you approach the dam's spillway, the path heads over to Little Buffalo Road and crosses it at some wooden steps. Cross the road, and pick up the trail continuing west as it enters the woods at a little creek. Lots of thicket in the area makes this a good place for spotting some of the many songbirds that visit the park. You are now on the Middle Ridge Trail (as denoted by the park map), although as soon as you enter the woods you'll cross a footbridge by a sign that refers to it as the North Side Hiking Trail. Nonetheless, it is well marked with red blazes—a good thing if you are hiking during the fall, as the abundance of oak and hickory leaves on the ground can make the path virtually invisible.

For the next 2.5 miles, the trail follows the direction of Middle Ridge to the west, climbing out of and back into hollows that divide the ridge toward Holman Lake. The walk is very pretty, through a forest of oaks and hickories with tall white pine trees on the ridges and hemlocks in the hollows, but it does have quite a bit of up and down to it. At about 1.5 miles, the trail descends an uncharacteristically steep hill on a nice path in the pines. Near the bottom, the trail turns sharp right into the hollow and across a footbridge, though a path continues straight out to the road. Keep your eyes open for the junction marked by blazes and turn right.

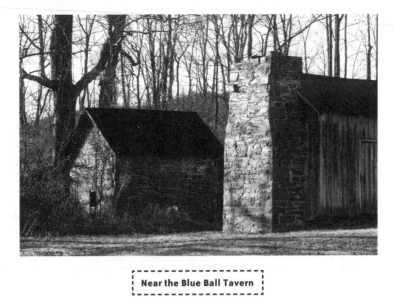

Near the Blue Ball Tavern

Cross Blackhill Road at 1.8 miles and climb a short hill. At the top of this hill, the path joins with a wide-open track through the woods. With loads of thicket on either side of the trail, this is a great area for bird-watching. At one point in a more open area, an infrequently used path heads off to the right to the top of the ridge, a couple of hundred feet away. If you are looking for wildlife, it may be worth the effort to drop your pack and take a peek up there. It seems prime territory for turkey and grouse as well as fox. At about 2 miles, you'll come to a large open meadow on your left that you walk beside for about 0.2 miles. The path drops into another hollow, crosses a footbridge, and climbs a short hill. At the top of the hill, you'll find two benches and a nice view back to the east over Holman Lake and the park.

From the benches, the trail continues a short distance to a very large oak tree. The trail makes a right turn into the woods here, while the track continues straight and downhill. The trail winds through the woods for about 0.1 mile, before crossing back over the track and descending to Little Buffalo Road by a gate and private road. Cross Little Buffalo Road, turn right, and walk west along its shoulder until you cross the bridge over Little Buffalo Creek. Just beyond the creek, step over the guardrail and walk down some steps to a wide track on the south side of the creek. The passage over the guardrail is marked by a sign with a white arrow and is directly beneath some large power lines. Follow the track along the creek, passing a large meadow on your right where you may spot a few deer browsing. In a couple of places the track will fork. Just follow the left forks staying near the creek. The walk along the creek features quite a bit of thicket and some impressive sycamore trees.

After about 0.5 miles along the creek, you'll come to a trail junction with a wide, grassy path heading up to the right. Turn right and follow that path a short distance to the Newport and Sherman's Valley Railroad grade marked by a white arrow. The white arrows indicate the path of a Volksmarch route around the park. Turn left and walk through a lovely pine forest for a short distance until you reach a junction of several trails heading off to the right at the base of a hillside covered with dense stands of thicket. A white arrow points up along one of the trails. Don't follow it. The trails that head off into the thicket are rather confused, and mostly seem to loop back to this spot. That said, the trails are worth exploring for a little while to see what you might see. As I was walking around the area trying to make sense of it, I happened to see a weasel chasing a squirrel out of its den, in addition to a multitude of birds.

From the hillside, continue along the railroad grade (now more of a service road), and follow it until you see some picnic tables and restrooms. The trailhead for the Buffalo Ridge Trail will be on the right, although the sign faces the opposite direction from which you are walking, so keep your eyes open. (If you cross a bridge over a small creek, you've gone too far.) Turn right on the white-blazed Buffalo Ridge Trail and follow it up a beautiful dark hollow, populated by tall pine, hickory, and hemlock trees. At the back of the hollow, cross a footbridge and climb to a service road. Cross the road and follow the trail as it traverses just below the crest of Buffalo Ridge for about 0.6 miles, at which point you'll pass a trail heading back west with a sign that says SHORTCUT TO MAIN AREA, about 100 yards east of a water tank.

As the trail descends from here, the walking gets rather rocky for about 0.25 miles. Then it improves, climbs back up to the ridge among large pine trees, and reaches a bench near the rocky ridge crest. This is a peaceful spot and worth planning as a rest spot on your hike. From the bench, follow the path along a ridge in a northeasterly direction, make a couple of switchbacks near its bottom, and descend a set of steps into the east picnic area at the base of the dam. The steps end at the railroad grade at an old railroad car. Turn right and follow the grade to the covered bridge, Clay's Bridge. Built in 1890, it originally crossed Buffalo Creek a mile west of its present location, providing a link to New Bloomfield for residents of the Sherman's Valley. Exemplifying Burr Arch construction, each interior side of the bridge features a wooden structural arch that spans the river. Once through the bridge, turn right onto a paved path and follow it for 0.25 miles back to the Blue Ball Tavern.

NEARBY ACTIVITIES

The obvious activities are at the state park, where you can explore some of the historical sites, picnic, swim, and fish. I highly recommend a walk from the east picnic area up the steps to the crest of the dam for a great view to the west. The park does a fine job with environmental programs and special events. During the Christmas season, the park decorates the east picnic area with lights and ornaments. During the fall, the park hosts the Old Fashion Apple Festival and activities on Halloween night.

TUNNEL TRAIL AND
IRON HORSE TRAIL LOOP   **32**

IN BRIEF

From the parking area on Hemlock Road, follow the Tunnel Trail to the abandoned railroad tunnel and descend toward Big Spring Run. Pick up the Iron Horse Trail and follow it east, crossing PA 274, and joining the old Path Valley Railroad grade. Follow the Path Valley grade back to the parking area.

DESCRIPTION

Constructed by the Youth Conservation Corps in the late 1970s, the Iron Horse Trail (IHT) forms a loop through the Tuscarora State Forest following the paths of two abandoned railroad grades. Although the trail is theoretically a rail-trail, it is considerably more rugged than any rail-trail you'll come across. It's a rocky knee-buster that requires good, sturdy footwear. Linking the Iron Horse Trail with the Tunnel Trail is the common excursion, though the latter is a nice, easy outing on its own. When completed as a loop, the Tunnel Trail is 1.85 miles long. The directions here provide information on both of the trails.

PART 1: TUNNEL TRAIL

From the information sign in the parking area, cross Hemlock Road and pick up the Tunnel Trail at a trail sign. Marked by blue blazes, the

KEY AT-A-GLANCE INFORMATION

LENGTH: Iron Horse Trail is 9.1 miles and the Tunnel Trail is 1.8 miles. If you join the two (the common excursion) and don't backtrack, the hike is 10.3 miles long.

CONFIGURATION: Loop

DIFFICULTY: Long and strenuous

SCENERY: Tuscarora State Forest land and much railroad history

EXPOSURE: Shade

TRAIL TRAFFIC: Iron Horse Trail is light and Tunnel Trail is moderate

TRAIL SURFACE: Dirt and rock

HIKING TIME: Allow 5–6 hours for the entire loop. The Tunnel Trail loop takes about an hour.

DRIVING DISTANCE: About 28.5 miles from intersection of PA 34 and PA 274 in New Bloomfield

ACCESS: Dawn–dusk

MAPS: USGS Blairs Mills and Blain; *Tuscarora Trail, Map J: Appalachian Trail, PA, to PA Route 641*

FACILITIES: Seasonal restrooms and water in picnic grounds at Big Spring State Park (parking area)

WHEELCHAIR TRAVERSABLE: No

SPECIAL COMMENTS: This is *not* your typical railroad-grade hike, as it is a rather stiff undertaking. The path is often rugged and climbs steep sections around private property.

Directions ———————➤

From PA 34 in New Bloomfield, follow PA 274 west for approximately 29 miles to Big Spring State Park. Turn left onto Hemlock Road at the park sign and park in the large parking area on the left.

GPS Trailhead Coordinates

UTM Zone (WGS84)   18T

Easting   273785

Northing   4460249

Latitude   N 40° 15′ 43.73″

Longitude   W 77° 39′ 36.65″

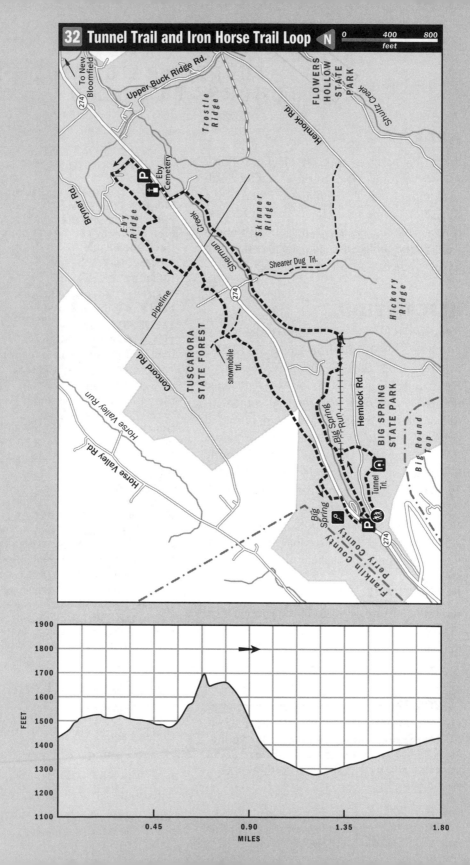

0   400   800
feet

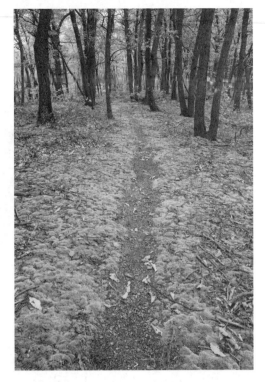

Along the Eby ridge

trail climbs into the woods, curves to the left, and contours the hillside. At about 0.25 miles, descend a set of steps and then turn right and climb a short rocky section. Shortly beyond, gain an old railroad grade and follow it straight toward the mountain. After about 100 yards, the grade ends at the entrance to the old railroad tunnel. Never completed due to lack of funds and geological complications, the tunnel was begun in 1803 in an attempt to extend the Newport and Sherman's Valley Railroad from its terminus at New Germantown into Franklin County. The tunnel is an interesting bit of railroad history and is worth the short detour to see it.

From the fence at the tunnel, walk back along the railroad grade and turn right at the first blue blaze on the trail. Walk downhill and, in a short distance, you'll cross Hemlock Road and enter a forest of small saplings. Continue walking downhill for another 0.2 miles and you'll reach the red-blazed Iron Horse Trail. Turn left to return to the parking area (0.3 miles) or right to continue the Iron Horse loop.

PART 2: IRON HORSE TRAIL

If you decide to skip the Tunnel Trail or leave it to the end of the day, hike out of the parking area to the east on a stone-edged gravel path marked by red and blue blazes and an Iron Horse Trail sign. After a short distance, the path bends to the left toward some picnic pavilions. At the bend, leave the main path and follow the blazes into the woods on a less defined track. As you leave the main day-use area, the trail follows Big Spring Run and soon passes a sign that marks the end of the Perry Lumber Company Railroad grade, abandoned in 1906. A short distance beyond, you'll pass the junction with the Tunnel Trail. Continue east along the railroad grade for just about a mile, crossing the creek twice over wooden footbridges. Although a wide path, the walking through this section is quite rugged, as the trail surface is formed by broken rock.

Just beyond the second bridge (about 0.8 miles from the Tunnel Trail), the obvious railroad grade continues straight down the valley, but the Iron Horse Trail turns uphill right to circumnavigate private property. The turn is marked by

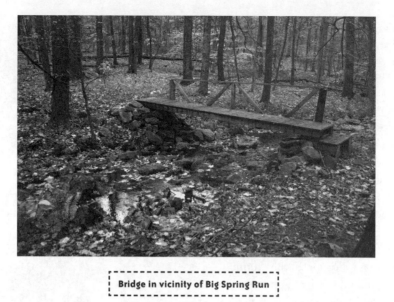

Bridge in vicinity of Big Spring Run

a sign and double red blazes. After a short climb, turn left on an obvious old railroad bed in a stand of maple and birch saplings. Follow the smooth path back down to Big Spring Run, crossing a tributary on the way. You can often hear hawks screeching in this area, and the forest supports a healthy deer population.

About 2 miles from the Tunnel Trail, you'll join the Perry Lumber Company Railroad grade again. Follow that for a short distance until it crosses the creek onto private property. Continue straight, staying south of the creek. At 2.2 miles, you'll pass a small private cabin and a sign that asks you to respect the owner by staying on the trail. Follow the cabin's access road to a gate and then out to a prominent dirt road at 2.4 miles. This road is the Shearer Dug Trail, and it provides access to some private cabins as well as the Rising Mountain Trail on the ridge to the south. Cross the road, enter the woods, and follow the path over two footbridges and across two pipeline clearings for about a mile to another prominent dirt road. An Iron Horse Trail sign is located here. Turn left and follow the road past a stand of pine trees to the highway. Just before the highway, turn right (east) into the woods and parallel the highway for about 0.25 miles before crossing to the Eby Cemetery on the north side of the road.

The trail proper reenters the woods through the brush at the southeast corner of the cemetery (right by the road), and parallels the road for about 0.5 miles. If you pick up the trail here, you are in for some of the worst hiking imaginable. At the time of this writing, the path near the cemetery was overgrown by thorn bushes fierce enough to destroy my sturdy pair of Carhartt overalls. To avoid such unpleasantness, walk east along the shoulder of the road for 0.4 miles to the eastern trailhead across from a parking area on the south side of the road. From that trailhead, marked by a sign, continue walking east for another 0.25 miles to another dirt road (Bryner Road) by a large clear-cut.

Turn left (north) and pass the clear-cut on your right and a private residence on the left. Beyond both of these, Bryner Road begins to climb slightly and bend to the right. At the point where the road bends left, the IHT enters the woods on the left, heading west now along the grade of the Path Valley Railroad. This is the railroad grade that was supposed to join the Newport and Sherman's Valley line with Franklin County to the west. Although that venture was never realized, the grade did extend as far as the site of the present Big Spring Park. In the early 1900s, the Perry Lumber Company used it to help move timber out of western Perry County.

The path along the top of the railroad grade for the next 0.6 miles is very pleasant. The woods are thick, making the setting feel remote. At 4.9 miles, the trail makes a sharp right turn and leaves the railroad grade to circumnavigate private property. Follow the red blazes uphill for about 0.3 miles to the crest of Eby Ridge by a couple of huge oak trees, where the trail makes a sharp left and drops down to a recent logging road. As you follow the road to the west, Conococheague Mountain will be in view to the north. At the crest of the road, veer left, pick up the red blazes again, and descend a very beautiful ridge along a moss-lined path through stands of pine trees surrounded by tall oaks. It would be difficult to imagine more pleasant walking, and the area is especially beautiful in the fall.

When you reach a clearing at a pipeline, turn left (south) and walk about 0.1 mile to a plastic white-and-yellow pipeline post. The trail enters the woods again at red blazes on the right and follows a railroad spur for about 100 yards before it ends abruptly at a small promontory. Continue following blazes through the woods, crossing a footbridge and then a drive for a private camp. Continue up switchbacks to regain the main railroad grade at a good area for spotting woodpeckers. Walk along the pleasant path as it traverses the hillside, avoiding the temptation to veer off on the occasional paths heading downhill. At 6.5 miles, the trail joins a dirt road. Turn right and follow it across another dirt road (marked as a snowmobile trail) and regain the railroad grade just beyond. A short distance beyond, you'll reach a significant fork in the trail and you'll want to stay left.

At about 8 miles, the trail makes a diagonal across an old road right above the highway near the state park. Just when you think it's all over, the trail turns uphill to once again circumnavigate a small plot of private land. Beyond that, follow red blazes through woods back to the highway and into the park. The parking area is just beyond the road.

NEARBY ACTIVITIES

Picnicking facilities are available at Big Spring State Park, and camping is available 6.5 miles away at Fowlers Hollow State Park. The Hemlocks Natural Area is located 3.1 miles south along Hemlock Road and is very much worth a visit (see page 144). Combining the short Tunnel Trail with a hike through the Hemlocks Natural Area would make for a very pleasant day.

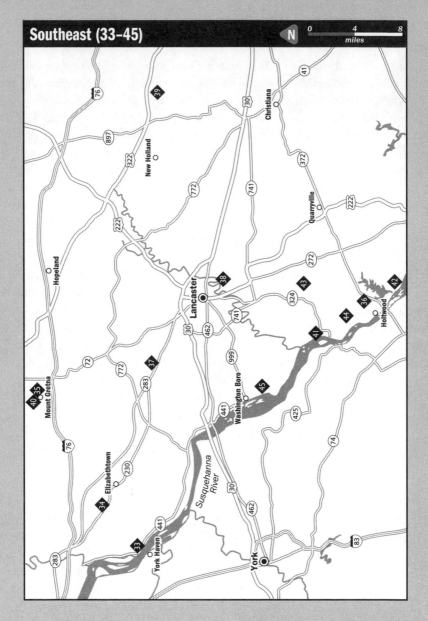

76
39
76
30
41
Christiana
897
322
New Holland
372
772
741
222
Quarryville
222
272
Hopeland
38
43
42
324
36
Lancaster
741
44
Holtwood
30
462
41
72
772
37
283
999
40 35
Mount Gretna
45
Washington Boro
441
425
76
74
Elizabethtown
230
34
Susquehanna River
30
462
441
33
83
York Haven
York
283

SOUTHEAST

33 CONOY CANAL TOWPATH TRAIL

KEY AT-A-GLANCE INFORMATION

LENGTH: 6.4 miles

CONFIGURATION: Out-and-back

DIFFICULTY: Easy walking

SCENERY: Old Pennsylvania Canal towpath; several old locks; Susquehanna River

EXPOSURE: Shade

TRAIL TRAFFIC: Light

TRAIL SURFACE: Dirt

HIKING TIME: 2.5–3 hours

DRIVING DISTANCE: 8.5 miles from PA 283 and PA 441 north of Middletown

ACCESS: 8 a.m.–dusk

MAPS: USGS York Haven

FACILITIES: Portable toilets at Kings Road and Bainbridge

WHEELCHAIR TRAVERSABLE: No

SPECIAL COMMENTS: An excellent hike for birding

IN BRIEF

This pleasant hike follows the route of the old Pennsylvania Canal along the remains of the towpath south from Falmouth boat launch to the parking area at Bainbridge and back.

DESCRIPTION

This little-known trail is interesting for both the access to local history and the wonderful birding opportunities it provides. According to Audubon Pennsylvania's *Susquehanna River Birding and Wildlife Trail Guide,* more than 229 bird species have been recorded along this trail, including birds of prey, such as the osprey, bald eagle, and screech owl; shorebirds such as herons, and black and wood ducks; and forest-dwelling songbirds, including thrushes, warblers, chickadees, and the cedar waxwing. Although the species aren't as abundant during the fall and winter, I find hiking the trail more pleasant during those seasons, as it can be rather buggy during the summer (hence the birds).

Currently the trail extends for approximately 4 miles from Bainbridge north to Conewago Falls, where Conewago Creek enters the Susquehanna River. The trail follows the old towpath for the Susquehanna branch of the Pennsylvania Canal, which ran between

---

GPS Trailhead Coordinates

UTM Zone (WGS84) 18T

Easting 354378

Northing 4442371

Latitude N 40° 7′ 8.59″

Longitude W 76° 42′ 32.06″

Directions

From PA 283, take the Fulling Mill Road/Union Street exit and follow PA 441 south through Middletown and then past Three Mile Island. Beyond Three Mile Island, keep your eyes open for Collins Road descending to the right. A Department of Fish and Game Falmouth Boat Access sign marks the turn. Turn right, cross the tracks, and park in the large parking area.

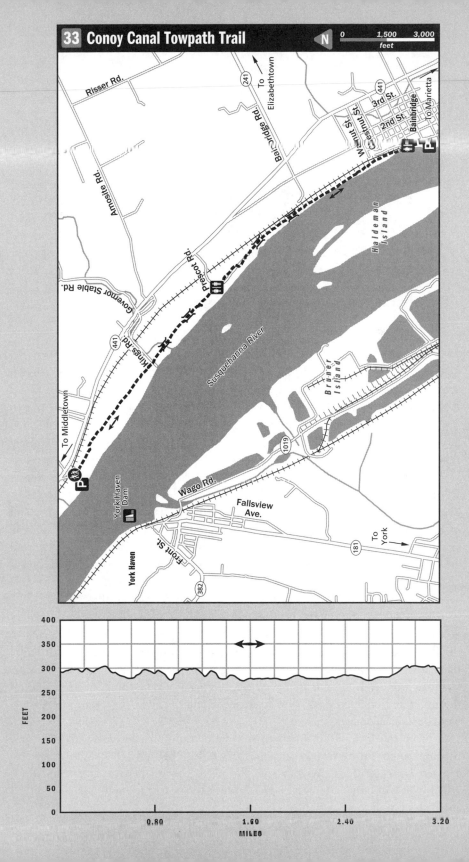

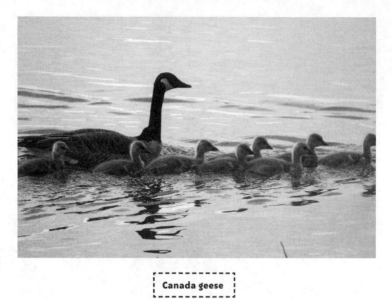

Canada geese

Columbia to the south and Clarks Ferry north of Harrisburg. Constructed in the 1820s and 1830s, this canal was part of an extensive system of canals and locks that provided transportation throughout the state. The canals were put to disuse with the development of the major train lines throughout Pennsylvania later in the 19th century. Remains of the canal and several locks are visible along this hike.

I find the most convenient access for this hike to be the boat launch area at Falmouth, located just downstream from the York Haven Dam. You can, however, begin from the south parking area located along the Susquehanna River at the end of Race Street in Bainbridge. From the Falmouth parking area, walk back out the entrance road and, just before reaching the railroad tracks, look for the trail entering the woods to the right (south). From the boat access, you actually begin about 0.4 miles south of the northern terminus at Conewago Creek. You can reach that by heading north on the trail from the other side of the road.

For this hike, follow the trail up a little hill into the woods and immediately you will reach the site of the Falmouth Lock. Although it is now filled with weeds, the lock is still an impressive bit of architecture that offers a sense of what barge navigators were working with 150 years ago. Whenever I see something like this I always wonder what it must have been like to build the thing, not to mention the miles and miles of canal that stretched along the river. The manpower must have been incredible.

From the lock, drop down to the main trail and continue walking south through some brushy woods. In about 0.3 miles, the trail veers slightly left and crosses a private drive. Walk across the drive toward a large grassy meadow, which you will pass on its west edge. Be sure to stick to the trail here, keeping a small stone wall to your right, as it is all private property.

The hike continues through fairly thick woods for some distance until it reaches Kings Road at just about 1 mile. At the road, you can walk over to the Susquehanna River to have a look around. Waterfowl often hang around along the shore, north and south of the clearing, and if you approach the river quietly, you may spot a wood duck or heron, or perhaps an eagle, in one of the tall trees.

From Kings Road, enter the woods along the trail and cross a couple of footbridges over small feeder creeks on the way. Use caution on all of the wooden footbridges as they can be very slippery. This is an especially nice section for birding. I had never seen a cuckoo before I started hiking along the Susquehanna River. Now it seems that I see them every time I do a river hike. I saw several through this section of the trail, and one had a nest within arm's reach of one of the footbridges.

After another 0.6 miles, the trail reaches a second private drive serving several more cabins. A portable toilet for the use of trail walkers is located on the right. You can walk along the drive if you like until you see a trail sign. Or if you look across the drive to your left a bit, you should be able to find a path entering the woods that continues along the top of the towpath running 50 yards or so east of the drive. The towpath here is grassy (someone even mows it on occasion) and in about 0.25 miles takes you to the site of the old Bainbridge Lock. Considerably smaller than the Falmouth Lock, this one is overgrown and filled with debris. It is still identifiable, however.

From the lock, walk to the private drive to the aforementioned sign, turn left, and at the end of the drive walk across the grass, veering slightly left to where the trail reenters the woods and picks up the towpath again. After a short distance, you'll reach a rather significant footbridge and then pass a swampy area that always seems to be teeming with birdlife. Notice the large sycamores through this section of trail.

For the next mile, the trail passes by a rather industrial section. A large power plant can be seen (and heard) across the river, and the backs of various businesses are seen on the left. The trail passes fairly close to the river in a couple of places, and the overhanging shrubs provide good cover for waterfowl. Just shy of 3 miles, the trail enters a clearing near some private homes on the left. Continue across the clearing staying high on the trail through the private property. When you reach the trees again, you will come to a dirt road, then a parking area with another portable toilet, and just beyond that the parking area at the end of Race Street in Bainbridge (3.2 miles). To return to your car, retrace the route.

NEARBY ACTIVITIES

The Susquehanna River in this area is a popular boating area, mostly for power-boats and touring kayaks.

34 CONEWAGO TRAIL:
Elizabethtown to Old Hershey Road

KEY AT-A-GLANCE INFORMATION

LENGTH: 4.2 miles

CONFIGURATION: Out-and-back

DIFFICULTY: Easy

SCENERY: Conewago Creek, farms, pleasant forest

EXPOSURE: More shade than sun

TRAIL TRAFFIC: Moderate

TRAIL SURFACE: Gravel and dirt

HIKING TIME: 1.5 hours round-trip

DRIVING DISTANCE: About 2 miles from central PA 743 and PA 230 in Elizabethtown

ACCESS: Dawn–dusk

MAPS: USGS Middletown and Elizabethtown

WHEELCHAIR TRAVERSABLE: Possible when dry

SPECIAL COMMENTS: Although it's a nice walk, there have, unfortunately, been some problems with assaults on this trail in the past, so it is safest to walk with a partner.

IN BRIEF

This easy hike traverses an old railroad grade that extends into Lebanon County, following the path of the Conewago Creek and passing by some beautiful corn and farm fields. It is especially pretty late in the day when the sun is low.

DESCRIPTION

Maintained by the Lancaster County Department of Parks and Recreation, the Conewago Recreation Trail is a 5-mile footpath that extends from PA Route 230 1.75 miles west of Elizabethtown to the Lebanon County line near the town of Lawn. At the 5-mile mark, the trail abruptly becomes the Lebanon Valley Rail Trail and continues east through Lawn for 12.5 miles (see page 188 for information on the Lebanon Valley Rail Trail).

For its length, the Conewago Trail follows the bed of the old Cornwall and Lebanon Railroad line alongside Conewago Creek, which flows just north of the trail. The Cornwall and Lebanon Railroad was built in the 1880s by iron magnate Richard E. Coleman, who used it to haul iron ore from his furnaces in Lebanon County to the mills in Steelton on the shore of the Susquehanna River. The rail line was abandoned after the floods from Hurricane Agnes in 1972. In 1979, Lancaster County acquired the

GPS Trailhead Coordinates

UTM Zone (WGS84) 18T

Easting 360217

Northing 4447303

Latitude N 40° 9′ 52.10″

Longitude W 76° 38′ 31.66″

Directions

From PA 283, follow PA 743 south into Elizabethtown. Turn right at the second traffic light (PA 230). Follow PA 230 for 1.75 miles. The parking area for the trailhead is on your right.

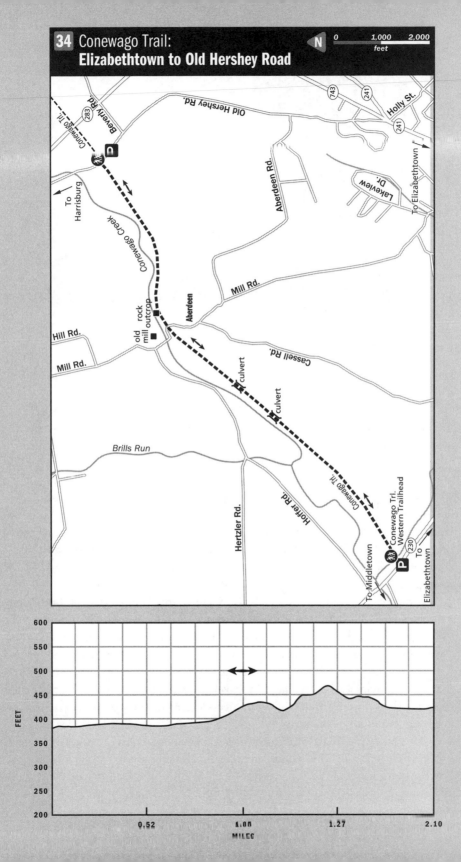

N

0   1,000   2,000
feet

Beverly Rd.

283

Conewago Trl.

Old Hershey Rd.

743

241

Holly St.

241

To Elizabethtown

To Harrisburg

Conewago Creek

Aberdeen Rd.

Lakeview Dr.

Mill Rd.

old rock mill outcrop

Aberdeen

Hill Rd.

Mill Rd.

Cassell Rd.

culvert

culvert

Brills Run

Hertzler Rd.

Hoffer Rd.

Conewago Trl.

Conewago Trl. Western Trailhead

P

To Middletown

230

To Elizabethtown

FEET

600
550
500
450
400
350
300
250
200

0.52   1.00   1.27   2.10

MILES

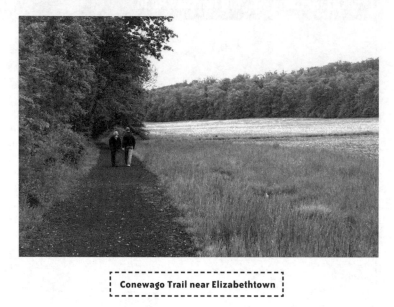

Conewago Trail near Elizabethtown

land that the railroad line followed, and in 1981 converted the land into a hiking and biking trail.

I discovered the Conewago Trail four years ago after spending two weeks in the hospital battling a serious illness. It was the perfect thing for me during the period of my recovery, and I walked it almost every day from September through November. The path is nearly level, as is the case with railroad grades, so the hiking is not very difficult. The path passes through sections of shade and sun, so while you are never getting roasted for long periods in the sun, you are also never under a dense canopy of trees for a long period either. Although the trail is popular with hikers, bikers, and runners, it never feels crowded and is an easy place to find some peace and solitude. Additionally, the scenery is lovely as the trail passes cornfields, old farms, and pretty sections of woods. Wildflowers abound in the spring; the colors of the trees and fields are magnificent in the fall.

Although the trail itself extends for 5 miles, this hike covers the first 2-mile stretch out and back from the parking lot on PA 230 near Elizabethtown to the Old Hershey Road at the 2-mile marker. This section of the trail provides easy access, plenty of parking, and avoids having to cross any major highways. Beyond the Old Hershey Road, the trail passes beneath PA 283 (very noisy) and shortly thereafter crosses PA 743 (a heavily traveled road). East of PA 743 are smaller road crossings where you can pick up nice sections of the trail, though the parking is limited at all of those.

This hike heads east from the parking lot along a cinder and gravel surface, immediately entering the woods. Here, you are surrounded by lovely hickory, beech, sycamore, and red-cedar trees. At 0.15 miles, the trail departs the woods and enters a clearing that serves as a crop field to the south of the trail. The field is often planted with corn, though some years it lies fallow. Several small oak trees dot the landscape to the right. The large field extends for a half mile to the east, is bounded by a forested hillside to the south, and provides for wonderful scenery at all times of the year. I highly recommend a walk near dawn or dusk when the sun is low because the light on this meadow can be quite picturesque. This is also a good place to spot white-tailed deer and wild turkeys en masse, as well as a variety of songbirds, including bluebirds and meadowlarks.

At 0.2 miles, the trail crosses a dirt farm road used to access the field to your right and the wild meadowland to the north of the trail. The trail continues bordered by a narrow stand of trees on the left and reenters the woods just past the 0.5-mile marker along the trail. Here, you'll be walking under a beautiful canopy of tall trees for the next 0.5 miles until the Mill Road crossing. The sunlight as it plays through these trees creates beautiful shadows on the path and on humid days creates hazy shafts that shine through the leaves. Along the way to Mill Road, the trail passes over two small side streams. In the woods alongside the trail are piles of the old railroad timbers, which are now home to chipmunks, spiders, ants, and other small critters.

At the Mill Road crossing, the trail runs close to a particularly rocky section of the Conewago Creek. It is worth walking over to the creek and the bridge on Mill Road (just to the north of the trail crossing) to have a look at the creek and the old mill building with its characteristic Pennsylvania Dutch architecture. Parking used to be available along the creek here, and the rocky stretch just upstream from the bridge used to draw plenty of people who came to wade and sun themselves on some of the large boulders clogging the creek. During the past year, however, the whole area along this section of the creek has been posted as private property and parking is no longer allowed. Please don't stray from the path except where it crosses roads.

From the Mill Road crossing, the trail climbs briefly and within 0.1 mile enters a cut through a rocky outcrop that obviously had to be blasted to run the railroad line through. Just beyond the outcrop, the trail crosses another small tributary to Conewago Creek and then follows the Conewago quite closely for another 0.25 miles before the creek meanders north. On the south side of the trail lies a large farm, the openness of which provides some nice views. The north side of the trail is wooded, much of the land owned by the Hershey Trust.

Within a quarter of a mile of the turnaround, two houses are set back in the woods. Shortly thereafter, you arrive at the 2-mile marker and the crossing with the Old Hershey Road. On the east side of the road, you'll find a small parking area with room enough for about three cars, and it can provide an alternate starting point for the hike. In the spring, some lovely wildflowers grow in the area of the parking lot, the colors of which are worth the walk itself.

NEARBY ACTIVITIES

Elizabethtown has several restaurants and all of the amenities that you might need. The Twin Kiss, located between the two traffic lights on 743, has good hot dogs, and Flavers, on the main drag through town, is a restaurant with nice outdoor seating by a small creek. On Saturday mornings, there is a large market on the right a couple of miles farther down PA 230 toward Middletown.

35 GOVERNOR DICK

ⓘ KEY AT-A-GLANCE INFORMATION

LENGTH: About 2 miles

CONFIGURATION: Loop

DIFFICULTY: Moderately strenuous

SCENERY: Excellent views of Lancaster, Lebanon, and Dauphin counties

EXPOSURE: Shaded

TRAIL TRAFFIC: Moderate–heavy

TRAIL SURFACE: Dirt and rock

HIKING TIME: 1–1.5 hours

DRIVING DISTANCE: About 13 miles from PA 283 and PA 743 in Elizabethtown

ACCESS: Dawn–dusk

MAPS: USGS Manheim

FACILITIES: Portable toilet at parking area; picnic tables on top of Governor Dick Hill

WHEELCHAIR TRAVERSABLE: No

SPECIAL COMMENTS: The lookout tower on top of Governor Dick Hill provides one of the best views in Lancaster County.

GPS Trailhead Coordinates

UTM Zone (WGS84)   18T

Easting   375521

Northing   4455894

Latitude   N 40° 14′ 38.99″

Longitude   W 76° 27′ 46.64″

IN BRIEF

This wonderful hike follows the path of an old railroad grade through the woods and then heads uphill to the observation tower via a dirt road. After stopping to take in the great views from the tower, you descend along a gentle path that traverses the hill until a short steep section drops down to the original trail.

DESCRIPTION

Governor Dick Hill is a popular hiking destination for people who live in the small townships around the southern Lebanon County hamlet of Mount Gretna. And for good reason: the 66-foot-tall observation tower on its summit offers a wonderful panoramic view of the surrounding countryside. On a clear day, you can see parts of Lancaster, Lebanon, Dauphin, York, and Berks counties.

First-time visitors invariably wonder about the origin of the name of the hill. It was named in the latter part of the 19th century for an African American woodchopper and charcoal burner who worked exclusively in this area. His name was Dick, and his co-workers referred to him as "Governor." The hill was named for him after he died.

Directions ⟶

From PA 283, follow PA 743 south toward Elizabethtown. At the first traffic light, make a sharp left turn (you will be going almost in the opposite direction) onto PA 241. Follow 241 for 7.75 miles until it ends in the town of Colebrook. Turn right onto PA 117. After 100 yards, PA 117 turns left toward Mount Gretna. Take this left and follow for 3 miles to the intersection with Pinch Road. Turn right on Pinch Road and follow for 0.5 miles to the parking area on your left.

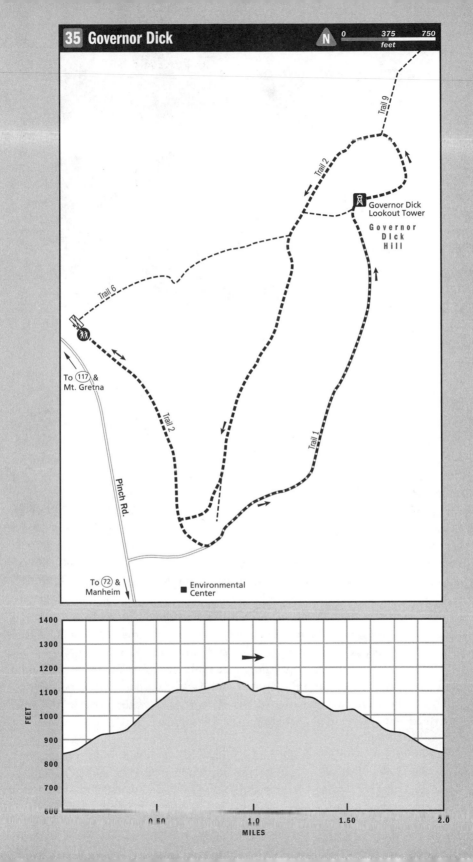

N

0   375   750
feet

Trail 9

Trail 2

Governor Dick
Lookout Tower

Governor
Dick
Hill

Trail 6

To (117) &
Mt. Gretna

Trail 2

Trail 1

Pinch Rd.

To (72) &
Manheim

■ Environmental
  Center

1400
1300
1200
1100
1000
900
800
700
600

FEET

0.50   1.0   1.50   2.0
MILES

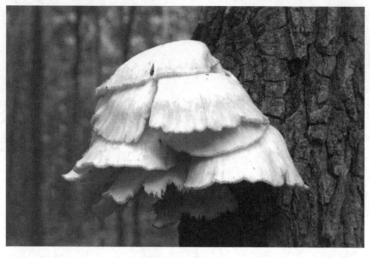

Shelf fungus

The 1,105 acres of woodland on which the hill lies was purchased in 1934 by Clarence Schock of the Schock Independent Oil Company (SICO), who donated the land to the Mount Joy school district in 1953. The SICO Foundation built the observation tower in 1954. The land has been deeded to be maintained in its natural state and used solely for recreational purposes. The Clarence Schock Foundation (formerly the SICO Foundation) still contributes funds to maintain the area, and is a generous contributor of scholarships for students attending local colleges.

The popularity of the area for recreational purposes, though, predates Schock's acquisition of the land. In 1889, the Cornwall and Lebanon Railroad completed the construction of the Mount Gretna Narrow Gauge Railway. The narrow gauge shuttled visitors between the station that the C&L Railroad had established at the present site of Mount Gretna and the summit of Governor Dick Hill, a 4-mile ride. The current trailhead and parking area on Pinch Road, in fact, lie at a site where the old railroad passed. With the area's pretty woodlands and lake, the Pennsylvania Chautauqua Society founded the town of Mount Gretna around 1890. It has been a popular summer resort for travelers since.

Many of the hikers on Governor Dick Hill tend to follow the same 1-mile path from the parking lot to the summit and back again. For the sake of variety, I tend to be inclined more toward the loop hike configuration, so the hike described here offers a slight variation from the standard, with just a few hundred feet added distance.

The main trail begins at the parking lot, where you will find trash cans and a portable toilet. Two yellow gates block old roadbeds that extend from the lot. Begin this hike by passing by the right-hand gate. The hike climbs gently on a wide but somewhat rocky track through a lovely forest of oak and hickory trees.

Keep your eyes open for birds along this hike. In one day during the spring, I spotted three pileated woodpeckers in these woods. As you climb, you'll notice many rough trails that take off into the woods. Most of these are the effects of mountain bikers and hikers who have cut between switchbacks. For the sake of the preservation of the area, I encourage you to stay to the main numbered trails. As of this writing, the Schock Foundation was evaluating the trails in the area and considering limiting usage of some for hiking only.

At 0.3 miles, you will reach a trail junction with numbered trail signs and a rough and rocky path heading uphill to your left. That path is Trail 2 and is the common route up. You will return via that path. For the purposes of this hike, though, continue straight past that junction along Trail 3 for another 150 feet until you come to the junction with an old dirt road. Another trail marker with the number 3 on it is located here, and at this point turn left and follow the road. The road climbs rather steeply for approximately 0.25 miles before it levels out for the remainder of the hike to the top of Governor Dick Hill, easily recognizable by the large observation tower. Do not neglect to climb to the top of the tower via a series of ladders inside it! The view is worth the bit of effort. Several picnic tables are available for having a snack in the meadow around the base of the tower.

For the descent, follow Trail 2 down the hill. Several trails take off in various directions from the top of the hill, so be sure that you get the right one. Trail 2 leaves the meadow below the tower to the north and is identified by a sign that says PINCH AND RT. 117. The trail proceeds on nice level ground curving to the right (northeast). After 0.1 mile, you will pass a small trail that enters from the right. Trail 2 bends sharply to the left, and in another 0.05 miles reaches a junction with a significant trail descending to the right. Continue straight on Trail 2 (turning right will take you to Route 117). This broad, easy-to-follow path traverses the side of Governor Dick Hill descending steadily but gently.

At 1.7 miles into the hike, you'll come to an unnumbered trail junction giving you the choice of continuing straight across the hillside or turning to the right and descending steeply along a rather rough section of trail. Take the right-hand path. The steep and rocky section is only a couple of hundred feet long and ends at the junction with the main trail that you passed an hour or so ago on your ascent. Turn right here and in ten minutes you are back at the car.

NEARBY ACTIVITIES

Mount Gretna is a little community that is worth exploring. During the summer, be sure to finish up your hike with a trip to the Jigger Shop for an ice cream or hamburger.

36 KELLY'S RUN

KEY AT-A-GLANCE INFORMATION

LENGTH: 5.2 miles

CONFIGURATION: Loop with a section of out-and-back to the Pinnacle Overlook

DIFFICULTY: Moderate

SCENERY: Kelly's Run natural area, Pinnacle Overlook, and Susquehanna River

EXPOSURE: More shade than sun

TRAIL TRAFFIC: Light

TRAIL SURFACE: Dirt with a short section of paved climbing from the river

HIKING TIME: 3–4 hours

DRIVING DISTANCE: About 5.6 miles from the intersection of PA 372 and PA 272 in Buck, PA

ACCESS: 8 a.m.–dusk

MAPS: USGS Holtwood; a map of the trail and recreation area is available at the parking lot.

FACILITIES: Restrooms and water at the recreation area

WHEELCHAIR TRAVERSABLE: No

SPECIAL COMMENTS: This is one of the most beautiful hikes I have ever done, though it may be impassable after heavy rain. Use care during hunting season.

IN BRIEF

This hike follows the Kelly's Run Trail from recreation area near Holtwood into Kelly's Run, where it picks up the Pinnacle Trail and makes a 1.4-mile out-and-back trek to the Pinnacle Overlook above the Susquehanna River. The route then follows Kelly's Run to the Susquehanna River and climbs to the top of the river escarpment along the paved, but disused, Old Pinnacle Road. At the top of the road, it follows trails through fields and woodlands back to the recreation area.

DESCRIPTION

The Kelly's Run Natural Area, through which this hike passes, is part of the 5,000-acre Holtwood Environmental Preserve. The environmental preserve was established for recreation purposes by Pennsylvania Power and Light, which operates the hydroelectric dam at Holtwood and also owns large tracts of land on each side of the Susquehanna River at Lake Aldred. Designated by the U.S. Department of the Interior as a National Recreation Trail, the Kelly's Run–Pinnacle Trail System takes you into the heart of the natural area and provides access to its extraordinarily beautiful hemlock and rhododendron–lined glen. The natural area has also been designated

GPS Trailhead Coordinates

UTM Zone (WGS84) 18S

Easting 387320

Northing 4410914

Latitude N 39° 50' 26.76"

Longitude W 76° 19' 1.13"

Directions ⟶

From PA 272 in Buck, travel west on PA 372 for 4.9 miles. Turn right on River Road and then left on Old Holtwood Road. The parking area is about 0.25 miles ahead on the right. A second, smaller parking area, at the trailhead, is located around the corner on Drytown Road. That area, though, is not open year-round.

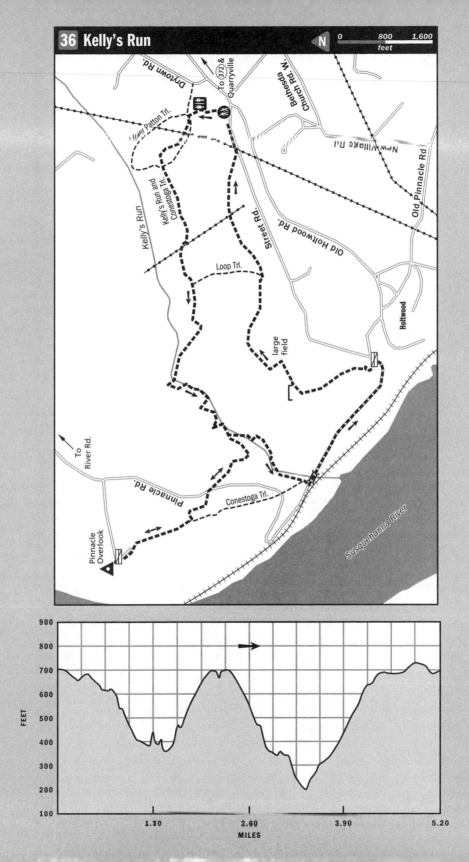

N

0   800   1,600
feet

To 372 &
Quarryville

Drytown Rd.

Bethesda W.
Church Rd.

Mill Patton Trl.

New Villore Rl.

Old Pinnacle Rd

Kelly's Run

Kelly's Run and
Conestoga Trl.

Street Rd.

Old Holtwood Rd.

Loop Trl.

large
field

Holtwood

To River Rd.

Pinnacle Rd.

Conestoga Trl.

Susquehanna River

Pinnacle
Overlook

FEET

900
800
700
600
500
400
300
200
100

1.30   2.60   3.90   5.20

MILES

by Audubon Pennsylvania as a featured site on the Susquehanna Birding and Wildlife Trail.

This hike begins by following the blue-blazed Kelly's Run Trail, which shares the path for a fair distance with the orange-blazed Conestoga Trail. The latter trail extends for 61 miles from Pumping Station Road in Lebanon County to Lock 12 in York County across the Norman Wood Bridge. The Kelly's Run trailhead is at the small parking area on Drytown Road, though that area is not open year-round. If it is closed, begin hiking from the main parking area by the ballfield on Holtwood Wood. The trail is easily picked up from a path heading into the woods behind the restrooms. Head west on the pleasant dirt trail as it begins its gradual descent into Kelly's Run. Pass some power lines and, at 0.25 miles, pass the junction with the yellow-blazed Oliver Patton Trail, a 0.75-mile loop through the upper part of Kelly's Run. Walk beneath a second set of power lines and at about 0.7 miles cross an interesting section of trail where it appears naturally paved by rocks. As you continue above Kelly's Run to its south, the red-blazed Loop Trail departs on the left (0.75 miles). Then you descend more steeply toward the creek.

At 1.1 miles, the trail crosses Kelly's Run and immediately afterwards a small tributary entering from the north. The path here would probably be impassable after heavy rains. This is an absolutely enchanting spot with tall hemlocks and oak trees, a large rock outcrop, and rhododendrons lining the steep-sided hollow. In late May and June the rhododendrons are in bloom, an event that adds even more to the spectacular scenery. Continue along the north side of the creek for another 0.4 miles to the junction with the Pinnacle Trail (white blazes). The Pinnacle Trail provides an out-and-back side trip of about 1.4 miles to an overlook above the Susquehanna River. Although the overlook can be reached by car, the walk out of Kelly's Run is lovely and offers some excellent opportunities for birding and wild-life viewing. Along this path I have seen many songbirds common to Pennsylvania as well as owls and many hawks. I have also seen a fox resting on the trail near the overlook.

To reach the overlook, turn right on the Pinnacle Trail and follow it uphill for about 0.15 miles, where it meets an unmarked trail heading to the right. Turn left and follow the path across two old roadbeds, the first of which is identified by a NO HORSES sign. At a third road of grass and dirt, turn right and follow the white blazes about 0.3 miles farther to the Pinnacle Overlook. The overlook offers a wonderful view of the Susquehanna River Valley to the north. Directly beneath you are several islands and the deepest part of Lake Aldred formed by the Holtwood Hydroelectric Dam. The overlook area has benches to rest on, a few picnic tables, and restrooms.

When you've had your fill of the scenery, retrace your steps back to Kelly's Run. Continue following the creek down toward the Susquehanna River, passing several rock outcrops, pools and drops in the creek, and more great scenery on the way. Just before reaching the Old Pinnacle Road at river level, the Conestoga Trail departs from the Kelly's Run Trail by a series of steps in the hillside heading north. Upon reaching the Old Pinnacle Road, a disused paved road, turn left and

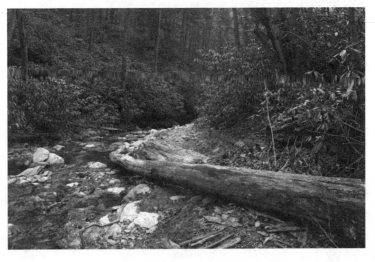

Kelly's Run

balance your way across the carcass of the old bridge over the creek—the spookiest part of the hike (take a deep breath and use the cable on the left for a handrail as you cross the rusted steel girders). Once across, follow the road uphill for a half mile to a gate. Keep your eyes open for bald eagles and osprey while you climb as they frequent this section of the river. Pass the gate and pick up the trail on the left by some blue blazes and a bench. The trail is wide track here and it climbs a ridge away from the river. After passing another bench, the trail levels out before reaching a large field.

Turn left and follow the edge of the field for a little more than half its width, to a trail post with a blue blaze on the left. Turn right and head for another post with a blaze out in the middle of the field. Cross the length of the field along a wide grass swath to the wide track at its far end. Enter the woods and pass the junction with the red-blazed Loop Trail at about 4.75 miles. Continue along the track for about another half mile back to the parking area, passing beneath the two power lines on the way.

NEARBY ACTIVITIES

Picnic facilities and a ball field are located at the recreation area. Just across the street is the Holtwood Arboretum. Small and informal, it displays several interesting tree species. A visit to the Holtwood Dam is certainly worth a drive down Old Holtwood Road to the level of the river. On the way down, you'll pass the entrance for the Face Rock Overlook on the left. Although the overlook is not the prettiest place in the world (it hosts myriad power lines and transformers), it offers a very impressive view of the ancient channels carved into the bedrock beneath the Susquehanna downstream from the dam. The area is also popular for viewing the spring and fall hawk migrations. Face Rock is open from 9 a.m. to dusk.

37 LANCASTER JUNCTION RECREATION TRAIL

KEY AT-A-GLANCE INFORMATION

LENGTH: 4.8 miles

CONFIGURATION: Out-and-back

DIFFICULTY: Easy

SCENERY: Upper Chickies Creek and Lancaster County farmlands

EXPOSURE: About half shade and half sun

TRAIL TRAFFIC: Moderate–heavy

TRAIL SURFACE: Cinders

HIKING TIME: 2–3 hours

DRIVING DISTANCE: Less than a mile from the Salunga exit on PA 283 west of Lancaster

ACCESS: Dawn–dusk

MAPS: USGS Columbia East and Manheim; a map of the trail is available online from the Lancaster County Department of Parks and Recreation at www.co.lancaster .pa.us/parks/lib/parks/Lancaster_ Junction.pdf.

FACILITIES: Restrooms and water at trailhead parking

WHEELCHAIR TRAVERSABLE: If dry

SPECIAL COMMENTS: A good hike with young kids. Excellent birding.

IN BRIEF

The trailhead for this hike is about 50 feet from the highway, but heading north it quickly quiets down, joins Chickies Creek, and follows the railroad grade for about 2.4 miles to Auction Road. Return via the railroad grade.

DESCRIPTION

Extending for about 2.4 miles from PA 283 outside of Salunga north to Auction Road, the Lancaster Junction Trail follows the grade of the old Reading–Columbia Railroad line. The trail is popular with hikers, bikers, and horseback riders, and it offers a nice outing for the kids. Hiking the trail provides you with some classic Lancaster County farmland scenery and lovely views of the upper stretch of Chickies Creek. The creek eventually drains into the Susquehanna River near Chickies Rocks, a large quartzite outcrop that overlooks the river about 7 miles directly southwest. The trail scenery is particularly attractive in the morning and late day when the sun is low and the shadows are long. Bordered by trees and brush, the trail is generally sheltered and makes for a good hike on a windy day. Common wild mammals that you may encounter are red foxes, groundhogs, and gray and ground squirrels. Bird activity is abundant in the thickets and woods lining the

GPS Trailhead Coordinates

UTM Zone (WGS84) 18T

Easting   379247

Northing   4439962

Latitude   N 40° 6′ 4.67″

Longitude   W 76° 25′ 0.15″

Directions

Take the Salunga exit off PA 283 west of Lancaster. Make the first right north of the bridge over 283 onto Champ Boulevard. Park at the end of Champ Boulevard.

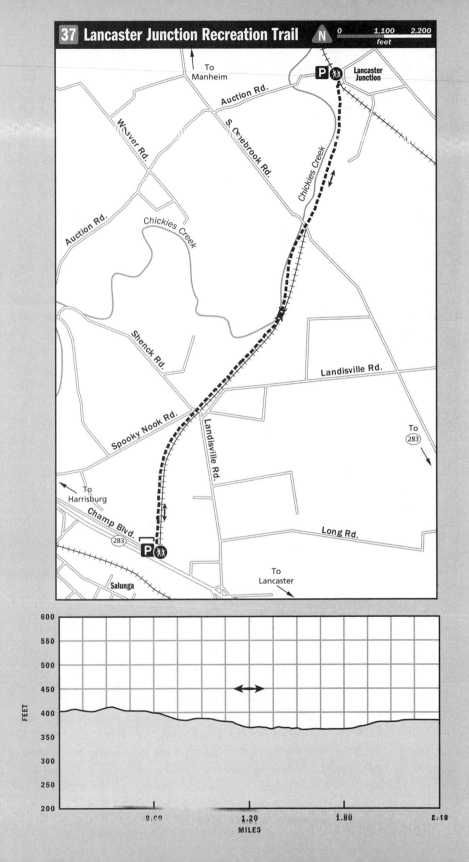

N

0   1,100   2,200
feet

To
Manheim

Auction Rd.

Weaver Rd.

S. Oakbrook Rd.

Chickies Creek

Lancaster
Junction

Auction Rd.

Chickies Creek

Shenck Rd.

Landisville Rd.

To
283

Spooky Nook Rd.

Landisville Rd.

To
Harrisburg

Champ Blvd.

283

Long Rd.

To
Lancaster

Salunga

FEET

600
550
500
450
400
350
300
250
200

0.60   1.20   1.80   2.40

MILES

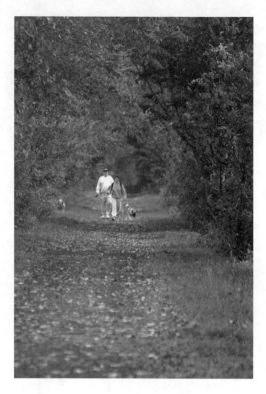

Hikers on the rail-trail

trail. Cardinals, bluebirds, warblers, chickadees, and catbirds are common. Hawks can often be sighted soaring above the farmlands, pheasant and grouse are occasionally spotted along the trail, and great blue herons frequent the creek waters.

From the southern trailhead on Champ Boulevard, head north along the trail, passing a metal bench after about 0.1 mile. Although the setting at the trailhead is rather noisy from highway traffic, after a quarter of a mile or so that is left behind and the environment is much more peaceful. For the first 0.5 miles, the trail proceeds directly north and then, by a large farm on the right, takes more of a northeasterly tack for the next 0.7 miles. At 0.65 miles, you'll cross Spooky Nook Road. Just before reaching the road, note the interesting stand of grassy plants 15 feet high or so on the left side of the trail. They appear to be a sort of cane, rush, or bamboo and though they seem out of place in central Pennsylvania I have also come across a dense stand of the same on the Lakeside Trail at Gifford Pinchot State Park (see page 243). A white cinder-block building at the road crossing is home to the Malmborg Flower Shop. If it is open when you pass, stop in and have a look around.

At 1.2 miles, the trail crosses a small stream over an old concrete bridge and parallels Chickies Creek quite closely. The creek is clear and placid along this stretch of trail as it winds among some tall oak and impressive sycamore trees. Signs of woodpeckers are obvious on the old trees. Just past the 1.5 mile mark, the trail crosses Colebrook Road. I walked for a distance in this area with a gentleman who lived nearby and who told me that occasionally the fish and game department releases ring-necked pheasants in the area. He had seen quite few, though he explained that the foxes tend to get them pretty quickly.

At 1.8 miles or so, you'll pass a grassy area to the left with some tall trees scattered about it and goats wandering around. Hawks often perch in the tall trees surrounding it. Soon after, the trail crosses a private farm road and a large produce farm on the right. Please keep to the trail as the road on either side is posted as private.

At 2.2 miles, you'll pass a second bench on the side of the trail, and just ahead, the gate at the parking area on Auction Road at the settlement of Lancaster Junction. A rail line enters from the southeast by a scenic old warehouse.

LANCASTER CENTRAL PARK:
Mill Creek Loop(s)

38

IN BRIEF

This pretty hike initially follows Mill Creek as it meanders throughout the park before it joins with the Equestrian Trail and passes some of the recreation areas in the park.

DESCRIPTION

Located 6 miles south of the city of Lancaster, Central Park is named for its location in the center of Lancaster County. Like many relatively urban parks, Central Park boasts quite a number of recreational facilities, making it a popular destination for people all around the county. The 544-acre park has ball fields, playgrounds, tennis courts, a pool, a fitness trail, equestrian trails, gardens, picnic pavilions, an environmental center, and, with five sites, the smallest public campground in the state.

The park is also rich in local history. In 1979, an ancient Indian burial ground was uncovered north of Golf Road near the microwave tower that this hike passes by. Robert Fulton conducted his first tests of the paddlewheel boat on the Conestoga River, which composes the northwestern boundary of the park. And one of the park byways, General Hand Road, is named for Edward Hand, George Washington's adjutant general, whose home is preserved in the park at the site of

KEY AT-A-GLANCE INFORMATION

LENGTH: 4.2 miles (1.5 miles on Mill Creek Trail loop and 2.7 miles on Conestoga–Equestrian trails loop)

CONFIGURATION: Figure-8

DIFFICULTY: Moderate

SCENERY: Mill Creek, Central Park environs

EXPOSURE: Slightly more sun than shade

TRAIL TRAFFIC: Light

TRAIL SURFACE: Mixed gravel, dirt, and grass with a short section of pavement

HIKING TIME: 45 minutes for Mill Creek Trail loop; 1.5 hours for Conestoga/Equestrian Trails loop

DRIVING DISTANCE: Approximately 7 miles south of PA 283 and PA 222 in Lancaster

ACCESS: Daily, dawn–dusk

MAPS: Park trails map available at park office; USGS Lancaster

FACILITIES: None at parking area; water, restrooms, and picnic areas available en route

WHEELCHAIR TRAVERSABLE: No

SPECIAL COMMENTS: This hike combines 3 trails throughout the park. Although each is easy to follow, care needs to be taken at some key junctions indicated in the text.

Directions ⟶

From US 30 just north of Lancaster, follow US 222 south for approximately 6 miles to Golf Road on the left. There is a sign for Lancaster Central Park. Turn left and follow Golf Road for 1.5 miles to the intersection with Kiwanis Road. Turn right and, just before the covered bridge, bear right into the parking area along Mill Creek.

GPS Trailhead Coordinates

UTM Zone (WGS84) 18T

Easting 390638

Northing 4430290

Latitude N 40° 00' 55.84"

Longitude W 76° 16' 56.21"

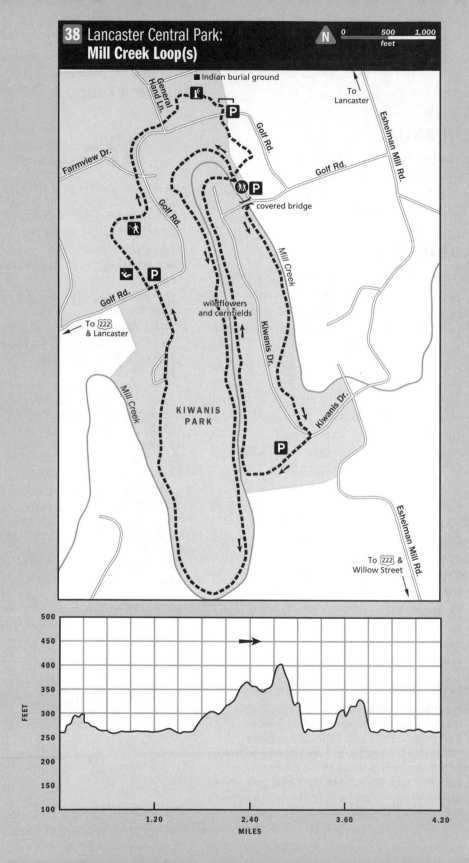

N

0   500   1,000
feet

■ Indian burial ground

To Lancaster

General Hand Ln.

Golf Rd.

Eshelman Mill Rd.

Farmview Dr.

Golf Rd.

Golf Rd.

P

P

covered bridge

Golf Rd.

P

Mill Creek

wildflowers and cornfields

Kiwanis Dr.

Kiwanis Dr.

Mill Creek

KIWANIS PARK

P

Eshelman Mill Rd.

To 222 & Lancaster

To 222 & Willow Street

500

450

400

350

300

250

200

150

100

FEET

1.20   2.40   3.60   4.20

MILES

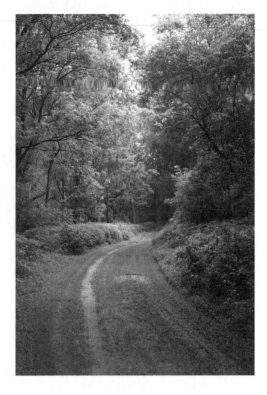

Mill Creek Trail

Rock Ford Plantation near the intersection of General Hand Road and Williamson Road.

Central Park is home to ten trails that are open to hiking, including a section of the Conestoga Trail System, which extends from northern Lancaster County south to the Mason Dixon Trail in York County. This hike follows four trails throughout the park and creates two loops, both of which are focused around Mill Creek, the small stream that forms the southern boundary of the park.

This hike begins at the center point of the two trail loops, at the covered-bridge parking area off of Kiwanis Road. The first loop, along the Mill Creek Trail through the Kiwanis Natural Area, is 1.5 miles long and takes about 45 minutes to complete. The second loop follows the Conestoga and Equestrian trails for most of their length and is approximately 2.7 miles long, taking about one hour and 20 minutes to complete. Putting both loops together is worth the effort, though if time doesn't permit, each offers a pleasant hike of its own.

PART 1: MILL CREEK TRAIL LOOP

Begin this section of the hike by walking over the covered bridge next to the parking lot. At 25 feet or so beyond the bridge, the trail drops down to river level via a steep but brief hillside to the left. The trail follows Mill Creek upstream in an open grassy area for 0.15 miles before passing power lines and entering the woods. Upon entering the woods, the trail is well marked with yellow blazes on the trees. The trail follows the level of the creek for a short distance before climbing up to the top of the peninsula that is home to the Kiwanis Natural Area. At 0.5 miles, the trail exits the woods at an intersection with Kiwanis Drive at a large picnic area with tables, a pavilion, restrooms, and water. The only route-finding difficulty you might have on this loop is here, trying to figure out where the trail reenters the woods.

To find the trail, cross Kiwanis Drive where it comes to a T-intersection just after you leave the woods. A large parking lot will be on your right, and you should walk along the grass next to the lot keeping it to your right. When you reach the corner of the lot, look downhill toward the woods, and you will spot the trail entering the woods marked by a yellow blaze. Once in the trees, the trail

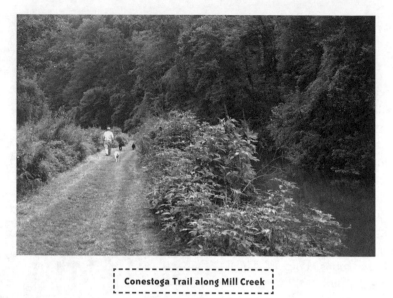

Conestoga Trail along Mill Creek

descends steeply, curving to the right (north), past the foundation of what appears to have been an old pump house, and down to the level of the creek. You have just passed over the top of the peninsula. When you reach the creek, pause to admire the large sycamore trees that line the banks. Cardinals and the occasional goldfinch add a splash of contrast to the lush green forest in the summer.

The trail now follows the creek (still upstream) around the peninsula's tip. At 1 mile, you will pass the junction with the Wildflower Trail. It climbs back over the peninsula and provides a slightly shorter excursion back to the covered bridge. Continue along the level of the creek around the peninsula and, at 1.5 miles, the trail will pass beneath the covered bridge. Hike back up to the road, walk through the bridge, and into the parking area.

PART 2: CONESTOGA LOOP

Leave the parking lot heading north, following white blazes on trees through a small grassy area beside the creek. You are now following the Scout Trail. In 0.1 mile, however, the trail comes to a junction with the Conestoga Trail System, which comes in from the woods on the right. The Scout Trail turns right here and shares the path with the Conestoga Trail for about 0.5 miles. Remember this spot, as it will be the end of the loop that you make.

Instead of turning right, continue straight ahead, staying at the level of the river along the Conestoga Trail, marked by salmon-colored blazes. The trail soon enters the woods and bends to the left following the direction of the creek. At 0.15 miles, the trail begins to show signs of being paved. Then it clearly turns into an abandoned paved road and begins to climb uphill. Be wary for the next bit of route finding: at 0.3 miles, the trail drops very steeply off the road to the left back to the level of the river. The sharp left turn is marked by salmon-colored arrows painted on the surface of the road and is easily missed.

Once you regain the level of the river, the trail is very obvious and becomes less precipitous. At 0.6 miles, the Conestoga Trail joins with the Equestrian Trail, which comes in from the right. Veer to the left here and enjoy the walk along the wide-open track, often grassy, as it passes through the Muhlenburg Native Plant and Wildflower Meadow, arguably the most beautiful spot in the park. For the next mile, the trail follows Mill Creek as it makes a long bend through the park. The far side of the creek rises up a steep forested hillside, while the side where the trail passes is open and gentle.

At approximately 1.6 miles, the trail leaves the creek and meets up with Exhibit Farm Road in an open grassy area flanked to the right by a large cornfield. A large rock with a salmon blaze marks the junction with Exhibit Farm Road. Follow the grass along the cornfield (there are trail signs) for another 0.2 miles until you reach the intersection of Exhibit Farm Road and Golf Road. Cross Exhibit Farm Road and then cross Golf Road. At this point, the Conestoga Trail turns left, paralleling Golf Road. Our hike continues straight (generally north) along the Equestrian Trail, passing a parking area to your right and then a playground on your left before entering a large grassy area with several large pine trees. Follow the line of pine trees to the end of the grassy area, turn right at another trail post in the northwest corner of the field, and follow the trail through a passage between some tall shrubs and trees next to the tennis courts.

At the end of this passage, the trail meets Golf Road, turns left, and follows the wide grassy shoulder of Golf Road for approximately 0.5 miles. Shortly, it crosses Farm View Drive and then General Hand Road. At 0.1 mile past General Hand Road, the shoulder gets very narrow and the trail climbs through a small, steep, wooded area approximately 100 feet back from the road. The trail emerges from the woods into a meadow with several trees and a large microwave tower on top. Head toward the tower following trail signs passing it on the right. Just beyond the tower (mile 2.4), you'll find a water fountain. From the fountain, the trail proceeds 0.1 mile over to a bench and a small parking area along Golf Road.

Here, the Equestrian Trail crosses the path of the Scout and Conestoga trails. The Equestrian Trail continues to follow the shoulder of Golf Road, while the Scout and Conestoga trails cross Golf Road and enter the woods at a tree marked with salmon and white blazes. Follow the path of these two trails into the woods, where they wind downhill for 0.2 miles to the grassy area where the loop began. The short passage through the woods is an ideal place to spot white-tailed deer.

NEARBY ACTIVITIES

Central Park provides all sorts of recreational activities, including a swimming pool, ball fields, a garden, and a campground. Downtown Lancaster is home to a host of shops, markets, and restaurants that are worth a visit. If you are hiking on Saturday, stop by the Central Market in town to pick up some snacks and drinks for a picnic in the park.

39 MONEY ROCKS COUNTY PARK

KEY AT-A-GLANCE INFORMATION

LENGTH: 4.5 miles

CONFIGURATION: Figure-8 with a section of out-and-back

DIFFICULTY: Moderate

SCENERY: Welsh Hills and nice views to the north from Money Rocks

EXPOSURE: Shaded

TRAIL TRAFFIC: Generally light

TRAIL SURFACE: Dirt and rock

HIKING TIME: 2.5–3 hours

DRIVING DISTANCE: 5.1 miles from US 322 and PA 23 in Blue Ball

ACCESS: Dawn–dusk

MAPS: USGS New Holland, Honey Brook; a trail map is available for download at www.co.lancaster .pa.us/parks/lib/parks/ MoneyRock12.pdf.

FACILITIES: None

WHEELCHAIR TRAVERSABLE: No

SPECIAL COMMENTS: Use caution when hiking during hunting season. Muzzle loading and archery seasons extend well into January.

IN BRIEF

This hike begins with a short walk from the parking area out to the Money Rocks Overlook, and then heads west on the Cockscomb Trail. From the Cockscomb area, it heads north and west along the hillside. At a T-intersection, it descends north to the Iron Horse Trail. After completing the Iron Horse Trail loop, this hike returns to the Cockscomb Trail, and completes that loop by climbing out of a hollow and along the ridge back to the Cockscomb outcrop.

DESCRIPTION

Located in eastern Lancaster County, the little-known Money Rocks County Park spans more than 300 acres in the Welsh Mountains of Pennsylvania, the second largest tract of forested land remaining in the county, the largest being the Furnace Hills along US 322 to the west (see page 86). This pleasant hike covers most of the trails in the park. It offers views of the surrounding countryside as well as opportunities to see ruffed grouse, wild turkey, and white-tailed deer, all of which are common to the park.

The trailhead for the white-blazed Overlook Trail, the first section of this hike, is located at the east edge of the parking area

GPS Trailhead Coordinates

UTM Zone (WGS84) 18T

Easting 416275

Northing 4438797

Latitude N 40° 5' 43.09"

Longitude W 75° 58' 55.94"

Directions

Follow US 322 east from the intersection with PA 23 in Blue Ball for 3.9 miles. Turn right onto Narvon Road (poorly marked). The parking area is 1.2 miles south on the right at a high point of the road.

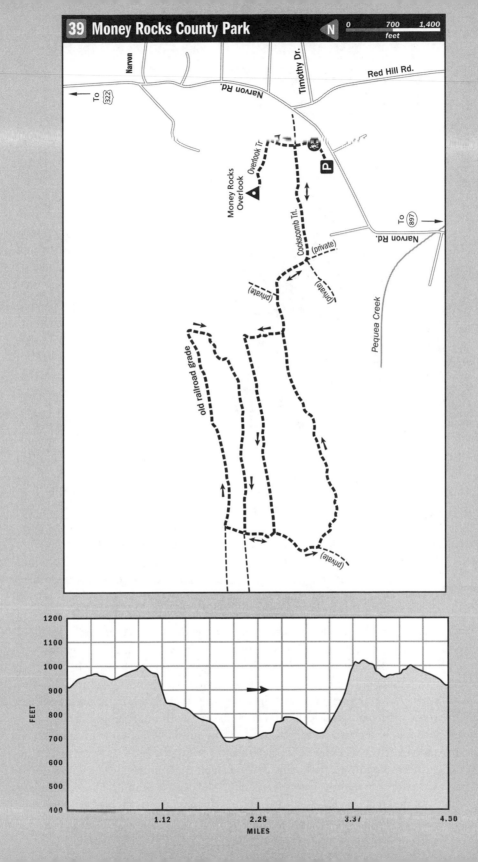

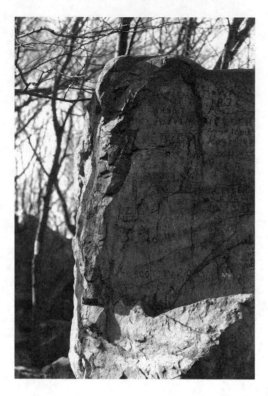

near a large wooden information sign. Begin by following the white blazes from the trailhead north along an old roadbed for about 0.3 miles to the Money Rocks Overlook, crossing the Cockscomb Trail (a roadbed marked by a prominent sign) en route. The overlook offers the best views on this hike of farms, towns, and distant wooded hills to the north. According to the Lancaster County Department of Parks and Recreation, legend has it that the rocks were so named because farmers from the Pequa Valley to the south hid their money among the rocks. Consisting mostly of a Chickies Formation white-and-pink quartzite formed by erosion of the softer rock surrounding it, the overlook sits atop cliffs and outcroppings ranging from 15 to 50 feet high. A metal railing safeguards one section of the cliffs, though care should be taken at all places when scrambling about the area. The best view and resting spots are located among the square boulders about 100 feet past the railing. Take note of the large rectangular boulder on the crest with names carved into it; some of them date back to the mid-1800s.

After enjoying the view, make your way back through the forest of white oak, black birch, and mountain laurel to the red-blazed Cockscomb Trail and turn right (west). This trail follows the flat ridge for about 0.3 miles to a junction with a dirt road that is posted with private property signs. Bear right and follow the red blazes over to the edge of the ridge where the Cockscomb Trail begins a gentle descent along the north-facing hillside. A short distance along the descent, you'll be able to spot the Cockscomb on the ridge crest to the left. Another smaller quartzite outcrop, the Cockscomb provides views mostly from late fall to early spring when the leaves are off the trees. In this area, about 1.1 miles into the hike, the Cockscomb Trail forks at a tree marked with multiple red blazes. Turn right and follow the trail down the steep, rocky hillside for a short distance to an old roadbed at the next level. Turn left and follow the road as it traverses the hillside. According to the park map, several small trails connect this section of the trail with the Iron Horse Trail several hundred feet downhill. Those trails are unmarked and much of the area surrounding the park is private land belonging to mining companies.

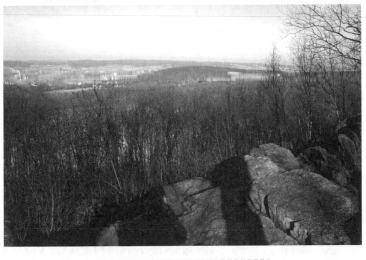

Welsh Mountains from the overlook

To be safe, follow the roadbed (the lower stretch of the Cockscomb Trail) for about 0.6 miles to a major **T**-intersection identified by a tall oak tree with double red blazes. The Cockscomb Trail, red-blazed and distinct, turns left uphill. To pick up the Iron Horse Trail, turn right and head downhill on an unmarked track that is more distinct in the spring and summer than fall and winter. Follow it for about 200 yards, staying right of a small watercourse. Soon you will reach a sign marking the Iron Horse Trail, marked by blue blazes. Continue past that sign on the now more prominent trail to a second sign at an old railroad grade. Turn right and follow the grade for 0.5 miles of very pleasant walking to a third Iron Horse Trail sign pointing uphill. Beyond the third sign, the grade passes onto private property barricaded by two large concrete blocks. Leave the grade and follow the trail uphill into the woods, crossing an old carriage road, and then reaching a second abandoned road with a trail sign onto which you'll turn right. This takes you back to the first Iron Horse Trail sign and the end of the 1.4-mile lower loop.

Trace your steps back up to the Cockscomb Trail, and follow it uphill into a pretty and dark hollow. Cross a creek and then continue about halfway up the hollow until you reach a fork in the trail. Continuing straight along the main track takes you into private property. Turn left and cut back across the hollow and gain the Cockscomb ridge by climbing a short steep section with timbers that serve more to retard erosion than to facilitate walking. Once upon the ridge, just below its crest to the south, about a mile of easy walking returns you to the car.

40 LEBANON VALLEY RAIL TRAIL:
Mount Gretna to Cornwall

 KEY AT-A-GLANCE INFORMATION

LENGTH: 8 miles

CONFIGURATION: Out-and-back

DIFFICULTY: Moderate

SCENERY: Oak and hickory forest, and some spots of railroad history

EXPOSURE: More shade than sun for the first 2 miles, and then it is mostly in the sun.

TRAIL TRAFFIC: Light during the week, moderately heavy on weekends

TRAIL SURFACE: Cinder and dirt

HIKING TIME: 3–4 hours

DRIVING DISTANCE: 12 miles from PA 283 and PA 743 north of Elizabethtown

ACCESS: Dawn–dusk

MAPS: USGS Manheim and Lebanon quads; a map of the trail is available online at www.lvrailtrail.com/maps.htm.

FACILITIES: None

WHEELCHAIR TRAVERSABLE: When dry

SPECIAL COMMENTS: The trail has been designated by Audubon Pennsylvania as a Susquehanna River Birding and Wildlife Trail.

GPS Trailhead Coordinates

UTM Zone (WGS84) 18T

Easting 374883

Northing 4456319

Latitude N 40° 14' 52.74"

Longitude W 76° 28' 15.84"

IN BRIEF

This hike follows the Lebanon Valley Rail Trail for 3.8 miles from the trailhead in Mount Gretna to the town of Cornwall. Along the way it passes by environs that are ideal for wildlife viewing. Just before reaching Cornwall, the trail crosses a scenic old railroad

DESCRIPTION

This hike follows the Lebanon Valley Rail Trail for 3.8 miles from the Mount Gretna Spur to the village of Cornwall. The rail-trail currently extends for 12.5 miles from the Lebanon–Lancaster county line 6.4 miles to the west of Mount Gretna to Whitman Road east of Cornwall. At the western terminus, the trail becomes the Conewago Trail and continues for another 5 miles into Elizabethtown (see page 164).

You can begin this hike in either Mount Gretna or Cornwall. I usually go from Mount Gretna simply because it is closer to where I live. I suspect that on a summer weekend, though, parking might be easier to find in Cornwall than in Mount Gretna, which gets rather crowded. Mount Gretna was established in 1892 as the site of the Pennsylvania Chautauqua, one of more than 200 Chautauqua communities established in the late 19th and early

Directions

From PA 283, follow PA 743 south toward Elizabethtown. At the first traffic light, make a sharp left turn (you will be going almost in the opposite direction) onto PA 241 and follow it for 7.75 miles until the town of Colebrook. Turn right onto PA 117. After 100 yards, PA 117 turns left toward Mount Gretna. Take this left and follow for 3 miles to the town of Mount Gretna. Park in the large public parking area on the right at the town center.

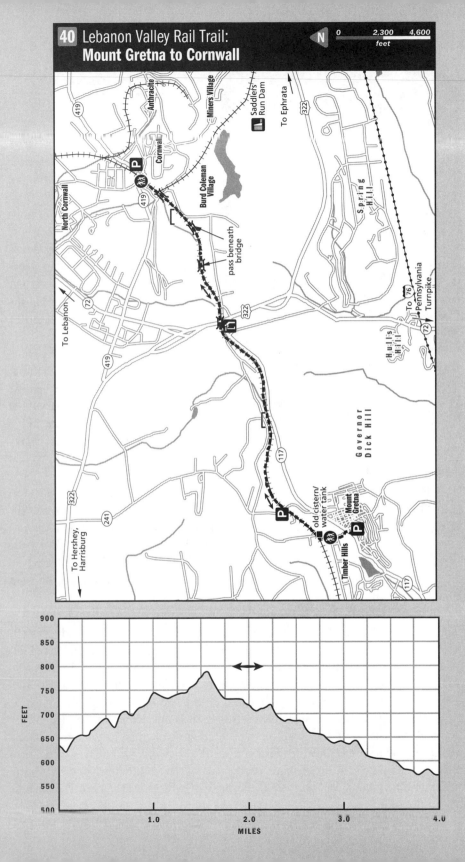

N

0   2,300   4,600
feet

To Ephrata

Anthracite

Miners Village

Saddlers
Run Dam

419

Cornwall

P

North Cornwall

Burd Coleman
Village

Spring Hill

419

To
Pennsylvania
Turnpike

76

72

To Lebanon

72

pass beneath
bridge

322

Hulls Hill

419

322

117

Governor Dick Hill

241

322

To Hershey,
Harrisburg

P

old cistern/
water tank

Mount Gretna

P

Timber Hills

117

MILES

FEET

900
850
800
750
700
650
600
550
500

1.0   2.0   3.0   4.0

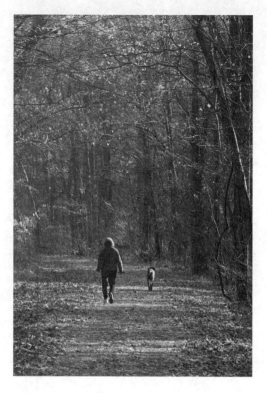

Along the trail near Mount Gretna

20th centuries. Founded at Lake Chautauqua in New York in 1874, the Chautauqua communities were dedicated to the self-education of people from all walks of American life. Each community held its own programs in the arts, sciences, and religion for guests and residents. The current town of Mount Gretna still bears that heritage, as its theater puts on performances during the summer and offers a highly regarded music series.

I begin this hike at the main parking area in Mount Gretna rather than at the trailhead proper because I am uncertain about the parking at the trailhead. Although there are no signs that prohibit parking, many private residences are located around the trailhead and parking nearby might infringe on the rights and privacy of property owners.

From the main lot in town, walk across PA 117 heading east and turn left onto Timber Road. Mount Gretna Pizzeria provides a good landmark for the turn, as well as a good slice of pie on your return. Follow Timber Road across a creek and continue a short distance to where it bends left. The trailhead for the Mount Gretna Spur of the rail-trail is on the right at the bend. The trail is paved initially and soon passes by what appears to be an old stone cistern on the right and a water tank on the left.

At 0.2 miles from the parking area, you come to the junction with the Lebanon Valley Rail Trail. Turn right and follow its level cinder track all the way to Cornwall. The rail-trail follows the path of the old Cornwall and Lebanon Railroad line that ran between Lebanon to the northeast and Conewago to the west. It was completed in 1883 by iron magnate Robert Coleman, and a bench acknowledging his historical significance is located on the Mount Gretna Spur.

The trail has been designated by Audubon Pennsylvania as a Susquehanna River Birding and Wildlife Trail, part of a network of trails in the Susquehanna basin that are acknowledged for bird and wildlife viewing. On the way into Cornwall, you'll find occasional benches on the side of the trail that provide wonderful locations for resting and watching, the next of which is just a tenth of a mile along the trail.

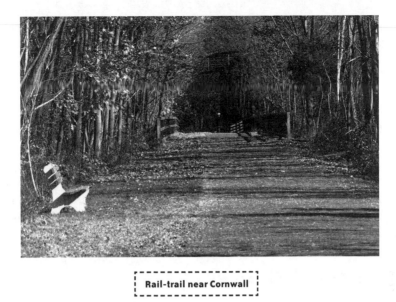

Rail-trail near Cornwall

At 0.6 miles, the trail crosses Butler Road outside of Mount Gretna, and just beyond the crossing you'll find the first trail-mileage marker (7) and another bench on the left. The trail is quite wide beyond Butler Road, because it has a mulch shoulder to the left that horseback riders are supposed to use. As you continue generally east along the trail, you will see many private residences through the woods.

At 1.75 miles, just past the crest of the railroad grade, you'll find a pair of benches. Old railroad ties that were discarded when the trail was developed lie in piles to either side of the path. Just beyond, a hollow drops off rather steeply to the north by a private residence. This is wonderful section for spotting birds. In particular, the woodpeckers and flickers seem to be abundant throughout this section of the trail.

At 2.5 miles, pass a bench and then cross over PA 3002 on a bridge. Between this bridge and the underpass at US 322 0.2 miles beyond, a dense thicket lines the trail to the north, and just beyond that is an open field. This is a superb stretch for bird sightings as several species of songbirds make their homes in this area, including cedar waxwings, nuthatches, warblers, chickadees, and juncos. After you pass beneath US 322, thicket lines both sides of the trail, and the bird-watching remains good. A decent pair of binoculars and a fair bit of patience can be helpful, as the birds tend to be small and very quick.

As you approach Cornwall, signs of development become more abundant. At 3.2 miles, the trail passes a large sump pond on the right. At 3.4 miles, it passes beneath a bridge and then by a private development on the north just outside the town of Cornwall.

Soon you'll pass by mile marker 10 and a bench; then walk across the old iron truss railroad bridge, which has been recently renovated. Just to the north of the bridge is the Cornwall Elementary School, with a couple of historic buildings on its property. Just beyond the bridge, the trail is paved and about 0.2 miles beyond that is the trailhead at PA 419 in Cornwall, the turnaround. Across the road, a large parking area is located just to the right of the trail. The parking area was the site of the old Cornwall and Lebanon Railroad Cornwall station, which burned in 1933.

In the 1800s, Cornwall was the source of a large deposit of high-grade iron ore, which accounted for the development of the railroad in this area. The original line, the North Lebanon Railroad, was completed in 1855. Industrialist Robert Coleman came in some years later and developed the Cornwall and Lebanon line, which provided competition to the North Lebanon RR. In 1972 the C and L was abandoned as a result of damage to the tracks from Hurricane Agnes, which also flooded the ore mines in Cornwall.

NEARBY ACTIVITIES

Mount Gretna is a summer resort with plenty of activities going on and recreational opportunities, including a beach and canoe rentals. The historic village is worth driving around to admire some of the quaint and unusual architecture. For food, try the Jigger Shop during the summer. The Hide-A-Way Cafe is located just beyond the town center heading east. Turn right onto Boulevard Street and it is on the left. It is open year-round and has an outdoor deck during the summer.

SHENKS FERRY WILDFLOWER PRESERVE

IN BRIEF

This hike covers all the trails in the Shenks Ferry Wildflower Preserve. It follows the main trail to the end of the hollow, and on the return it crosses the creek and follows an old path through the woods above Grubb Run.

DESCRIPTION

I had repeatedly seen signs for the Shenks Ferry Wildflower Preserve as I was exploring the glens and trails along the lower Susquehanna River in Lancaster County during the fall of 2006. A visit to the area was quite inviting, though I decided to put it off until the spring, figuring that would be the best time to visit. I spent the whole winter thinking of the place, conjuring images of blue skies, open meadows filled with grasses and flowers. I picked a week-day in mid-April, got up early on a rainy morn-ing and drove down to the preserve. What I found was remarkable, though not at all what I expected.

The wildflower preserve is located in something of a dark forested glen along a creek (Grubb Run) just before it flows beneath

Directions

From Lancaster, follow PA 324 south to New Danville. When PA 324 turns, continue straight onto New Danville Pike into Conestoga, where it becomes Main Street. Pass through the town and at an obvious fork in the road, bear left onto River Corner Road. Cross River Road and pick up Shenks Ferry Road. At Green Hill Road, turn left and follow it downhill beneath a stone tunnel to the railroad tracks at the river. Turn left at the tracks and follow Green Hill Road south. The trailhead is about 0.5 miles on the left. Park along the road.

KEY AT-A-GLANCE INFORMATION

LENGTH: About 2 miles

CONFIGURATION: Loop or out-and-back (the most popular)

DIFFICULTY: Easy if you hike out and back, moderate if you do the loop

SCENERY: Beautiful hollow filled with wildflowers

EXPOSURE: Shade

TRAIL TRAFFIC: Can get very busy

TRAIL SURFACE: Dirt

HIKING TIME: 1–3 hours or more, depending on how much time you spend looking at the wildflowers

DRIVING DISTANCE: 12 miles from PA 72 and US 222 in Lancaster

ACCESS: Dawn–dusk

MAPS: USGS Safe Harbor; a map of the preserve is available at the trailhead.

FACILITIES: Portable toilet along the trail

WHEELCHAIR TRAVERSABLE: Possible if dry

SPECIAL COMMENTS: The main trail along Grubb Run would be good for kids and is probably wheelchair accessible. If doing the loop, which involves crossing Grubb Run, the trail is a bit more rugged and not well maintained.

GPS Trailhead Coordinates

UTM Zone (WGS84) 18S

Easting 383182

Northing 4417810

Latitude N 39° 54′ 8.36″

Longitude W 76° 21′ 59.64″

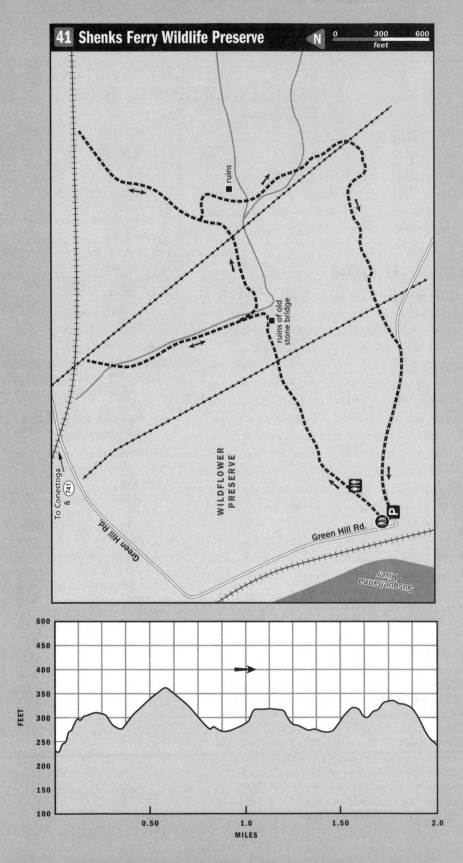

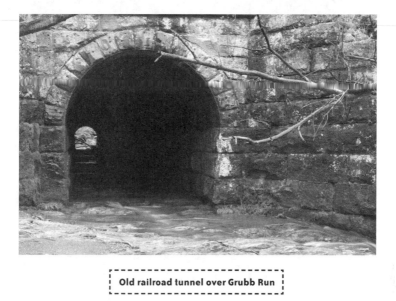

Old railroad tunnel over Grubb Run

the railroad tracks and into the Susquehanna River. Your first indication of approaching something special comes when you reach the level of the river and begin driving south next to the railroad tracks. When I first visited in April, the hillside on the left was completely covered (no exaggeration) in bluebells—more than I had even seen in one place before. After parking the car at Grubb Run, I was pretty amazed at the variety of plants and flowers I saw as I walked along the trail: jack-in-the-pulpits, fiddlehead ferns, trillium, Dutchman's-breeches, columbines, more bluebells. The flowers were everywhere.

The wildflower preserve is part of the Holtwood Environmental Preserve in southern Lancaster County, which also, incidentally, is home to the Kelly's Run Trail and Nature Preserve a few miles farther south (see page 172). Shenks Ferry Wildflower Preserve is a small tract of land, only about 50 acres according to the life list and trail map you can pick up at the trailhead. But the area provides habitat for more than 70 species of spring wildflowers and another 60 species that bloom throughout the summer months.

This hike covers most of the trails in the sanctuary. Begin hiking at the trailhead on Green Hill Road, identified by a sign with a map and photographs of some of the indigenous wildflowers. Follow the wide dirt path back into the hollow. As you walk above Grubb Run, a hillside rises to your left and descends to the creek on your right. In late April, the hillside to your left is covered with Virginia bluebells and white trillium.

After about 0.1 mile or so, you pass beneath a power line and at about 0.25 miles, you'll reach the ruins of an old stone bridge and a culvert that passes beneath the path. A side trail departs to the left and follows a small tributary for about 0.2 miles up a small hollow to a power line and old railroad grade. In early spring, the hollow is filled with Dutchman's-breeches (a common and beautiful

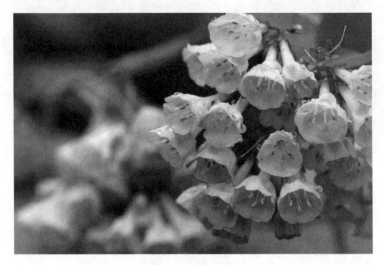

Virginia bluebells

white-and-yellow early-spring flower) and a variety of yellow composites. I also found it to be a good place to see a wild turkey.

After the side trip, return to the main trail, turn left, and continue walking in an upstream direction. You'll pass some power lines quite soon that cross over the main creek at the confluence of Grubb Run and a significant tributary entering from the southeast. Beyond those power lines, Grubb Run flows over long bedrock shelves, giving the stream a distinctive character. Follow the main trail for about 0.35 miles to its end at an old stone tunnel through which Grubb Run flows beneath an old railroad grade (1.1 miles including side trip).

From the tunnel, you can either backtrack along the path to the trailhead or you can make a loop of the hike. To do the latter, follow the trail back to the power lines that cross the confluence of the creek and its tributary. The trail map indicates that a side trail crosses Grubb Run just downstream from the confluence. I was unable to locate that path and found the following to be a good alternative: just before reaching the power lines, several trails descend to the level of the creek upstream from the confluence. This is probably the easiest place to cross Grubb Run, though it is necessary to walk in the water. Cross the creek at it shallowest point and follow the obvious trail around the tip of the peninsula formed by the two streams. As you round its end, you'll come to the ruins of an old homestead against the hillside of the hollow from which the tributary runs. This small hollow is extremely beautiful, as it is carpeted with a variety of wildflowers.

From the ruins, cross the tributary near the end of the peninsula to a gain an obvious trail ascending the hillside along a small steep creek parallel to the power-line cut. Many unusual wildflowers can be found along that little steep creek. It is the only place that I have found the small white miterwort, with its geometrically unique and complex petals. Follow the trail uphill for a short distance, crossing to the right side of the creek. At the top of the climb, the trail makes a sharp right turn beneath the power line at several signs posting private property. At the power line, the path becomes less distinct and somewhat overgrown. Cross the power-line cut, and when you enter the woods again, turn right following a faint path back down toward Grubb Run. After a short distance, you'll reach a wide path onto which you will turn left. Although the path is quite obvious here, it is frequently obstructed by deadfall.

Soon the trail reaches another power line in the vicinity of a private residence. The trail becomes quite indistinct here. Pass beneath the power line and as you enter the woods again, follow the path(s) of least resistance out to Green Hill Road, just 100 feet or so to your left. Alternately, you can walk beneath the power line over to Green Hill Road, though the terrain is quite swampy. Turn right on Green Hill Road and follow it a short distance downhill to your car.

NEARBY ACTIVITIES

The two towns closest to the preserve are Conestoga and Safe Harbor. Conestoga, the home of the Conestoga wagon, has a museum and historical society. It also features the Conestoga Wagon Restaurant on Main Street, which serves great food. The staff is also very friendly.

Just north of the hydroelectric plant on River Road in Safe Harbor, you'll find the Conestoga River Park. It has picnic areas and a playground. From there, the drive east along the shore of the Conestoga River is quite lovely.

42 SUSQUEHANNOCK STATE PARK

KEY AT-A-GLANCE INFORMATION

LENGTH: 2.15 miles

CONFIGURATION: Balloon

DIFFICULTY: Easy, with 1 climb

SCENERY: Wonderful views of Susquehanna River, rhododendrons, Wissler Run valley, and abandoned homesteads

EXPOSURE: Mostly shaded

TRAIL TRAFFIC: Light

TRAIL SURFACE: Dirt

HIKING TIME: 1.5–2 hours

DRIVING DISTANCE: About 10.2 miles from intersection of PA 372 and PA 272 in Buck

ACCESS: Dawn–dusk

MAPS: USGS Holtwood; a park map with all of the trails listed is available at the park.

FACILITIES: Seasonal restrooms and water

WHEELCHAIR TRAVERSABLE: No, though the first overlook is accessible by wheelchair.

SPECIAL COMMENTS: Break-ins have occurred at the parking area. Be sure to take all valuables with you or to store them out of sight.

IN BRIEF

This hike links several of the park trails to make a pleasant outing. It begins with a stroll out to the Hawk Point Overlook and then follows the Overlook Trail to the Wissler's Run Overlook. From there, it heads north on the Fire Trail for a short distance before descending into a hollow on the appropriately named Rhododendron Trail. It follows this trail out of the hollow and down to Wissler Run. Departing Wissler Run, it follows a small tributary past the Neel Foundation site to the Holly Trail, where it turns left and returns to the Fire Trail near the Wissler's Run Overlook.

DESCRIPTION

Named for the Native American tribe that inhabited the area before the development of the region by English settlers, Susquehannock State Park is another of those remarkable locations in the river hills southeast of Lancaster known for its wonderful scenery and opportunities to see wildlife and wildflowers. The park has been designated by the Audubon Society as part of a global network of places recognized for their outstanding value for bird conservation. Along the edge of the escarpment above the Susquehanna River, you can see bald eagles (many of whom nest in the area), osprey,

GPS Trailhead Coordinates

UTM Zone (WGS84) 18S

Easting 389697

Northing 4406744

Latitude N 39° 48′ 12.67″

Longitude W 76° 17′ 18.64″

Directions

From PA 272 in Buck, follow PA 372 west for about 5.7 miles to River Road (a sign for the park is located on the left before River Road). Turn left on River Road, cross the dam, and turn right on Furniss Road. Turn right on Silver Spring Road and right again on State Park Road on a bend. Use caution when leaving the park as the entrance is blind to cars approaching from the south.

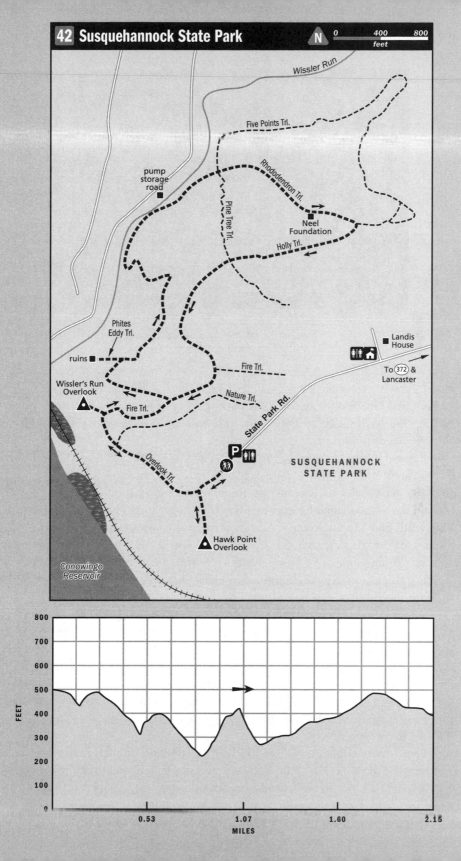

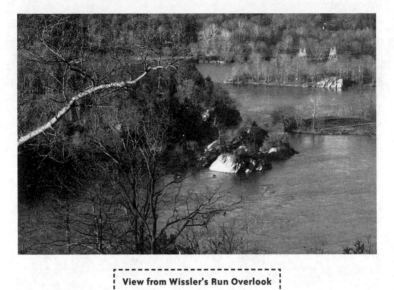

View from Wissler's Run Overlook

turkey and black vultures, a wide variety of hawks, and visiting seabirds. In the woods, you'll encounter many small species such as warblers, woodpeckers, sap-suckers, and bluebirds. If you visit the park at a time when the park office is open, pick up the *Field Guide to the Natural History of Susquehannock State Park* to help you identify its diverse natural features.

Begin this hike at the main parking area and follow the gravel path southwest to the Hawk Point Overlook. The overlook provides a nice start to the hike with an expansive view of the Conowingo Reservoir (the most southern impoundment lake on the Susquehanna River formed by the Conowingo Hydroelectric Plant in Maryland) and Mount Johnson Island to the south. Mount Johnson Island was the first bald eagle sanctuary established in the world, and the birds are common visitors to the environs of Susquehannock State Park. The overlook features a spotting scope and a bird identification chart that will help you to distinguish between the vultures, eagles, and osprey you may see from this point.

After visiting the Hawk Point Overlook, take the gravel path back toward the parking lot and pick up the Overlook Trail as it heads north out of the day-use area along the edge of the river escarpment. The trail follows a wide-open track marked with orange blazes and as it begins to descend among tall trees to Wissler's Run Overlook. This second overlook provides you with a great view upstream to the north toward Lake Aldred and the Holtwood Dam. Beneath you flows Wissler Run as it empties into the river by a storage plant, and several small islands dot the lake immediately west.

From this overlook, walk back to a trail junction just uphill from the overlook and turn left onto the Fire Trail. Traverse the hillside and climb slightly for about 0.25 miles to a junction with an old roadbed descending to your left. This is the Rhododendron Trail and you'll turn left on it and follow it into Wissler Run. As you descend, you'll see that the trail is appropriately named. Dense stands of rhododendron line the track on both sides for its entire length. In June and July, when the rhododendrons are in bloom, the trail is a remarkable sight. After 0.1 mile or so, you'll reach a sharp bend to the right and just beyond that a trail junction at the crossing of a small creek bed. If you turn left on the trail and continue along it for 100 yards or so, you'll come to the ruins of an old homestead on the left, just above the level of Wissler Run. You can walk down to have a look or just continue along this hike following the Rhododendron Trail to the right from the junction toward a rock outcrop on the hillside. The trail traverses just beneath it.

Soon you'll climb out of the hollow at a ridge in the woods. Descend the ridge back toward Wissler Run, following switchbacks down to the creek. On the way, you pass several interesting outcrops of sandstone with occasional layers of white quartzite or limestone slicing through them. Now at the level of the creek, you are once again surrounded by rhododendrons. This is a particularly enchanting spot with the creek tumbling over small ledges as it winds its way to the river. From the creek, follow the Rhododendron Trail upstream and then eventually into a hollow formed by a small tributary. At about 1.35 miles, you'll come to a trail crossing. The Five Points Trail heads off to the left and the Pine Tree Trail turns right. Continue straight on the Rhododendron Trail and in about 0.2 miles you'll reach the Neel Foundation. According to the park brochure, this site was the homestead of a veteran of the Revolutionary War, Thomas Neel. The foundation of the house still remains, though little more. Take note of the enormous hickory tree beside it.

Pass by the homestead site and shortly you'll reach the junction with the Holly Trail. Turn right on the Holly Trail and follow it back to the Wissler's Run Overlook. On the way, you will cross the Pine Tree Trail, where you continue straight, and then join with the Fire Trail, onto which you turn right just before reaching the Wissler's Run Overlook.

NEARBY ACTIVITIES

The park has many picnic areas, a playground, and several ball fields, as well as group camping area. North of the park and north of PA 372 along River Road is the Shenks Ferry Wildflower Preserve. It is definitely worth a visit during the spring and summer.

43 TROUT RUN AND STEINMAN RUN NATURE PRESERVES

KEY AT-A-GLANCE INFORMATION

LENGTH: Complete hike is 4.5 miles; several possibilities for shorter variations exist.

CONFIGURATION: Out-and-back

DIFFICULTY: Easy–moderate with the exception of the 0.5 mile-stretch in the Trout Run ravine that is moderately difficult

SCENERY: Trout Run and Steinman Run Nature Preserves, streams flowing through wooded hollows

EXPOSURE: Shade

TRAIL TRAFFIC: Light

TRAIL SURFACE: Dirt; rocky in Trout Run

HIKING TIME: About 3 hours

DRIVING DISTANCE: 13.6 miles from PA 283 and PA 72 in Lancaster

ACCESS: Dawn–dusk

MAPS: USGS Conestoga; a *Pennsylvania Gazetteer* can be helpful for locating the various parking areas.

FACILITIES: Portable toilets at the Clearview Road parking area

WHEELCHAIR TRAVERSABLE: No

SPECIAL COMMENTS: This hike crosses Trout Run either 4 or 6 times in the first half mile. The first half mile may be impassable after periods of heavy raid or due to icy conditions in cold weather.

IN BRIEF

This first part of this hike follows Trout Run to the south through its small, rocky gorge. At the confluence with Steinman Run, the hike continues south along that creek through the Steinman Run Nature Preserve to the upper reaches of the creek, where it makes a loop and then returns.

DESCRIPTION

The Trout Run Nature Preserve is a 124-acre tract of land owned by the Lancaster Conservancy. The Steinman Run Nature Preserve is a 264-acre tract adjacent to it to the south. The two natural areas differ in character in that Trout Run consists primarily of a wooded, steep-sided ravine through which the creek flows. Steinman Run, on the other hand, consists of more open, rolling woods. Both areas provide habitat for quite a bit of wildlife and both host an impressive array of spring and summer wildflowers.

From the parking area on Pennsy Road, follow the path over the old railroad grade that passes over the stone tunnel and descend the other side to the level of the creek. Once you reach the creek, you'll see prolific blue blazes, many of which are painted over old yellow blazes. You are now in a small gorge,

GPS Trailhead Coordinates

UTM Zone (WGS84)   18S

Easting   389909

Northing   4419282

Latitude   N 39° 54′ 59.34″

Longitude   W 76° 17′ 17.30″

Directions ———————→

From Lancaster, follow PA 272 south to Smithville. Turn right (west) on Pennsy Road. The parking area and trailhead are 2 miles ahead on the left. Look for an old stone railroad tunnel over Trout Run and a brown Lancaster Conservancy sign. Parking is limited.

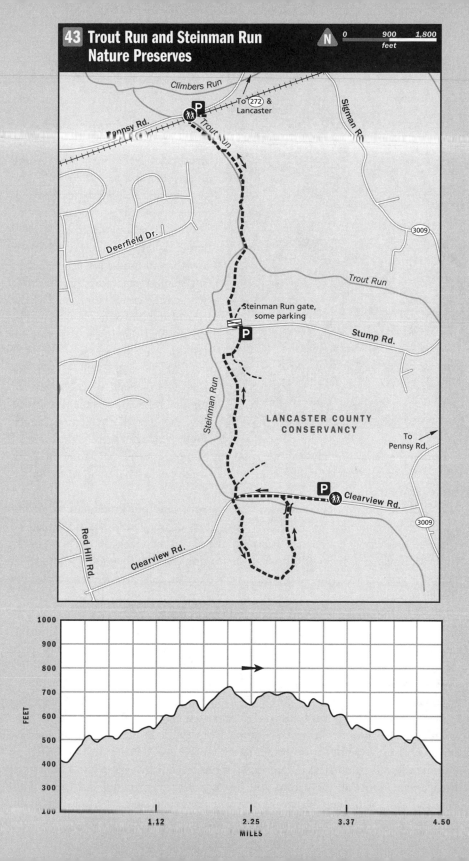

N

0   900   1,800
feet

Climbers Run

To 272 &
Lancaster

Sigman Rd.

Pennsy Rd.

Trout Run

3009

Deerfield Dr.

Trout Run

Steinman Run gate,
some parking

Stump Rd.

Steinman Run

LANCASTER COUNTY
CONSERVANCY

To
Pennsy Rd.

Clearview Rd.

3009

Red Hill Rd.

Clearview Rd.

1000
900
800
700
600
500
400
300
100

FEET

1.12   2.25   3.37   4.50
MILES

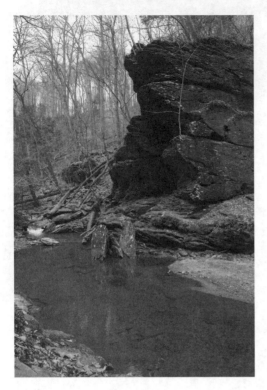

filled with ash, hickory, birch, and hemlock trees. Follow the blazes south along the west side of the creek, and at about 0.25 miles the blazes indicate your first of several creek crossings. At the time of this writing you could cross over a large, rather slick log. For what it is worth, you might just as well look for shallow water and get used to wading the creek here, as all of the rest of the crossings require you to do so. Bear this in mind if you are considering a hike in the winter.

After crossing the creek, follow its east bank of the creek for another 0.25 miles to the next crossing, the first of three in 0.1 mile. Here, you are entering the steepest section of the Trout Run ravine. Outcroppings of moss-covered sandstone line both sides of the creek, which tumbles over boulders into pools where you might spot a native brown trout.

Cross to the west bank and walk past a rock outcrop. Immediately beyond the outcrop is the next crossing. This one (and consequently the next) can be bypassed by following a narrow footpath just above the creek on the west bank. The path traverses a steep hillside, but the footing is generally good and the steep section is very short. Either stay to the west bank or cross to the east and follow the flat ground for 100 feet and cross back to the west. Follow the west bank for a couple of hundred yards and again you will come to another crossing back to the east bank of the creek. This one is obligatory as it allows you to circumnavigate a large cliff along the west bank. The creek here is steep and rocky and quite scenic. It is a pretty spot especially in May and June as the forest has a beautiful understory of mountain laurel.

Follow the east bank for couple of hundred yards to the confluence of two streams: Trout Run from the east or left and Steinman Run from the west. Cross Trout Run one more time just upstream from the confluence. This is the last stream crossing (without a footbridge) until you return. You are now entering the Steinman Run Natural Area. After crossing the creek, turn around and look back downstream into the gorge that you just came through. This is an especially beautiful spot, with the two creeks entering your field of view from either side

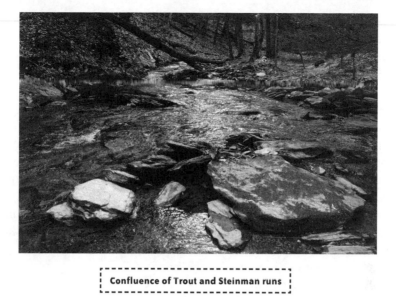

Confluence of Trout and Steinman runs

of the periphery of your vision, and Trout Run flowing away from you over boulders around a large cliff.

From the confluence, the trail bends to the right and follows Steinman Run through the woods to the east of the creek. The walking for this part of the hike is on much more secure ground and is pleasant through a pretty second-growth forest. At about 0.85 miles, you enter a large flat area in the woods and then pass a trail junction with a lavender-blazed path heading off to your left. I was unable to ascertain where this path leads. Just beyond, you'll find the gate at Stump Road. From this point you can return, providing you with a hike of about 2 miles more or less, or you can continue on for another 2.5-mile loop through the Steinman Run Natural Area.

Turn left on Stump Road and follow it for about 100 yards to a large parking area on the right. The blue-blazed path continues past the right of two wooden gates and follows an old roadbed a couple of hundred yards to a branch in the trail. The main path continues to the left, but our hike—and the blazes—descend to the right. Follow the hollow of Steinman Run, staying above and a couple of hundred feet east of the creek, which now flows through private property. Walking in this forest of saplings and young oak, ash, hickory, and birch trees offers great scenery.

Follow the path for about 0.7 miles, crossing a small tributary to the creek, and then an old roadbed, until you come to a second roadbed. Turn right and descend down to the creek where it flows beneath Clearview Road, now disused. Note the enormous oak tree on your right as you descend and the prominent maple at the intersection with Clearview Road. From the junction, you can walk out to the south trailhead and parking area, about 0.25 miles to your left, or you can make the 0.9-mile loop through the southern section of the Steinman Run Nature Preserve. Doing the latter is worth the effort.

Turn right on Clearview Road, cross the creek, and immediately turn left following the blue-blazed trail as it now climbs up a small ridge on the west side of Steinman Run. The path ascends the ridge and then descends back to Steinman Run in a lovely section of its valley. Although forested, the area around the creek feels open and is generally flat, and makes great habitat for deer. At about 0.5 miles from Clearview Road, you reach the first of two footbridges—a nice place to sit and rest. Cross the bridge and follow the path along the creek. In about 100 yards the trail forks. Stay to the left and continue following the creek for about 0.25 miles to a second footbridge over a small tributary. Another 100 yards takes you back to Clearview Road between Steinman Run and the parking area. The blue blazes end here.

Turn right and walk about 200 yards to visit the parking area, which has a portable toilet and a nice view near a large farm. Or turn left and walk about 200 yards to get back to the bridge at Steinman Run where you will pick up the trail and follow it back to the car.

If you have two cars, you can run a shuttle between the parking areas at Clearview Road and Pennsy Road. If you do this, the hike would walk best from Clearview to Pennsy, south to north. If beginning at Clearview Road, be sure to turn right on the old roadbed just before Steinman Run. A prominent old maple tree marks the intersection. You'll see blue blazes here.

NEARBY ACTIVITIES

See profile for the nearby Shenks Ferry Wildflower Preserve (page 193).

TUCQUAN GLEN NATURE PRESERVE 44

IN BRIEF

This beautiful hike follows the south bank of Tucquan Creek, through its glen filled with hemlock and rhododendron, to the railroad bridge at the Susquehanna River. The route crosses the creek via the bridge, ascends a short steep gulley up the escarpment, and picks up the old Tucquan Glen Road over a promontory and back down to the creek.

DESCRIPTION

Certainly the jewel site of the Lancaster Conservancy, the 336-acre Tucquan Glen Nature Preserve in Martic Township provides a gem of an excursion. Although not a long hike, you get a lot of great scenery packed into the mile-long gorge of this tributary of the Susquehanna River. The creek has understandably been designated a Pennsylvania Scenic River. The forest along the sides of the glen consist of tall mature poplars, white and pin oaks, and hickory trees. Hemlocks, white pines, and rhododendrons line the banks of the steep creek as it tumbles over large boulders forming deep

KEY AT-A-GLANCE INFORMATION

LENGTH: 2.3 miles

CONFIGURATION: Loop

DIFFICULTY: Moderate

SCENERY: The beautiful gorge of Tucquan Glen

EXPOSURE: Mostly shaded

TRAIL TRAFFIC: Light during the week; can be very busy on summer weekends.

TRAIL SURFACE: Dirt; rocky in places

HIKING TIME: 1.5–2 hours

DRIVING DISTANCE: About 23 miles from PA 283 and PA 272 in Lancaster

ACCESS: Dawn–dusk

MAPS: USGS Holtwood

FACILITIES: None

WHEELCHAIR TRAVERSABLE: No

SPECIAL COMMENTS: Several cars have been broken into at the parking area. Be sure to take all valuables with you or secure them in your trunk.

Directions ⟶

From Harrisburg and the north, the easiest route is to take PA 283 to Lancaster. Follow PA 272 south to the town of Buck and head west on PA 372 toward Holtwood. Follow 372 for 4.9 miles to SR 3017, River Road. Turn right and follow for 2.65 miles. Two small parking areas are located on the west side of the road directly across from the Tucquan Woodworks building. If those are full, a larger area is located about 100 yards south on the east side of the road.

From York and the west, pick up PA 372 and follow it east across the Susquehanna River for 2.3 miles from the river to SR 3017. Turn left.

GPS Trailhead Coordinates

UTM Zone (WGS84) 18S

Easting 385464

Northing 4413521

Latitude N 39° 51′ 49.89″

Longitude W 76° 20′ 21.04″

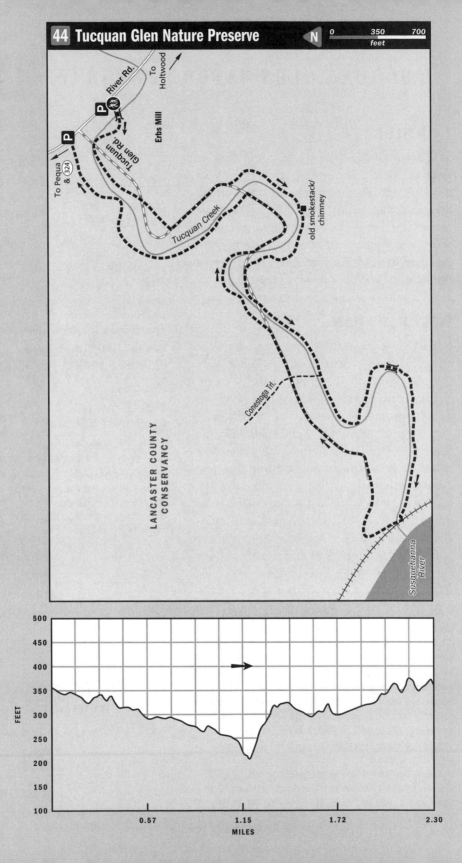

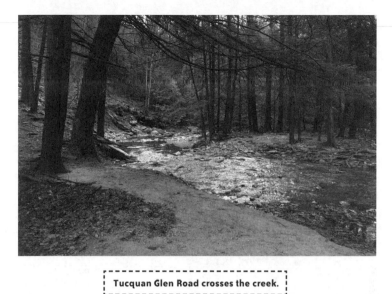

Tucquan Glen Road crosses the creek.

pools and steep drops. In late May and June, when everything is in bloom, the place is amazing. According to the *Susquehanna River Birding and Wildlife Trail Guide* published by Audubon Pennsylvania, Tucquan Glen is home to more than 40 species of wildflowers as well as 21 species of ferns. The glen is also home to great horned owls and is frequented by white-tailed deer.

A couple of notes of caution: First, the rocks can be quite slippery along the trail, so use care to avoid any nasty slips. Although accessible year-round, the rocks can get covered with ice and the route along the south side of the creek may become impassable. The preserve is open to hunting, so be sure to wear blaze orange during hunting season and consider hiking on Sunday.

This hike walks best in a clockwise direction. From the parking area, cross the creek over a small wooden footbridge. The trail is marked for its entire length with blue blazes, and it veers to the right once you cross the bridge. As you enter the preserve, you'll come to the remains of the old Tucquan Glen Road and the trail follows it for a short distance until the road crosses the creek. You'll notice blue blazes over on the north side of the creek. Those mark the path on the other side, but there is no need to cross until you get to the Susquehanna River. Follow the creek through an extraordinary area of pine and hemlock. At about 0.5 miles, the gorge narrows and the trail passes through a rock outcrop via some narrow ledges and then crosses a small side creek. Just beyond the creek, the ruin of a large stone chimney stands on the side of the trail.

Continue along the creek and, at approximately 0.8 miles, you'll notice some red blazes enter from the north side of the creek at an unlikely place to cross. This is a section of the 61-mile-long Conestoga Trail, and it shares the path with the Tucquan Glen Trail along the south bank of the creek. From this point to the river, you'll follow red and blue blazes. About 0.9 miles into the hike, the gorge becomes much narrower, and the creek becomes steeper and more choked with boulders. The trail

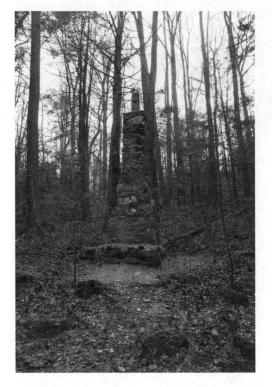

hugs the south hillside, and it crosses a wooden footbridge along a particularly exposed section of rock above a large pool at the base of a cliff. The scenery from the footbridge to the river is outstanding. Beyond the bridge, the valley gets tighter and tighter and the creek more choked with large sandstone boulders. At 1.2 miles, the gorge opens up and the trail reaches the railroad along the Susquehanna River. From here, the Conestoga Trail continues south climbing up the escarpment above the river.

The second half of this hike is rather different in character from the first, as it generally follows the old roadbed for a good part of the way back to the car. For a good portion of the walk it stays above the level of the creek providing views into the glen from above. To complete the loop, cross the creek via the railroad bridge. About 30 feet beyond the bridge, the trail heads directly up a short, steep gulley by a blue blaze. The path improves very quickly, makes a switchback, and joins the old roadbed for a short climb up to a promontory above the creek. This is a particularly nice place to sit for a while. If you walk out to the edge of the promontory (use caution!), you'll get a nice view back into the glen at its most rugged point. From the promontory, the road descends pleasantly back down to the level of the creek. At 1.5 miles, it crosses the Conestoga Trail, and at 1.85 miles, the old road crosses the creek. Stay on the north side of the creek and follow the footpath along the bank back to River Road.

NEARBY ACTIVITIES

The Holtwood Environmental Preserve to the south has a park with recreation facilities and is home to the Kelly's Run Natural Area. The nearby Pinnacle Overlook offers a place to picnic, and a fine view of Lake Aldred on the Susquehanna River and the mouth of Tucquan Glen. To get there, head south on River Road a short distance and turn right onto Pinnacle Road and follow the signs to the overlook. During the spring and summer, the Shenks Ferry Wildflower Preserve, a couple of miles to the north, cannot be beat. Take River Road to the north and follow signs.

TURKEY HILL 45

IN BRIEF

This mostly shaded hike follows an escarpment above the east bank of the Susquehanna River. The first mile proceeds rather steeply through a forest of pawpaw trees before reaching a meadow near the top of Turkey Hill. From there the hiking is less strenuous through a forest of oak, maple, and hickory trees out to the main overlook.

DESCRIPTION

I learned about the Turkey Hill Trail from my friend, Ad Crable, who is the outdoors editor at the *Lancaster New Era*. He told me about the wonderful views of the Susquehanna River that can be had from the trail and that was enough to spark my interest. So on a reasonably cool Monday in August, my 7-year-old son, Jackson, and I shouldered our packs and began the trek. In retrospect, I would say that this is not a good hike for young children. For a good mile of the route, the trail climbs steeply and traverses a hillside that descends precipitously toward the river. I spent a fair amount of time making sure that Jackson was paying careful attention to what he was doing.

Nonetheless, we had quite a remarkable hike. We spotted three bald eagles, two of them

KEY AT-A-GLANCE INFORMATION

LENGTH: 4 miles

CONFIGURATION: Out-and-back

DIFFICULTY: Moderately strenuous

SCENERY: Views of the Susquehanna River

EXPOSURE: Mostly shade

TRAIL TRAFFIC: Light

TRAIL SURFACE: Dirt

HIKING TIME: 2–2.5 hours

DRIVING DISTANCE: 6.2 miles from US 30 and PA 441 in Columbia

ACCESS: Dawn–dusk

MAPS: USGS Safe Harbor

FACILITIES: None

WHEELCHAIR TRAVERSABLE: No

SPECIAL COMMENTS: This moderately strenuous hike offers wonderful views of the Susquehanna River as well as great opportunities for bird-watching. The stand of pawpaw trees is itself worth the visit.

Directions

From US 30 east of York, PA, take the first exit east of the Susquehanna River at signs for PA 441 and 462. Follow PA 441 south for 4 miles into Washington Boro, where it ends at the intersection with PA 999 and turns into River Road. Check your odometer here. Follow River Road south for 1.9 miles from the intersection with 999. The parking area is on the right in the brush and is identified by a large brown Lancaster Conservancy sign.

GPS Trailhead Coordinates

UTM Zone (WGS84) 18S

Easting 375754

Northing 4425153

Latitude N 39° 58′ 2.69″

Longitude W 76° 27′ 17.39″

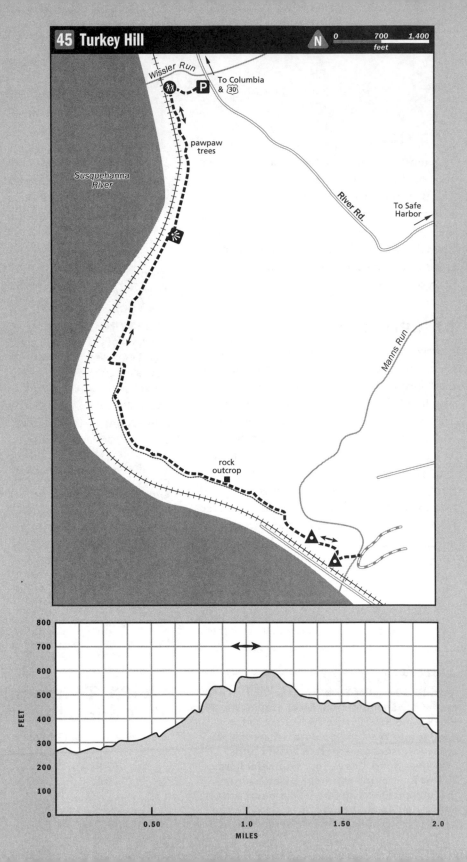

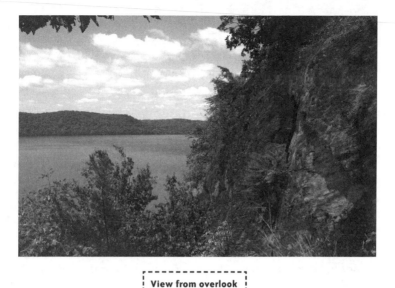

View from overlook

not a quarter mile from the parking lot; saw hundreds of butterflies of many varieties, including monarchs, swallowtails, sulphurs, and blues; and discovered a yellow-billed cuckoo tending to her nest just a few feet from the trail. Additionally, this hike passes through the largest forest of pawpaw trees in the world north of the 39th parallel (north, that is, of roughly Annapolis, Maryland). Known for their fruit, which has a sweet flavor and a banana-like consistency, these thin, broad-leafed trees are clustered quite thickly along the first mile of this hike. On our trek, we found plenty of fruits, but none that were ripe in mid-August.

The Turkey Hill Trail extends from a small parking lot with enough space for four or five cars, just off of PA 999 south of Washington Boro, for 3 miles to another parking area just outside of Creswell, Pennsylvania. The trail is maintained by the Lancaster Conservancy, and judging by the amount of cobwebs stretched across its width, the trail sees little traffic. The trail is marked along its length with blue blazes.

This hike covers the first 2 miles of that trail, from the northern terminus to the wonderful overlook above the Susquehanna River and Manns Creek at the 2-mile marker. Yes, it is a shorter hike to the overlook from the south end of the trail; however, access from the south does not afford all of the expansive views of the Susquehanna that you get from the north, nor does it offer the interest of the pawpaw trees. Additionally, I would say that our good fortune with eagle sightings had everything to do with the fact that we hiked in from the north along the river.

The first challenge of this hike is locating the trailhead and parking area south of Washington Boro—follow the directions carefully, as it is easy to miss. At the parking lot, you'll find a yellow gate in front of a dirt road and just uphill from that a footpath identified by a boulder at its beginning. Both the road and footpath take you to the trailhead proper near a clearing and an old railroad bed in about 0.1 mile, the footpath being slightly more direct. From the clearing, the trailhead is to the left (south) and is marked by a large trail sign and a rather waterlogged map.

The trail begins climbing as soon as it enters the woods and does so for most of the next mile, at times rather steeply. At about 0.3 miles, the trail enters the pawpaw trees, which become rather abundant at times after 100 yards or so. At 0.4 miles, the trail begins to climb more steeply across a precipitous hillside. In places the edges of the trail have eroded, making it rather thin, but if you are careful with your footing, you should have no problems. In the midst of this steep section, a large log with a blue blaze lies across the trail in the vicinity of an old talus field. Although the hillside is rather steep here, ample room is available to have a seat and enjoy the first of many glorious views of the river below.

After continuing to climb, the trail emerges from the woods at 1 mile from the car (the mile marker for the trail is about 0.1 mile farther on). A wooden sign marks the point where the trail leaves the woods, which can be helpful for finding your route on the way back. Here, the trail turns to the right (south) and follows a fence line until it very obviously enters the woods again at a corner of the fence 0.2 miles later. All along this meadow you are in the vicinity of Turkey Hill proper, the top of which is behind the fence on private land. There are no views of the river from the grassy meadow, but the walking is nice and flat.

As you enter the woods, the trail descends steeply until it crosses a small waterway and begins to level out. We spotted the cuckoo and her nest in the vicinity of this waterway. The trail soon begins to climb again, passes by a rocky outcrop, and leaves the woods once again at a fence line. Turn right and follow the fence to its corner, where the trail again enters the woods on an abandoned roadbed that quickly gives way to a footpath. At 1.8 miles from the car, the escarpment above the Susquehanna River becomes more of a narrow hogback, and the trail passes just beneath a rocky outcrop to its east. Scrambling up to the rocks is worth the effort as the view from 400 feet above the level of the river is quite striking.

Continuing on from there, the trail descends gently for 0.2 miles until it comes to a large overlook above the river. We spotted our third bald eagle as we stepped onto the overlook—it flew from a tree beside the overlook—and watched as it fished on the river below us. To the north of the overlook, tall cliffs frame your view of the river, and to the south, the ridge drops very steeply to Manns Creek. This is the turnaround for the hike, and it is a wonderful place to rest, have a snack, and enjoy the view. If you are so inclined, you can hike down to Manns Creek, where you will find the 2-mile trail marker and a lovely little pool just downstream from the point where the trail crosses the creek. At the time of this writing, however, a tree that was nearly impassable lay across the trail between the overlook and creek crossing.

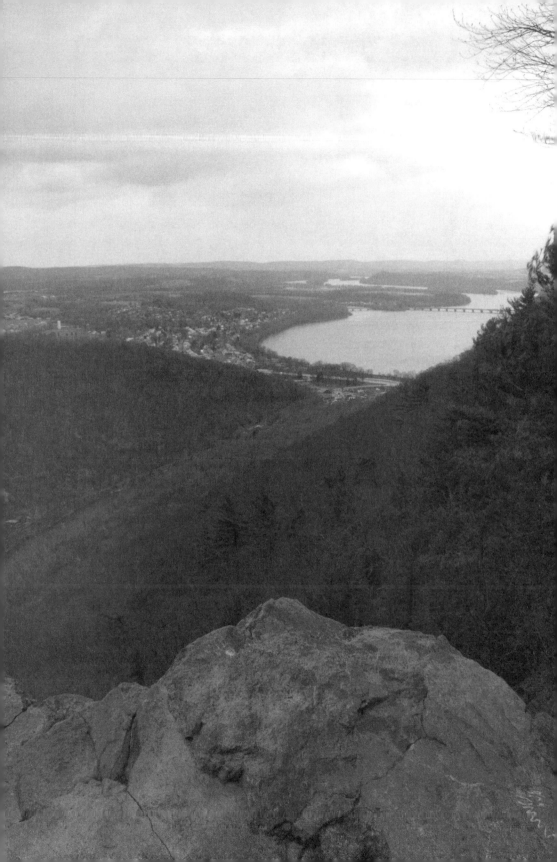

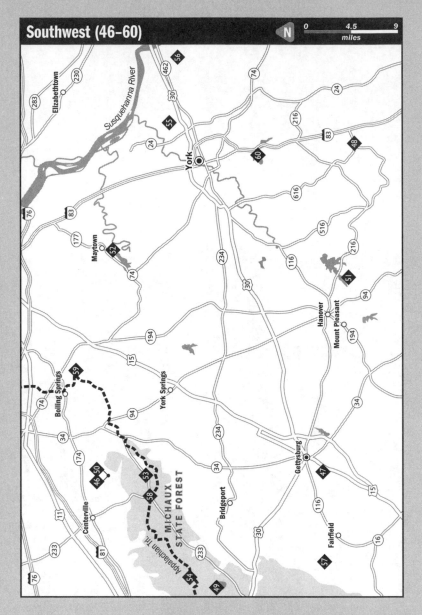

Elizabethttown

230

283

Susquehanna River

56

462

30

74

24

55

216

24

York

60

83

48

616

76

83

177

516

Maytown

52

216

74

234

116

51

194

94

Hanover

Mount Pleasant

194

15

York Springs

234

Gettysburg

Bolling Springs

59

94

34

74

34

174

Centerville

46·50

53

MICHAUX STATE FOREST

58

Bridgeport

34

47

15

111

116

Fairfield

233

81

Appalachian Trl.

30

16

57

76

233

54

49

SOUTHWEST

46 BUCK RIDGE TRAIL

KEY AT-A-GLANCE INFORMATION

LENGTH: About 6 miles one-way

CONFIGURATION: One-way or out-and-back

DIFFICULTY: Moderate

SCENERY: Kings Gap and Pine Grove Furnace parks, lovely woods and meadows

EXPOSURE: Mostly shade

TRAIL TRAFFIC: Light

TRAIL SURFACE: Dirt

HIKING TIME: 3 hours one-way

DRIVING DISTANCE: About 8 miles from Interstate 81 and PA 233 south of Carlisle

ACCESS: Dawn–dusk

MAPS: USGS Dickinson; Michaux State Forest public-use map; a trail map is available at the Kings Gap and Pine Grove Furnace visitor centers.

FACILITIES: Water and restrooms available in parks near both trailheads

WHEELCHAIR TRAVERSABLE: No

SPECIAL COMMENTS: Done as a one-way excursion from Kings Gap to Pine Grove Furnace State Park, this hike requires 2 cars. An out-and-back trip of about 12 miles makes a nice day trip, though it is best begun from the southern trailhead at Pine Grove Furnace.

GPS Trailhead Coordinates

UTM Zone (WGS84) 18T

Easting 306986

Northing 4440561

Latitude N 40° 5′ 35.60″

Longitude W 77° 15′ 51.00″

IN BRIEF

Beginning at Kings Gap Environmental Education and Training Center, follow the Buck Ridge Trail south, along Buck Ridge. The trail descends for most of its length to Pine Grove Furnace.

DESCRIPTION

Stretching between the Kings Gap Environmental Education Center to the north and Pine Grove Furnace State Park to the south, the Buck Ridge Trail offers a wonderful hike through the South Mountain Province of south-central Pennsylvania. The trek follows old logging roads that take you through open fields and dark hollows.

The hike can be done either as a one-way trip or as an out-and-back excursion. If you hike it one-way, you'll want to begin at Kings Gap because the trail walks better from north to south. You'll need to spot a car at the parking area across the street from the visitor center at Pine Grove Furnace State Park. Or you can take advantage of one of the Buck Ridge Brunch programs offered periodically by the staff at Kings Gap. The program includes an interpretive hike, brunch at the mansion at

Directions

From Interstate 81, take exit 37, Newville, and follow PA 233 south for 2.3 miles to Pine Road. Turn left onto Pine Road (signs for Kings Gap Environmental Education and Training Center) and follow it for another 2.3 miles to Kings Gap Road (sign for Kings Gap). Turn right and follow the winding road up to the mansion area. The parking area, with several trailheads, is on the left, just before the loop at the mansion area begins.

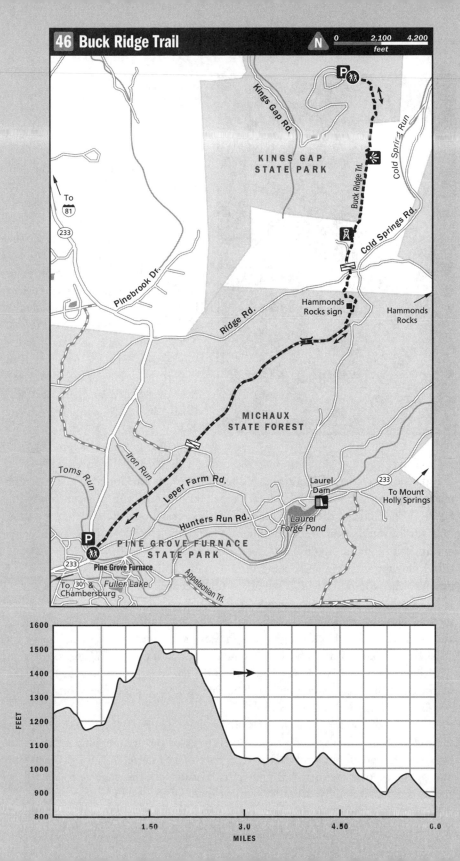

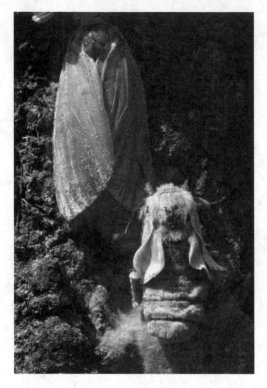

Gypsy moths

Kings Gap, and a ride from Pine Grove Furnace back to Kings Gap.

Although a little on the long side, an out-and-back trip on the Buck Ridge Trail (BRT) provides a reasonable day trip. Personal experience, however, has taught me that for an out-and-back excursion, you would do well to begin at the south trailhead at Pine Grove Furnace because Kings Gap is considerably higher in elevation than Pine Grove. The parking area and trailhead at Pine Grove Furnace are located on the northeast corner of the intersection of PA 233 and Hunters Run Road, across the street from the visitor center.

Hiking from Kings Gap to Pine Grove, you'll begin at the parking area on the left, just before the loop for the mansion area begins. Several trails begin from this parking area and an information sign provides a good landmark for identifying it. From the car, follow the Scenic Vista Trail out the old roadbed south and east along the clearing for about 200 yards. You'll soon reach the junction with the Maple Hollow Trail, which continues straight, and you'll see a post marked with BRT. Turn right at the junction following the BRT and Scenic Vista Trail as the path descends toward a hollow into the woods. The BRT is marked for its length with orange blazes.

At about 0.5 miles into the hike, the BRT departs from the Scenic Vista Trail to the left along another old road. Stay to the left, following the orange blazes, and begin to ascend Buck Ridge through a pretty understory of huckleberry and blueberry. About 0.5 miles beyond the junction, you'll pass a trail off to the right that descends to the Pond Day Use area and then the 1-mile marker. From that marker, the BRT makes two climbs. The first is steep but not very long, the second is quite long but not very steep.

Just shy of 2 miles, the trail levels out on the top of Buck Ridge, and you'll pass through a forest of mostly oak trees. When I visited the area in June of 2007, the gypsy moths had all but stripped the trees bare of all foliage. To look at one of my photographs, you'd swear it was midwinter. Fortunately, the damage to the foliage is only temporary and by later that summer many of the leaves had grown back.

After walking along the ridge for a short distance, you'll pass a marker on the right, indicating that you are at 1,540 feet of elevation. The hike is pretty

Iron Run

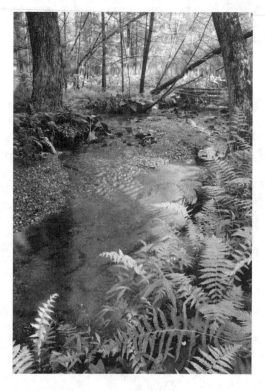

much downhill for the next 4 miles. Descend from the ridge, pass the 2-mile marker, and then pick up a wide open service road onto which you'll turn left.

Continue along the road for a short distance until you reach a forest-road gate. Pass the gate and cross over a significant forest road, following the orange blazes into woods on the far side. The trail winds downhill for a distance, at times moderately steeply, and it comes to a fork where you will stay right. Just beyond, you'll reach a side trail and a sign pointing the way to Hammonds Rocks. Resist the urge to visit the rocks. Although they afford a nice view, they are much easier to reach by car. Continue downhill for a distance, to where the trail meets an old washed-out logging road. Turn right and continue descending, passing the 3-mile marker in a short distance. Cross a small creek over a footbridge and continue through the woods for another half mile before entering more of an open clear-cut area for about a mile. The area has plenty of thick brush that makes good habitat for a variety of birds.

At about 4.5 miles you'll pass an iron gate with a BRT sign just beyond it. Walk out to the road, cross it, and enter the woods just to the left of a private drive. After circumnavigating the property, you'll come to another old logging road—the Leaf Trail Road—where you'll stay left. Just beyond the junction is the 5-mile marker. Follow this for about a mile to a significant dirt road just beyond some private residences. Turn right, walk about 200 feet out to the main road (PA 233) and turn left. About 200 feet along is the parking area for the south trailhead. Across the street, you'll see the ranger station and just beyond that is a general store that sells supplies and refreshments.

NEARBY ACTIVITIES

Pine Grove Furnace State Park has swimming areas, a campground, and places to picnic. Kings Gap has several picnic areas and provides a host of interpretive and educational programs.

47 GETTYSBURG NATIONAL MILITARY PARK

KEY AT-A-GLANCE INFORMATION

LENGTH: 7 miles

CONFIGURATION: Loop

DIFFICULTY: Moderate

SCENERY: Rural farm country, hardwood forests, streams, military monuments and memorials

EXPOSURE: More sun than shade

TRAIL TRAFFIC: Generally light

TRAIL SURFACE: Dirt

HIKING TIME: 4 hours

DRIVING DISTANCE: 5 miles from intersection of US 15 and US 30 east of Gettysburg

ACCESS: Dawn–dusk; parking at the amphitheater parking area is available during the summer.

MAPS: USGS Fairfield and Gettysburg

FACILITIES: Restrooms and refreshments available at the visitor center, portable toilets along trail

WHEELCHAIR TRAVERSABLE: Some sections

SPECIAL COMMENTS: This hike is more of a naturalist's excursion through the military park rather than an informative historical hike.

IN BRIEF

This hike route mostly follows the path of the horse trail through the southern part of the military park. As a result, it tends to see rather little traffic, although it doesn't pass by as many of the heritage sites as the Billy Yank or Johnny Reb trails (see page 224 for more information).

DESCRIPTION

Although known for its numerous military monuments commemorating the soldiers who fought here for three days in July of 1863, Gettysburg National Military Park is perhaps less well known for its natural history. The park is part of Audubon Pennsylvania's Susquehanna River Birding and Wildlife Trail, and, in addition to the historical setting, the scenery it provides of open farmland and wooded hollows is quite delightful. I have found it to be a wonderful place for wildlife viewing, having seen foxes and a wide variety of birdlife on my visits there. This hike description provides an outing in the park that offers you more exposure to its secluded areas and less to the more popular historical sites.

This is not to diminish the value of the park for its contribution to American heritage and history. Several useful guides to the park

GPS Trailhead Coordinates

UTM Zone (WGS84) 18S

Easting   306775

Northing   4408617

Latitude   N 39° 48′ 20.13″

Longitude   W 77° 15′ 25.77″

Directions

From US 15 east of Gettysburg, follow US 30 west through the center of town. At the traffic circle, head south on Business 15 to PA 116 west (one block south of the circle). Turn right onto PA 116, and then left onto Southwest Confederate Avenue. Begin the hike at the amphitheater parking area, about 2 miles south on the right.

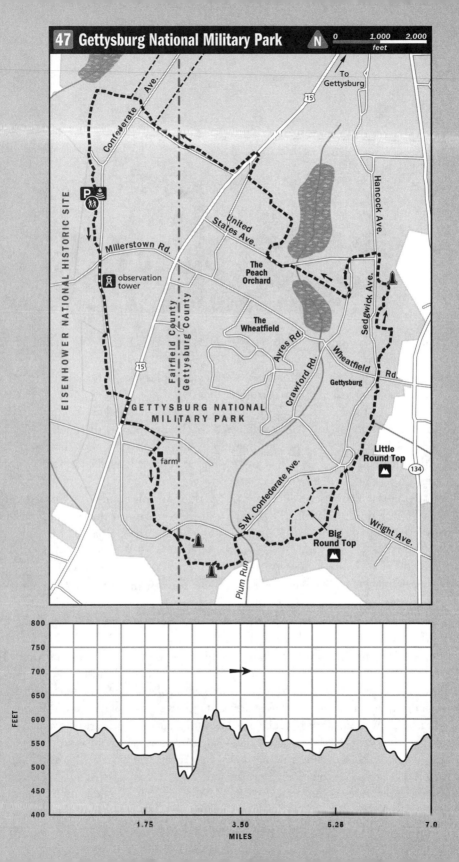

N

0   1,000   2,000
feet

To
Gettysburg

15

Confederate Ave.

Hancock Ave.

P

EISENHOWER NATIONAL HISTORIC SITE

Millerstown Rd.

United
States Ave.

observation
tower

The
Peach
Orchard

Sedgwick Ave.

Fairfield County
Gettysburg County

The
Wheatfield

Ayres Rd.

Crawford Rd.

Wheatfield   Rd.

15

Gettysburg

GETTYSBURG NATIONAL
MILITARY PARK

farm

Little
Round Top

134

S.W. Confederate Ave.

Big
Round Top

Wright Ave.

Plum Run

FEET

800
750
700
650
600
550
500
450
400

1.75   3.50   5.25   7.0

MILES

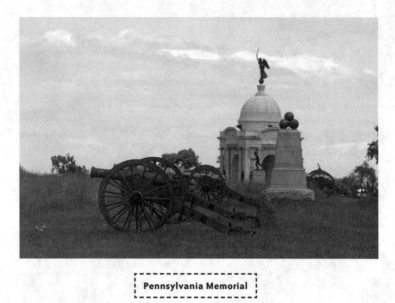

Pennsylvania Memorial

and its historical sites and monuments are available at the visitor center, located on Emmitsburg Road and across from the Gettysburg National Cemetery. Hikers interested in visiting historical sites would do well to purchase a copy of the *Gettysburg Heritage Trail Guide* published by the Boy Scouts of America. It has directions for and interpretive information on the 9-mile Billy Yank Trail and the 3-mile Johnny Reb Trail, as well as other shorter walks. It is available at the visitor-center bookstore.

Begin this hike at the amphitheater parking lot on Southwest Confederate Avenue. Pick up the gravel path about 20 or 30 feet west of the parking lot and turn left, heading south. The hike begins by winding through a short section of hardwood forest before the path reaches Millerstown Road. Cross Millerstown Road and then cross left over SW Confederate Avenue and take a walk up to the top of the observation tower for an excellent view of the surrounding country-side. To the north and east, you look out over the farms and woodlands that compose the battlefield area. To the south and west, you can see the peaks of South Mountain 15 miles distant.

After visiting the tower, return to the trail on the west side of Southwest Confederate Avenue and continue south as it enters a forest of tall oak trees. This is a good place in the early morning to look for owls, and during the day you can find woodpeckers and thrushes in the area. After a short distance, the path comes out of the woods and crosses SW Confederate Avenue by some of the park's characteristic wooden barricades. Walk across the road, around the small farmhouse, and over toward the corner of Emmitsburg Road (Business 15) and Southwest Confederate Avenue. Cross Emmitsburg Road onto a dirt road heading east and downhill through farm country toward the lowlands around Plum Run and several farms. After about 0.25 miles, you'll come to a gravel track heading off toward a farmhouse to the right and a sign indicating that only authorized vehicles are allowed to continue along the main dirt road beyond that point.

Turn right onto the gravel track (you'll see a sign indicating that this is the horse and footpath) and follow it around the farmhouse to its drive. Turn left and then pass the barn to its right. Please be respectful of the residents and move through the property quickly and quietly.

Beyond the barn, the trail enters a beautiful lowland area, a good spot for wildlife viewing. If you are a photographer, this is a great place for a long lens and a tripod. Among the reeds and grasses you may spot warblers (I have seen several cerulean warblers here), cardinals, bluebirds, and perhaps some woodland mammals. Soon the path reaches Southwest Confederate Avenue and a sign indicating that horses should turn left at the shoulder. Instead, cross the road and enter the woods on a footpath. In about 100 feet or so, you'll reach a fork in the trail. The hike continues to the right, but if you turn left, you'll come to a couple of state and regimental memorials and monuments on top of a small rise. Continuing south along the main trail, you'll soon come to another fork. Again the left fork will take you to several memorials and monuments atop a small rise. The right fork (the path of this hike) descends into a beautiful hollow filled with mature poplars, hickories, and catalpas before coming back out to the road next to a stone bridge over Plum Run. Turn right and follow the shoulder over the bridge and then cut back into the woods on the horse path just beyond. The trail gets a little murky for a short distance as it begins traversing around Big Round Top, passing two junctions with a trail that makes a loop over Big Round Top to the left. If you go up to the summit, you'll find several monuments, though the view from the top is not particularly good. You would do well to continue along the trail over to Wright Avenue at the base of Little Round Top.

After crossing Wright Road, follow the significant path as it climbs up over Little Round Top. This hill was the site of a furious battle beginning on July 2, 1863. Many memorials have been erected near its summit commemorating those who fought and died. From the top, you'll be able to get a good vantage of the extent of the terrain and the battlefield as it stretches out to the north and west.

From Little Round Top, follow the horse path (which passes just east and below the crest of the hill) to the north for a distance until you reach the corner of Wheatfield Road and Sedgwick Avenue. Cross Wheatfield and continue north along the shoulder of Sedgwick and follow the path into the woods again when you reach the Major John Sedgwick Equestrian Monument. You'll follow the trail through the woods for about a half mile to the monument erected for Kearny's New Jersey Brigade atop a hill. From the monument, walk downhill to Sedgwick Avenue and follow it north to the intersection with United States Avenue by the G. Weikert House. Cross Sedgwick and follow the shoulder of United States Avenue to the west. You'll have a wonderful view of the Pennsylvania Memorial and several cannons to the north from here. After a short walk along United States Avenue, the path leaves the road to the left and makes a short circuit through Plum Run. This is a very pretty section of trail that should not be missed. As the trail winds through open fields and then a stand of trees, it passes by a long network of wooden barricades through some lowlands. This is another excellent area for viewing wildlife.

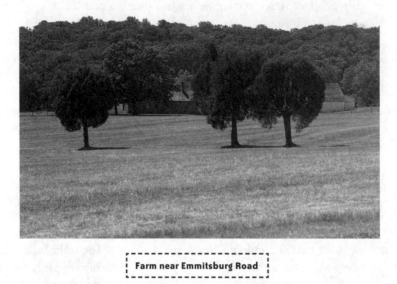

Farm near Emmitsburg Road

The path returns to the road in the area of the Trostle Farm. Turn left and follow the shoulder around the farm and then turn right onto the gravel path by a sign commemorating the site of Bigelow's Last Stand. Follow the path as it winds around through open fields providing lovely rural views and the opportunity to see kestrels, which appear to nest in this area, and red-tailed hawks. The Pennsylvania Monument stands prominently on the eastern horizon. Soon, the path reaches Emmitsburg Road. Cross the road, and follow the path through open farmland to the left (south), eventually bending back to the west toward a red farmhouse and barn. You'll be able to see the observation tower off to the southwest as you cross this wide-open stretch of farmland.

Follow the trail between the farmhouse and the barn (a roost for hundreds of barn swallows) and continue directly west along the path. As the trail enters the woods again, you will reach a junction, marked by a sign, indicating that you can follow the path straight or make an additional spur to the right (north). If you turn right, you'll add 1.75 miles to the hike by visiting the Virginia Memorial. Our hike, however, continues straight out to Southwest Confederate Avenue. When you reach the road, you can either turn left and follow the shoulder for 0.25 miles to the amphitheater parking area, or you can continue straight across the road and follow the path past a field and to a second junction with the north spur of the trail. At the junction, turn left and walk south to the amphitheater parking area.

NEARBY ACTIVITIES

You should definitely stop by the visitor center to view the exhibits on the history of the battle. There you can get information on an automobile tour of the park (well worth doing) and on visiting the Gettysburg National Cemetery. The town of Gettysburg, along Business 15, has restaurants and shops galore.

HERITAGE RAIL TRAIL:
Railroad to Glen Rock

48

IN BRIEF

This hike follows the Heritage Rail Trail from the town of Railroad to Glen Rock and back.

DESCRIPTION

Consisting of 176 acres, York County's Heritage Rail Trail County Park is a linear park that extends from the Colonial Courthouse and Memorial Park in York city for 21 miles to the Maryland state line. According to the park Web site, the railroad line was originally the path of the Northern Central Railroad, which provided transportation between Washington, D.C., and upstate New York. The county acquired the land, which was devastated during Hurricane Agnes in 1972, from the Pennsylvania Department of Transportation in 1990 and opened the trail in 1999. The county is considering extending the trail an additional 5 miles to the north to the John C. Rudy County Park. The attractive trail passes through rolling farm country and woodlands for most of its length, and it passes by several historic sites. The trail sports mileage markers every mile and plenty of benches for resting and soaking up the scenery. It is quite heavily used by cyclists, especially on weekends, and is open to equestrian travel as well. I chose to hike this section of the trail because I understand that it

i KEY AT-A-GLANCE INFORMATION

LENGTH: 7 miles

CONFIGURATION: Out-and-back

DIFFICULTY: Easy

SCENERY: Farms and rolling countryside

EXPOSURE: Half sun, half shade

TRAIL TRAFFIC: Moderate–heavy

TRAIL SURFACE: Packed gravel

HIKING TIME: About 3 hours

DRIVING DISTANCE: 2 miles from Interstate 83 and PA 851 south of York

ACCESS: 8 a.m.–dusk

MAPS: USGS Glen Rock; a map is available at ycweb server.york-county.org/Parks/RailTrail.htm.

FACILITIES: Portable toilets at trailhead; convenience store and restaurants in Glen Rock

WHEELCHAIR TRAVERSABLE: Yes

SPECIAL COMMENTS: A nice hike for bird-watching

Directions

Take Exit 4 (Shrewsbury/PA 851) off Interstate 83. Follow PA 851 west for 2 miles into the town of Railroad. The parking area is on the right across the road from the Jackson House Bed and Breakfast (which looks delightful) and just before crossing the tracks.

GPS Trailhead Coordinates

UTM Zone (WGS84) 18S

Easting 354426

Northing 4402664

Latitude N 39° 45′ 41.30″

Longitude W 76° 41′ 58.10″

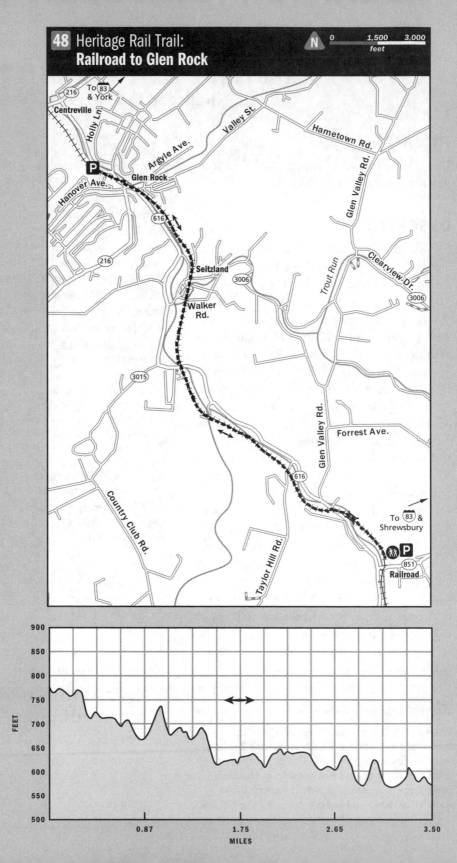

To (83)
& York
(216)
Centreville
Holly Ln.
P
Hanover Ave.
Glen Rock
Argyle Ave.
Valley St.
Hametown Rd.
Glen Valley Rd.
(616)
(216)
Seitzland
(3006)
Trout Run
Clearview Dr.
(3006)
Walker Rd.
(3015)
Country Club Rd.
Glen Valley Rd.
Forrest Ave.
(616)
Taylor Hill Rd.
To (83) &
Shrewsbury
P
(851)
Railroad

FEET

900
850
800
750
700
650
600
550
500

0.87   1.75   2.65   3.50
MILES

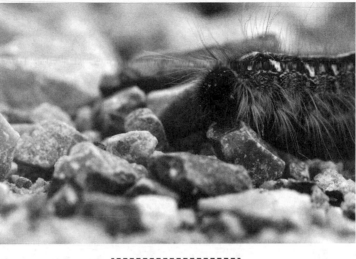

Caterpillar along the trail

is less heavily traveled than other sections. Nonetheless, you should still expect fairly heavy traffic on the weekends.

Hummingbirds, catbirds, robins, eastern towhees, nuthatches, and Baltimore orioles are popular birds that you may see along the hike. And this section of trail follows Codorus Creek South Branch for most of its length, which provides additional habitat for waterfowl such as ducks and the occasional heron.

This hike begins at the parking area in Railroad at the 3-mile marker on the trail. From the trailhead, walk north along the gravel path. The trail shares the route with an active railroad line. Although passing trains are infrequent, you should use caution not to walk on the tracks and when making crossings. As you walk north, you will soon pass over a creek and then make the first track crossing. Just beyond is a bench. The trail winds its way north for about a mile to the 4-mile marker. About 100 yards beyond the marker, you'll find three shaded picnic tables to the left (west) of the trail. This is quite a pretty spot among the tall hickory trees, jack pine, and mountain laurel, and is a worthwhile place to plan a picnic or snack stop.

About 0.5 miles beyond the picnic table, you'll find an interpretive sign on the left of the trail with information about the railroad line, and just beyond that the trail passes over a creek, a tributary of Codorus Creek South Branch. Just beyond the overpass is another bench on the side of the trail. From this point, the trail bends to the northeast and then crosses the tracks again just before reaching the 5-mile marker. Soon you'll reach a road crossing at Seitzland. And within the next mile, you will cross a road by the 6-mile marker, the first of three road crossings in Glen Rock. At the second crossing, keep your eyes open for the Mignano Bros. Ristorante on the left, which has good food and serves ice cream. You'll pass a minimart on the right before the next crossing, and just beyond on the left is

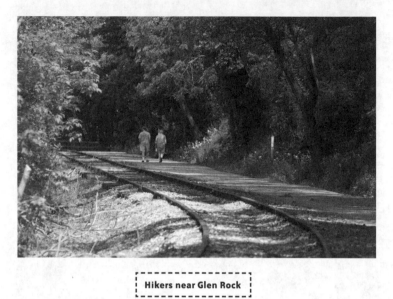

Hikers near Glen Rock

the parking area in Glen Rock. From the parking area, turn around and walk back to Railroad. Should you choose to begin the hike at Glen Rock, please be sure to follow parking restrictions.

NEARBY ACTIVITIES

Captain Bob's Crab Restaurant is directly across the tracks from the trailhead at Railroad. A trip from Railroad to New Freedom, 2 miles to the south, is worth the drive. The trailhead there is at the site of the old New Freedom rail station, which is on the National Register of Historic Places. The station has a museum (open on Saturdays) and a cafe, as well as restrooms and water. Directly across the street from the museum, you'll find the Hodle Tavern with a bar and full menu and patio seating. If shopping is your game, the Shrewsbury Markets in nearby Shrewsbury have plenty to keep you occupied for quite some time.

HOSACK RUN LOOP

IN BRIEF

This hike follows the Greenwood Trail for several miles before joining with the Appalachian Trail (A.T.). It pick ups the A.T. and follows that into Quarry Gap, past the Quarry Gap Shelter, and onto the ridge above. From the ridge, the hike follows the Hosack Run Trail down into a beautiful and remote rhododendron-filled ravine and then rejoins the Greenwood Trail a mile or so from the trailhead.

DESCRIPTION

This hike is without a doubt my favorite hike in the South Mountain Province of central Pennsylvania. The walking is very pleasant; the trails aren't especially crowded; the distance is very manageable; the scenery is excellent. If you do this hike in late June or early July when the rhododendrons are in bloom, you are in for a real treat. In the fall, the colors can't be beat. And even in the summer, the hike tends to stay cool.

Begin this hike at the parking area for the wheelchair-access ramp by the northwest corner of the Lone Pine Run Reservoir. The trailhead is across the road and begins by passing by a forest gate. The initial trail, the Greenwood Trail, is a biking, hiking, and

KEY AT-A-GLANCE INFORMATION

LENGTH: 6.2 miles

CONFIGURATION: Balloon

DIFFICULTY: Moderate

SCENERY: Pretty, open woodlands; steep and rugged rhododendron-filled ravines

EXPOSURE: More shade than sun

TRAIL TRAFFIC: Light

TRAIL SURFACE: Dirt

HIKING TIME: 3 hours

DRIVING DISTANCE: 21.7 miles from Interstate 81 and PA 233 south of Carlisle

ACCESS: Dawn–dusk

MAPS: USGS Caledonia Park; Michaux State Forest public-use map; *Appalachian Trail, PA Route 94 to US Route 30 (Sections 12 and 13)*

FACILITIES: None

WHEELCHAIR TRAVERSABLE: No

SPECIAL COMMENTS: My favorite hike in South Mountain

Directions

From Interstate 81, take Exit 37 (Newville/Pa 233). Follow PA 233 south for 20 miles to Milesburg Road. Turn right on Milesburg Road and follow it 1.7 miles to the parking area at the wheelchair-access ramp on the right at Lone Pine Run Reservoir. The trail begins at the forest road gate across the street.

GPS Trailhead Coordinates

UTM Zone (WGS84) 18S

Easting 290157

Northing 4424011

Latitude N 39° 56′ 24.79″

Longitude W 77° 27′ 21.04″

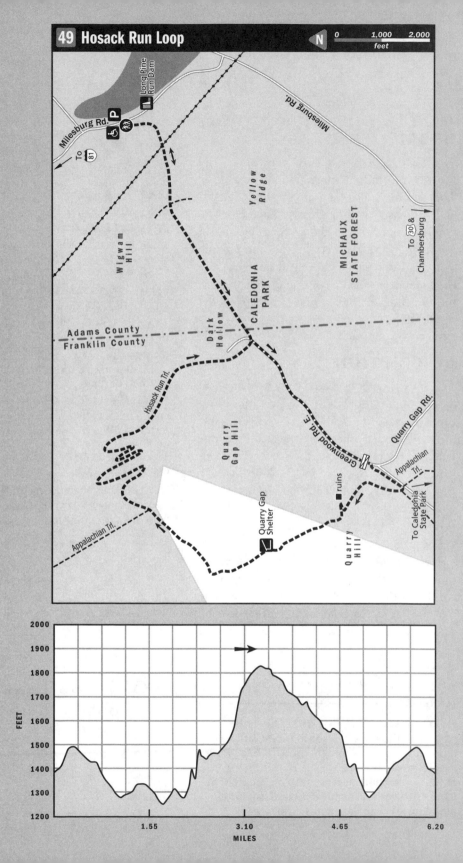

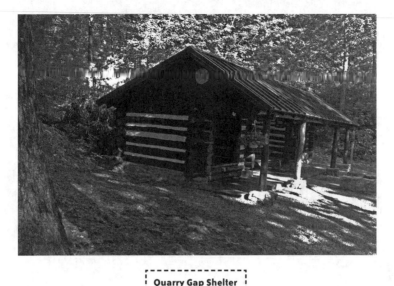

Quarry Gap Shelter

equestrian trail. It is blazed in blue as far as the Appalachian Trail. Follow the Greenwood Trail, an old haul road, up a hill and around to the right, then out to a power line. The power line clearing is a good place to see wildlife, especially deer and fox, and to watch for birds in the many boxes along its edges.

Pass the power line and follow the path down a gentle grade to the crossing of a path that is unmarked and not on any map. Continue straight downhill. The track gets a little washed out and rocky in this area for a short distance, but never becomes too unpleasant. At about 1.2 miles, you'll cross a small creek in an area that is thick with rhododendrons, and about 150 feet beyond that is the junction with the Hosack Run Trail, identified by a labeled post. This begins the loop part of the hike.

Continue straight along the Greenwood Trail past a deer exclosure on the left, through some pretty, open pine woods and meadows. This is great habitat for deer, which are abundant, as well as foxes, rabbits, and other woodland wildlife. After about 0.7 miles, you'll cross a second little creek and just beyond that you'll find a forest gate at Quarry Road. Pass the gate and follow the trail across the road and into the woods on the other side. According to the Michaux State Forest map, the trail is now called the Locust Gap Trail. According to the Appalachian Trail map, the entire trail from the reservoir is called the Locust Gap Trail. Whatever its proper name, all you have to do is to continue following the blue blazes as the trail climbs gently from the road.

In about 0.25 miles, you'll reach the Appalachian Trail, onto which you will turn right, heading north. After a short distance, the A.T. is crossed by a forest gate and the ruins of some old buildings are located on the right side of the trail. Follow the A.T. up into Quarry Gap, a steep and rocky ravine filled with dense rhododendrons. At times the foliage is so thick that the bushes form a tunnel over the trail. Walk another 0.25 miles beyond the gate, and you'll reach the Quarry Gap Shelter.

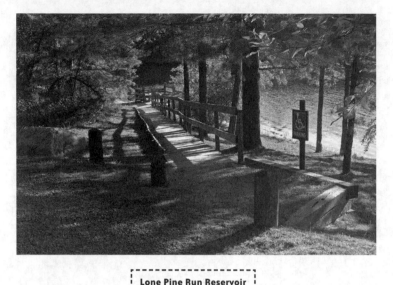

Lone Pine Run Reservoir

This shelter is unlike any other that I've come across in Pennsylvania. A caretaker has carried potted flowers in from nearby Caledonia State Park. Pennsylvania Dutch welcome signs are mounted at each end of the shelter. It is clean, freshly painted, and situated in a lovely spot.

Continuing beyond the shelter, the A.T. gets rather rocky for a short distance and then crosses a creek at a log. Beyond the creek, the quality of the trail improves dramatically but the walking gets quite a bit more steep. After a bracing climb of 0.5 miles, the trail levels out and about 200 feet beyond the leveling point the Hosack Run Trail (blue blazes) departs to the right at a trail sign (3.3 miles).

Follow the Hosack Run Trail through the woods and into the hollow below via a series of switchbacks down a steep hillside on a good trail. The path is in excellent condition and is well blazed. At just about 4 miles, you'll reach the bottom of the hill and are now in the appropriately named Dark Hollow. The steep-sided gap is filled with hemlock and some of the thickest rhododendron I've ever seen. This is a very beautiful and remote area, filled with the sounds of woodpeckers and thrushes, and much wildlife hiding in the brush. You'll head down the hollow from here, following the trail as it traverses above the thick bushes around the creek. Soon the trail drops down and crosses the creek in the area of a large boulder field on the left. Not far beyond it crosses back over the creek in an area of some enormous deadfall. Beyond that, you'll soon return to the Greenwood Trail (5.1 miles). Turn left and follow it back to the car.

NEARBY ACTIVITIES

Two state parks are located on PA 233 nearby and both have swimming and picnicking facilities. They are Pine Grove Furnace State Park to the north and Caledonia State Park just a couple of miles south of Milesburg Road.

KINGS GAP LOOP HIKE **50**

IN BRIEF

Beginning at the trailhead for the Scenic Vista Trail and Buck Ridge Trail, follow the Scenic Vista Trail to the Pond Day use area. From there, follow the Watershed and Boundary trails along the perimeter of the park and ascend back to the trailhead from Kings Gap Hollow via a walk along the Ridge Overlook Trail and Maple Hollow Trail.

DESCRIPTION

Unique among Pennsylvania state parks, the Kings Gap Environmental Education and Training Center is oriented more toward activities and programs that promote a greater understanding of the natural world than toward purely recreational purposes. The center consists of 1,454 acres of scenic woodlands that are home to several day-use areas, 16 miles of hiking trails, a visitor center, and a majestic 32-room mansion situated on a mountaintop in the South Mountain region of south-central Pennsylvania. The center provides a host of educational opportunities year-round, including environmental-education programs for high-school students and teachers, weekend interpretive programs, and backcountry hikes.

KEY AT-A-GLANCE INFORMATION

LENGTH: 6.3 miles

CONFIGURATION: Loop

DIFFICULTY: Moderate

SCENERY: Kings Gap Environmental Education and Training Center and great views of the Cumberland Valley

EXPOSURE: Mostly shade

TRAIL TRAFFIC: Light

TRAIL SURFACE: Dirt

HIKING TIME: 3–3.5 hours

DRIVING DISTANCE: About 8 miles from Interstate 81 and PA 233

ACCESS: 8 a.m.–dusk

MAPS: USGS Dickinson; a trail map is available at the Kings Gap visitor center and online at www.dcnr .state.pa.us/stateparks/Parks/ kingsgap.aspx.

FACILITIES: Water and restrooms available at visitor center

WHEELCHAIR TRAVERSABLE: No

SPECIAL COMMENTS: The trails on this hike can be quite rocky in places, so a sturdy pair of boots is advisable.

Directions

From Interstate 81, take exit 37, Newville, and follow PA 233 south for 2.3 miles to Pine Road. Turn left onto Pine Road (signs for Kings Gap Environmental Education and Training Center) and follow for another 2.3 miles to Kings Gap Road (sign for Kings Gap). Turn right and follow the winding road up to the mansion area. The parking area, with several trailheads, is on the left, just before the loop at the mansion area begins.

GPS Trailhead Coordinates

UTM Zone (WGS84) 18T

Easting 306986

Northing 4440561

Latitude N 40° 5′ 35.60″

Longitude W 77° 15′ 51.00″

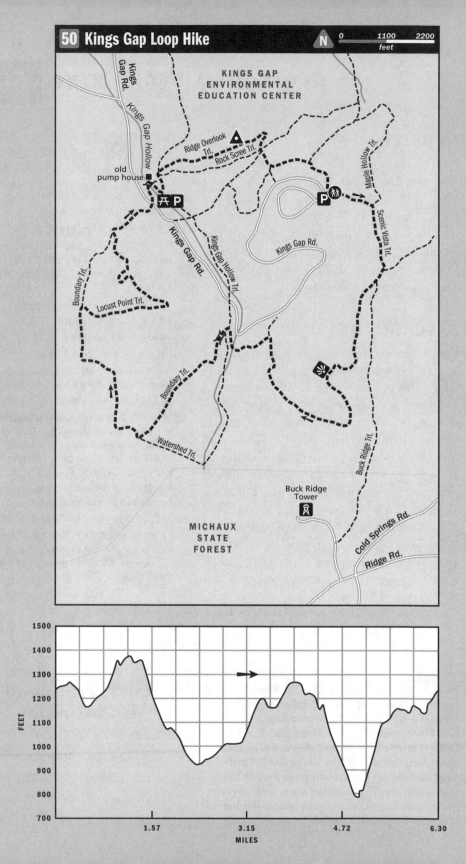

The mansion and the views of the surrounding terrain are worth the visit in and of themselves. This hike, though, provides access to some of the more remote regions of the park, offering some wonderful scenery and excellent views.

Begin this hike from the parking area by following the red-blazed Scenic Vista Trail to the east through a clearing. This trail shares the path with the Maple Hollow and Buck Ridge trails initially. After about 0.25 miles, follow the red blazes to the right (south), leaving the Maple Hollow Trail behind. The trail descends toward a hollow into the woods, and after another 0.25 miles the Buck Ridge Trail departs to the left. Continue along the Scenic Vista Trail for a little more than a half mile to the Scenic Vista Overlook (1.1 miles), where you will find a couple of nice benches and an even nicer view into Kings Gap Hollow to the west.

From the overlook, follow the trail over a ridge and through a splendid, silent forest down into Kings Gap Hollow. At just about 2 miles, the route makes a sharp left turn, although the obvious path appears to continue straight. Make the left (there is no sign) and follow the red blazes down a trail that looks like a watercourse to the program pavilion at the Pond Day Use Area (about 2.2 miles). The pavilion is dedicated to the memory of Frank E. Masland, whose family once owned the mansion. You'll find restrooms at the day-use area, and plenty of benches and tables to take a rest and have a snack.

From the pavilion, head downhill and slightly to your right to the obvious information board at the road. Here, you will find a sign that points the way to the Boundary Trail and Watershed Trail along the Kings Gap Trail. Follow the latter downhill for a short distance to the junction with the Boundary and Watershed trails, which follow a common path to the left. The junction is well marked. Turn left, and just ahead (50 yards) you'll find a sign at a small bridge over the creek that says WATERSHED TRAIL, 1.8 MILES. Cross the bridge, and stay to the left following the Watershed Trail (purple blazes) toward the Boundary Trail.

Continue on the Watershed Trail for about 0.75 miles, passing several small side trails, to a T-intersection. The Boundary Trail (green blazes) goes to the right here while the Watershed Trail heads left. Turn right onto the Boundary Trail, so named because it follows the boundary of the park lands. You'll immediately pass a sign facing the opposite direction that says END OF BOUNDARY TRAIL. Follow green blazes uphill and along a straight logging road through pretty, open woods to a forested ridge, where you'll find the junction with red-blazed Locust Point Trail (3.7 miles). Turn right and follow that uphill.

The Locust Point Trail makes a side trip of about a mile over a lovely wooded hillside that has a nice viewpoint about 0.6 miles along. Before reaching the viewpoint, the trail makes a sharp left turn and heads downhill. The turn is well blazed, but worth paying attention to, as a side trail there will take you out to a clearing. Follow the Locust Point Trail until it returns you to the Boundary Trail, where you will turn right and follow that down to the park road at a picnic bench and parking area (4.9 miles).

From the picnic bench, cross the road angling downhill and follow the sign for the Kings Gap Hollow Trail (slightly to the left) toward the creek below.

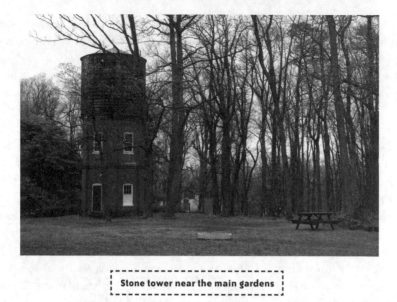

Stone tower near the main gardens

Shortly you will reach a pretty footbridge. Cross the creek and then turn right onto a wide trail. (If you turn left, you'll come to the remains of an old pump house downstream a hundred feet or so.) After turning right, you will quickly reach the junction with the Ridge Overlook Trail (purple blazes) to your left by some large boulders in the woods. Follow that trail up to the ridge. Just as you attain the ridge and the terrain flattens out, the Ridge Overlook Trail crosses the Rock Scree Trail. Continue straight along the ridge for about 0.75 miles to the overlook, identified by a sign. You'll have a wonderful view of the Cumberland Valley to the north and west from here. Looking to the southeast, you should be able to make out the mansion on the hillside above you.

Continue along the ridge to the east for a short distance, where the trail makes a switchback and descends the ridge to the west into a hollow. Soon the Ridge Overlook Trail joins the Rock Scree Trail. Then, just beyond, it crosses the Forest Heritage Trail. Continue straight past a deer exclosure on the left. Just beyond that, you will reach a second crossing of the Forest Heritage Trail (lime green blazes). Turn left here and follow the Forest Heritage Trail for a short distance to the Maple Hollow Trail (yellow blazes). Turn right. In a hundred feet or so, the Maple Hollow Trail makes a sharp left and then emerges into a small clearing that offers a view to the north. Follow the trail along a forest cut from the clearing to the right, which will return you in a couple of minutes to the parking area.

NEARBY ACTIVITIES

Kings Gap offers many environmental programs as well as wonderful places to have a picnic. Visit the mansion, the gardens, and the visitor center just uphill from the parking area.

MARY ANN FURNACE TRAIL LOOP 51

IN BRIEF

Following the white-blazed Mary Ann Furnace Trail, this hike makes a loop through the woods along the southwest shore of Lake Marburg.

DESCRIPTION

The Mary Ann Furnace Trail consists of a 3.5-mile network of trails in three loops on the south shore of Lake Marburg at the lake's western end. This 2.5-mile hike follows the white-blazed main loop around the perimeter of the trail network. Lake Marburg is a large (1,275-acre) man-made water impoundment that is popular with fishermen who angle for bass, crappie, perch, muskellunge, and catfish. The lake's construction was a cooperative project between the H. P. Glatfelter Paper Company located in Spring Grove, which needed the water for industrial purposes, and the Commonwealth of Pennsylvania, which administrates the lake for recreational purposes. The lake is home to a large and varied population of waterfowl, and it is quite common to see Canada geese, wood ducks, teal, and herons along its 26 miles of shoreline.

Directions ⟶

From Interstate 83 in York, follow US 30 west for 7.5 miles to PA 116 west. Follow PA 116 for 12 miles to PA 216 just before reaching Hanover. Turn left on PA 216 and follow it for about 3 miles, crossing Lake Marburg. Turn right onto Dubbs Church Road. Follow that for 1.85 miles to SR 3070, Black Rock Road. Turn right and follow for about a mile. The trailhead and parking are on the right just beyond the bridge over Codorus Creek West Branch at a wetlands area.

ⓘ KEY AT-A-GLANCE INFORMATION

LENGTH: 2.5 miles

CONFIGURATION: Loop

DIFFICULTY: Easy

SCENERY: Pretty walk in the woods; nice views of Lake Marburg

EXPOSURE: Mix of sun and shade

TRAIL TRAFFIC: Moderate

TRAIL SURFACE: Dirt

HIKING TIME: 1.5 hours

DRIVING DISTANCE: About 25 miles southwest of York

ACCESS: Dawn–dusk

MAPS: USGS Hanover; a map is included in the recreation guide for Codorus State Park, available at the park office and at www.dcnr .state.pa.us/stateparks/Parks/ codorus.aspx.

FACILITIES: None at the trailhead but plenty in the state park

WHEELCHAIR TRAVERSABLE: No

SPECIAL COMMENTS: The hike can get a bit buggy in the summer.

GPS Trailhead Coordinates

UTM Zone (WGS84) 18S

Easting 334708

Northing 4403997

Latitude N 39° 46′ 11.53″

Longitude W 76° 55′ 47.58″

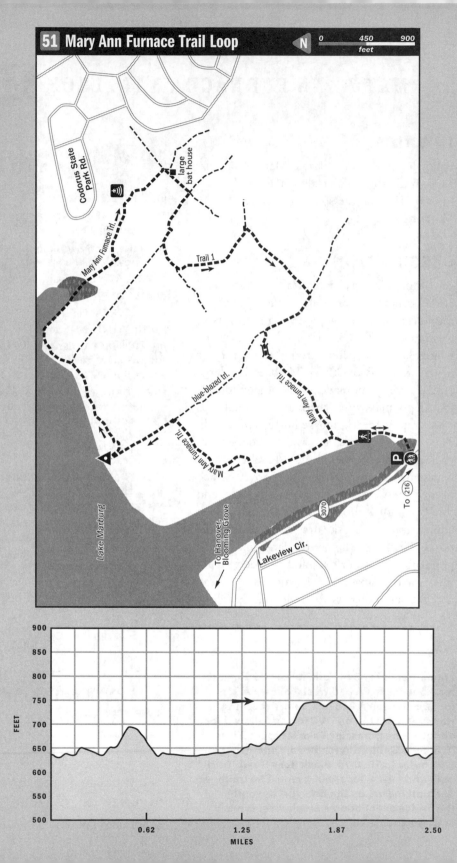

N

| 0 | 450 | 900 |

feet

Codorus State Park Rd.

large bat house

Mary Ann Furnace Trl.

Trail 1

blue-blazed trl.

Mary Ann Furnace Trl.

Mary Ann Furnace Trl.

Lake Marburg

To Hanover, Blooming Grove

3070

Lakeview Cir.

P

To 216

900
850
800
750
700
650
600
550
500

FEET

0.62   1.25   1.87   2.50

MILES

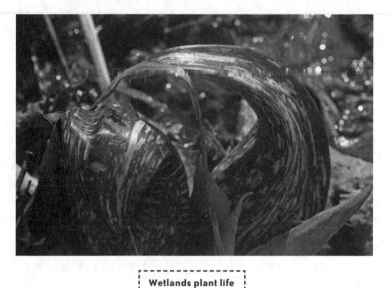

Wetlands plant life

The park's woodlands are home to deer, pheasant, rabbits, squirrels, and other small game.

The hiking trail is named for the Mary Ann Forge and Furnace that was located on nearby Furnace Creek, the westernmost feeder stream to Lake Marburg. The furnace was founded in 1761 by Mark Bird and George Ross, an attorney from Lancaster, Pennsylvania, and a signer of the Declaration of Independence. The furnace produced cannons, cannonballs, and shot used by the Continental army under George Washington's command. A historic plaque was erected at the site of the Iron Master's house on Black Rock Road near the trailhead by the Daughters of the American Revolution in 1949.

From the parking area on Black Rock Road, walk across the footbridge over Codorus Creek West Branch and follow the path around a small cove through a wetlands area. On a spring morning, this cove is filled with the songs of spring peepers. As you bend around the back of the cove, you'll come to a long boardwalk. Cross the boardwalk and climb a little hill where you will find a fork in the trail with a sign for Trails 1 and 2. Follow the arrow toward Trail 1, heading to the left. At about 0.6 miles, the trail comes to a T-intersection at a grassy road. Turn left and follow the path down to the shore of the lake. Just before reaching the shore, the trail makes a 90-degree right turn, though you can walk down to the lake to a pretty vantage point.

From the bend, the trail parallels the shore of the lake through an attractive forest of cedars. Just shy of a mile into the hike, enter a small clearing with a trail approaching from the right and a sign for the Mary Ann Furnace Trail. Continue straight, staying near the shore of the lake. Soon the trail bends to the right and enters a second secluded cove: Wonder Cove. Continue to the back of the cove and follow the small hollow beyond, passing a short section of boardwalk.

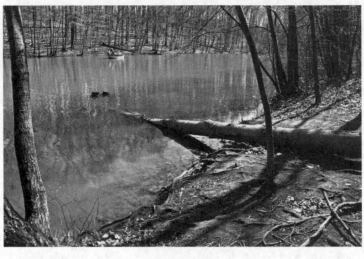

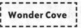

Wonder Cove

Soon you'll climb a hillside, passing beneath the park amphitheater and grassy picnic area—a nice place to stop and hang out for a while. After passing the amphitheater, descend a wide grassy path to a large open meadow at the head of the hollow to a crossing with an old dirt road. Turn right on this road, and take note of the large bat box on the left side of the trail just after you turn. Cross the creek through a muddy section of trail and climb a short hill to another trail crossing (1.5 miles).

Turn right at the crossing and contour around a hillside past a couple of old wooden posts. In a short distance, you'll reach a field on top of a hill at another Mary Ann Furnace Trail sign. A yellow-blazed trail enters the woods directly ahead, and a white-blazed trail enters the woods about the 20 feet to the left (south) of it. Bear left and follow the white blazes into the woods. Wind through the woods until you come to the edge of the hillside field. This spot offers a nice view of the hills in this part of the park.

Follow the trail until it forks and then turn right, following it along the boundary of private property to the left. When you reach a T-intersection, turn right again and descend into a small hollow. At 2.1 miles, a blue-blazed trail heads off straight, and you want to bear left, staying with the white blazes across a small creek. Climb a small hill that seems steep relative to the other grades on this walk. After cresting the hill, descend for a short distance until you reach the trail junction near the boardwalk in the first cove. Turn left, and the parking area is just five minutes along.

NEARBY ACTIVITIES

Codorus State Park, through which the trail passes, offfers facilities for many kinds of recreational activities, including fishing, swimming, boating, camping, and picnicking.

PINCHOT LAKE LOOP 52

IN BRIEF

This hike generally follows the path of the Lakeside Trail indicated on park maps around Pinchot Lake.

DESCRIPTION

This hike tends to follow what the Gifford Pinchot State Park brochure refers to as the Lakeside Trail around Pinchot Lake, although this hike incorporates a couple of side trails to circumnavigate the campground area. In places the hike passes through some of the busiest areas of the park, and in other places the most remote. It's a great hike that encompasses some beautiful country and affords some fine opportunities for viewing wildlife.

Begin this hike by exiting the parking area at Boat Mooring Area 2 to the southeast, walking past the handicapped parking space along a paved path toward the restrooms. Just past the restrooms, look to your right and you will see a sign that says LAKESIDE TRAIL. Take this trail, which initially follows the lakeshore through cedar and hickory trees beneath the cabin area.

At about 0.5 miles, the trail meets a road and angles to the left through a field of wild-flowers where it splits into two grassy paths. Both take you to the far side of the field, where the trail reenters the woods on dirt. A quarter

KEY AT-A-GLANCE INFORMATION

LENGTH: 8.5 miles
CONFIGURATION: Loop
DIFFICULTY: Moderately strenuous because of length
SCENERY: Gifford Pinchot State Park environs; wonderful views of the lake and woods
EXPOSURE: Mostly shade
TRAIL TRAFFIC: Medium–light
TRAIL SURFACE: Varies from dirt and rocky to paved in places
HIKING TIME: 4–5 hours
DRIVING DISTANCE: About 9 miles from Interstate 83 and PA 177 south of Harrisburg
ACCESS: Dawn–dusk
MAPS: USGS Wellsville and Dover; maps of the park with the trail outlined are available at the Park Office, though the hike here varies slightly from the Lakeside Trail that is indicated on that map.
FACILITIES: Restrooms and water available at various locations along the first 5 miles of the hike
WHEELCHAIR TRAVERSABLE: No
SPECIAL COMMENTS: Use discretion about completing this hike following a heavy rain. At approximately 7 miles, the path crosses a creek that would be impassable with much water in it.

Directions

From Harrisburg, follow Interstate 83 south to Exit 35, Lewisberry, PA 177. Follow PA 177 south for 6.9 miles to Mount Airy Road. The park office for Gifford Pinchot State Park is at the corner on the left. Turn left and follow the road about a half mile to the parking area at boat mooring #2.

GPS Trailhead Coordinates

UTM Zone (WGS84) 18T

Easting 339404

Northing 4438660

Latitude N 40° 4′ 58.47″

Longitude W 76° 53′ 1.04″

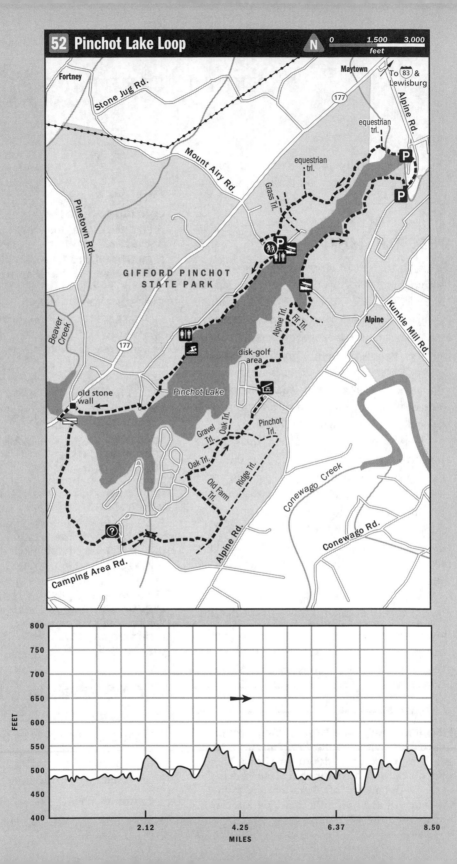

52 Pinchot Lake Loop

N

0   1,500   3,000
feet

Maytown

To 83 &
Lewisburg

Fortney

Stone Jug Rd.

177

Alpine Rd.

equestrian
trl.

Mount Airy Rd.

equestrian
trl.

Grass Trl.

Pinetown Rd.

GIFFORD PINCHOT
STATE PARK

Beaver Creek

177

Alpine Trl.

Fir Trl.

Alpine

Kunkle Mill Rd.

disk-golf
area

old stone
wall

Pinchot Lake

Gravel Trl.

Oak Trl.

Pinchot Trl.

Oak Trl.

Old Fam Trl.

Ridge Trl.

Conewago Creek

Alpine Rd.

Conewago Rd.

Camping Area Rd.

FEET

800
750
700
650
600
550
500
450
400

2.12   4.25   6.37   8.50

MILES

of a mile or so beyond that, you'll reach the Quaker Race Day Use Area, with its picnic pavilions, a swimming beach, and a concession stand that are open during the summer. When you reach the recreation area, hop on the paved path by the first set of restrooms and follow it past the swimming beach to its end at a pavilion. Walk toward the woods between two large sycamore trees and you'll see a Lakeside Trail sign where it enters the woods. The trail immediately crosses a small footbridge, curves to the left, and climbs gently. As you enter the woods, admire the interesting and beautiful stand of cane to the right.

When you reach a maintenance building, turn right on the dirt road and follow it for a couple of hundred feet until you see a Lakeside Trail sign on the left near a gate on the road. Turn left on the trail and follow it for about 0.4 miles to a spruce tree and a maintenance access gate. The trail veers left and then past an old stone wall onto PA 177 at the intersection with Pinetown Road. Turn left and walk the shoulder across the bridge over the lake.

A prominent blue blaze has been painted on the end of the bridge's guardrail, and there is a sign for the Lakeside Trail. For the most part, this hike follows the blue blazes along the south side of the lake. Enter the woods here and follow the lakeshore for a short distance through a forest of maple and oak trees. Soon the trail bends right and climbs uphill from a junction with a trail to the left. As it levels out, the trail widens and appears to be an old bridle path as it heads to the southwest. Eventually the trail passes by a road and large meadow, both of which are on the right.

Just shy of 3 miles, this hike comes to an open area surrounded by pine trees with a small cedar tree with a blue blaze on your left. A grassy path comes in from the right and the trail appears to continue straight. Turn right onto the grassy path and shortly you will come to the campground access road. Cross the road and enter the woods at the Lakeside Trail sign. The campground kiosk will be to your left. It has vending machines and information.

At this point, the park map shows the Lakeside Trail turning immediately to the left and cutting through the campground, whereas continuing straight takes you along the Ridge Trail. I was unable to locate the junction, so I continued to follow the blazes along the Ridge Trail. At 3.6 miles, the trail reaches a T-junction by a telephone line. Be sure to turn left here. The walking is really lovely along an old roadbed a fair bit above the lake. In another 0.2 miles, you'll reach the junction of the Ridge Trail and the Old Farm Trail.

Here, you have some choices. The blue blazes continue straight along the Ridge Trail, and you can follow them to the junction with the Pinchot Trail that joins the Gravel Trail atop a small hill with a log bench near the lake (about 0.7 miles). At that point, you'll turn right. Or you can turn left on Old Farm Trail (slightly shorter option), which descends to the edge of the campground where it meets the Oak Trail (about 0.25 miles). Neither trail is marked, but a sign on the left says NO PETS ALLOWED IN CAMPING AREA. Turning left brings you to a meadow and small playground. Turn right here and follow the gravel path (which is both the Old Farm Trail and Oak Trail) up a gentle hill, noting the shagbark hickory growing in this area.

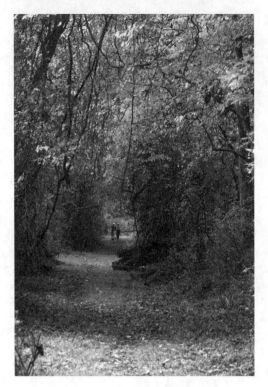

Following this latter option, at 4.3 miles you'll reach another trail junction where the Old Farm Trail turns right and heads back uphill and the Oak Trail continues straight to a significant junction 0.2 miles ahead. Here, the Gravel Trail enters from the left and crosses the Oak Trail. Turn right and follow the Gravel Trail by a sign that advises CAUTION: STEEP GRADE. The grade is neither very steep nor very long, though. At the top is the log bench and the junction with the Pinchot Trail.

Take the Gravel Trail as it heads downhill, following the blue blazes. At 4.8 miles, the path enters an open grassy area, and comes to a signpost with a bicycle symbol pointing to the woods on the left. Enter the woods and then cross the access road to the Conewago Recreation Area. The path continues by a disk-golf course to the left and a large pavilion with a restroom to the right. At 5 miles the trail veers left and then forks. A blue blaze on a tree indicates that this hike heads uphill to the right following the Alpine Trail.

Another 0.4 miles and the Midland Trail enters from the left. Turn right onto the Midland Trail and immediately cross a little footbridge. Soon you pass the Fir Trail on the right, and then reach a T-junction with the Boulder Point Trail. Turning left will take you to Balanced Rock, a geological formation along the lakeshore. Turning right keeps you on the Lakeside Trail as it circumnavigates a secluded cove where I saw a heron feeding.

At 5.8 miles, the trail reaches Boat Mooring Area 3. Follow the lakeshore past a cul-de-sac and a canoe-storage rack. You'll find a Lakeside Trail sign by a picnic table on the right. Continue through the woods right next to the lake. At this point, the hike enters a secluded section of the park as it follows the boulder-strewn lakeshore.

At 7 miles, the trail reaches the northeast end of the lake at the dam. Although you can't walk across the dam, take a walk out on it for a wonderful view. From the dam, descend an old gravel road into a parking area by Beaver Creek, the outflow from the lake. Walk out of the parking area and cross the bridge on a paved sidewalk. As soon as the pavement ends, you'll see a blue blaze on the guardrail. Step over it and walk down some steps. Walk through woods parallel to the road until

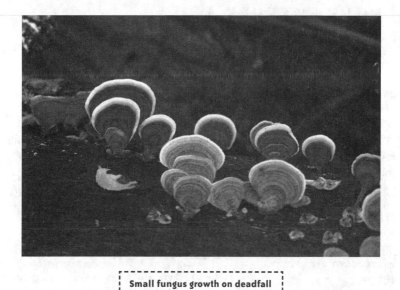

Small fungus growth on deadfall

the trail climbs and heads to the left away from the road. Soon it climbs a series of wooden steps before reaching a parking area by the dam. A sign indicates that the Lakeside Trail follows the fence southwest around the dam's spillway. This is the last of the trail signs.

As soon as the trail meets the level of the lake again, you'll find a beautiful spot at a cove for relaxing on the left. Just beyond that the trail crosses Rock Creek where the creek tumbles over small ledges. Beware: the creek would be impassable after heavy rain. The blue blazes end at the creek.

Cross the creek and climb generally uphill to the left. At 7.3 miles, the path meets the Equestrian Trail. Turn left and watch for woodpeckers in this area. The trail parallels the lakeshore, though above it a fair distance. Stay on this trail for what feels like a long 0.6 miles. At times the track gets very rocky and follows watercourses that climb away from the lake. At 8 miles, you'll reach a significant, though unmarked, trail junction just beyond a heavily washed-out section of the Equestrian Trail. The junction is easily identifiable by the footbridge immediately left of the Equestrian Trail.

Turn left and follow the path through the woods for the next 0.35 miles until you reach the paved park road. En route, you'll pass a trail crossing marked by a NO HORSES sign and then a grassy cut in the woods that leads to a park-maintenance area to the left. When you reach the paved road, turn left and walk into the parking lot.

NEARBY ACTIVITIES

Gifford Pinchot State Park offers all sorts of activities, including a swimming area, several boat launches, fishing, a disk golf course, picnic pavilions, and a campground.

53 POLE STEEPLE AND MOUNTAIN CREEK

KEY AT-A-GLANCE INFORMATION

LENGTH: 4.2 miles

CONFIGURATION: Loop

DIFFICULTY: Moderate

SCENERY: Pine Grove Furnace State Park environs, a great view from the summit of Pole Steeple, halfway point of Appalachian Trail

EXPOSURE: Mostly shaded

TRAIL TRAFFIC: Moderately heavy

TRAIL SURFACE: Dirt

HIKING TIME: 2–3 hours

DRIVING DISTANCE: About 9 miles from PA 233 and Interstate 81

ACCESS: Dawn–dusk

MAPS: USGS Dickinson; Pine Grove Furnace State Park map

FACILITIES: None at the parking area; restrooms and water are available nearby at Laurel Lake.

WHEELCHAIR TRAVERSABLE: No

SPECIAL COMMENTS: Use caution atop the cliffs at Pole Steeple.

IN BRIEF

After the short ascent of Pole Steeple, a quartzite outcrop along a mountain ridge, this hike picks up the Appalachian Trail and follows it west down to Railroad Bed Road. After joining the road, the hike follows Mountain Creek Trail along the creek, through wetlands, back to the parking area.

DESCRIPTION

From the parking area, walk across the road, the old South Mountain Railroad grade dating back to the time of the forge and furnaces in the valley, to the trailhead marked by a sign and blue blazes just left of some private residences. The trail is wide with good footing as it climbs rather steeply at first through a forest of pine and fir trees, many of which show signs of woodpecker feeding. At about 0.5 miles, the trail forks and blue blazes go in both directions. If you take the right fork, the trail climbs more gently as it makes switchbacks along the steep hillside. The left path takes a direct route up the hill. Both join again where the terrain levels out just above the fork and just below the cliffs of Pole Steeple. Follow the path a short distance to a trail junction at a saddle on a ridge with a sign pointing right to the Appalachian Trail and a bench (0.65 miles). Turn left

---

GPS Trailhead Coordinates

UTM Zone (WGS84)   18T

Easting   306310

Northing   4434465

Latitude   N 40° 2′ 17.41″

Longitude   W 77° 16′ 13.08″

Directions

Take exit 37, PA 233, from Interstate 81 and follow 233 south for about 8 miles to the park office at the intersection with Pine Grove Road. Turn left on Pine Grove Road and follow that east for 1.5 miles to Railroad Bed Road, just beyond the Laurel Lake (aka Laurel Forge Pond) day-use area. Turn right. The parking area is on the right just above the outlet to the lake across from a couple of private cabins.

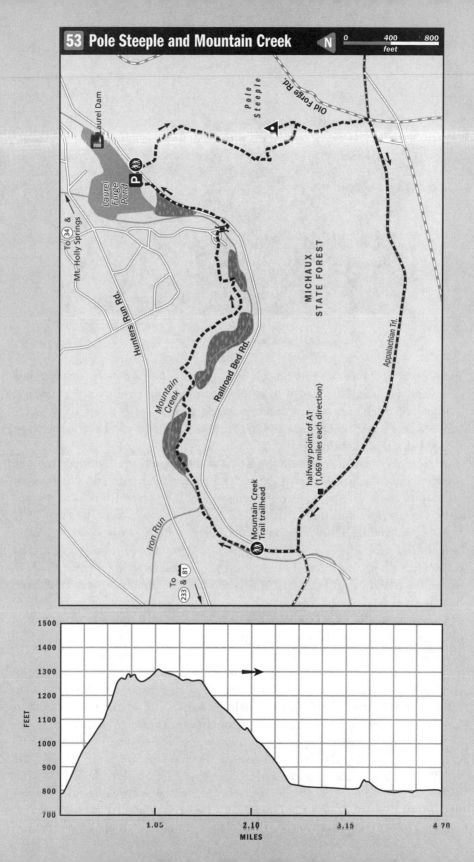

53 Pole Steeple and Mountain Creek

N

0   400   800
feet

Laurel Dam

Pole Steeple

Old Forge Rd.

Laurel Forge Pond

P

To 34 &
Mt. Holly Springs

Hunters Run Rd.

Mountain Creek

Railroad Bed Rd.

MICHAUX STATE FOREST

Appalachian Trl.

halfway point of AT
(1,069 miles each direction)

Mountain Creek Trail trailhead

Iron Run

To 233 & 81

FEET

1500
1400
1300
1200
1100
1000
900
800
700

1.05   2.10   3.15   4.70
MILES

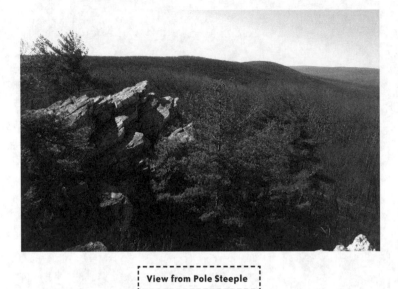

View from Pole Steeple

and follow the blazes to Pole Steeple (0.8 miles). The hike to this overlook is deservedly popular. Surrounded by stout table mountain pine trees, Pole Steeple is a quartzite rock outcropping about 75 feet high. It offers excellent views of the Sunset Rocks Ridge to the north and the Pine Grove Furnace State Park, including Laurel Lake, directly below.

From Pole Steeple, return to the saddle and follow the trail south up a gentle rise to the Appalachian Trail (A.T.) at about 1 mile. At this point, the climbing for the day is done. The trail junction forms the hub of several trails radiating as spokes in different directions. The A.T. crosses directly perpendicular to the Pole Steeple Trail and the Old Forge Road cuts a diagonal in from across the A.T. and downhill to your left. Turn right onto the A.T., here an old roadbed marked by white blazes, and descend a pleasant grade for 1.5 miles to the railroad grade in the valley. At about 1.3 miles, you'll pass the halfway point on the A.T., marked by a prominent sign. From here, the A.T. extends 1,069 miles north to the summit of Mount Katahdin in Maine and south to the summit of Springer Mountain in Georgia. Just beyond the halfway point, you'll pass a clearing surrounded by pines and in a few minutes reach Railroad Bed Road by Mountain Creek.

From the A.T., the most direct route back to your car—and the most common—is along the paved road with the cars. A more pleasant alternative is to follow the Mountain Creek Trail through the woods just north of the road. This less-traveled path follows and crosses Mountain Creek through wetlands and provides considerably more opportunity for viewing wildlife than the road. Mountain Creek is habitat for beaver and mink, though both are rather elusive. But you'll never have a chance of encountering either if you follow the road. At this writing, the creek had recently flooded, making the trail a little indistinct in a few places, particularly near the end where it rejoins the railroad grade; however, the view of the flood debris itself is worth the trek. The trail is well marked with red blazes the entire length, and with some care at the end, you should have no trouble following it.

To make this 1.5 mile excursion, turn right on Railroad Bed Road and after about 100 yards you'll see a trailhead on the left identified by a sign that says FOOT TRAFFIC ONLY. Turn left onto the trail and follow the red blazes generally along the course of the creek through the woods. About 0.75 miles from the trailhead, the trail crosses the creek at a good log crossing, obviously constructed since the floods. I've often seen white-tailed deer bedded down in the area north of the creek. At about 1.4 miles, the trail enters a small clearing at the edge of the creek, and then veers left away from the creek into a wetlands area. Finding the route gets a little tricky around here, as the blazes seem to disappear for a short distance. Look to your left, away from the creek, and you should see a small footbridge over a braided stream, which at the time of this writing was in disrepair due to the flood. Balance over the bridge into the wetlands area, and you should begin to see blazes again. After about 25 yards, you'll cross another stream braided over some timbers. Just beyond these timbers, the obvious trail continues straight; however, keep your eyes trained to your right for the red blazes and a less distinct path onto which you will turn right (about 20 feet beyond the timbers). Follow this to the cul-de-sac at the end of Ice House Road and a good bridge over Mountain Creek. The trail gets much more well defined in the area of Ice House Road.

If you should miss the path, you will come quickly to a presentation area with benches and a fire ring beneath some cabins on a small hill. These are all part of a YMCA camp. Turn back and look for the junction. If you still have difficulty locating it, return to the presentation area and pass it through the woods, keeping it to your left, following the hillside with the cabins above. You will meet the trail within 50 yards or so near the bank of creek. Cross the good bridge over the creek, turn left on the road, and follow it for 0.25 miles back to your car.

NEARBY ACTIVITIES

Pine Grove Furnace State Park is a wonderful place with loads of activities. It has two lakes with swimming areas, picnic areas, biking and hiking trails, and the site of the old Pine Grove Furnace. It also has a wonderful campground. Your best bet is to stop by the park office at the intersection of PA 233 and Pine Grove Road for a park map and information on current events.

54 ROCKY KNOB

KEY AT-A-GLANCE INFORMATION

LENGTH: 4.3 miles

CONFIGURATION: Loop

DIFFICULTY: Easy–moderate

SCENERY: Mountain-laurel highlands and beautiful view of Lone Pine Run Reservoir

EXPOSURE: Mostly shade

TRAIL TRAFFIC: Moderate

TRAIL SURFACE: Dirt

HIKING TIME: 2–2.5 hours

DRIVING DISTANCE: 18.5 miles from Interstate 81 and PA 233 south of Carlisle

ACCESS: Dawn–dusk

MAPS: USGS Caledonia Park; Michaux State Forest public-use map; *Appalachian Trail, PA Route 94 to US Route 30 (Sections 12 and 13)*

FACILITIES: None

WHEELCHAIR TRAVERSABLE: No

SPECIAL COMMENTS: A popular hike in South Mountain that never gets too crowded.

GPS Trailhead Coordinates

UTM Zone (WGS84) 18S

Easting 291534

Northing 4428194

Latitude N 39° 58′ 41.59″

Longitude W 77° 26′ 28.67″

IN BRIEF

This hike follows the Rocky Knob Trail from Ridge Road south over Sier Hill to a saddle beneath Rocky Knob. From the saddle, the hike descends into a hollow and follows an old Civilian Conservation Corps (CCC) road back to the trailhead. An additional spur leads through the lower hollow from the junction with the CCC road out to a trailhead on Birch Run Road to the south.

DESCRIPTION

If you have any doubts about what mountain laurel looks like, this hike should alleviate those doubts forever. In late May and early June, the woods are filled with blossoms unlike any place I have seen before. During the summer, the forest is thick with the understory. Come autumn, the terrain begins to thin out a little bit and the trees put on a brilliant display of color.

This hike begins by following an old roadbed south from the parking area. The road was constructed by the CCC in 1937 in an attempt to make a connecting road between Ridge Road to the north and Birch Run Road to the south. The project was unsuccessful,

Directions

From Interstate 81, take Exit 37 (Newville/ Pa 233). Follow PA 233 south for 14 miles to Shippensburg Road. Turn right on Shippensburg Road and follow it up the ridge for 2.5 miles to Ridge Road on the left. Turn left and follow Ridge Road for 2 miles to the parking area. The parking area is on the right and it has room for five or six cars. The trailhead is directly across the road, identified by a forest usage sign. Just past the trailhead on Ridge Road is a wooden milepost marked Number 10.

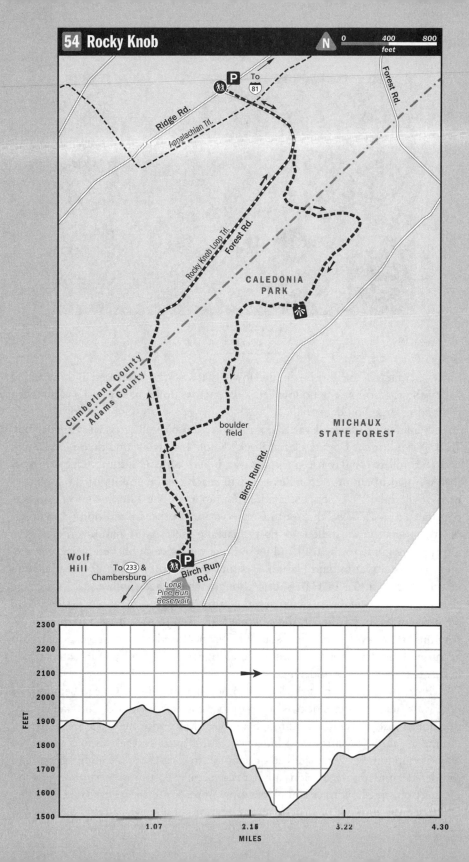

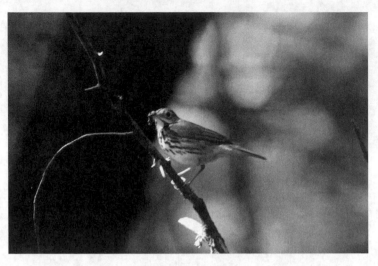

Ovenbird

however, due to the terrain in the lower part of the unnamed hollow along which the road runs. The hollow gets very narrow down below and its flanks are covered in large boulders.

A couple of hundred yards along the road, you will cross the Appalachian Trail. A sign for the orange-blazed Rocky Knob Trail is located there, explaining that the trail is for day-use purposes and hikers only. Continue straight across the A.T. and in about 0.25 miles you will reach the beginning of the loop section of the hike by a signpost marked Number 1. The Rocky Knob Loop was constructed in 1977 by the Youth Conservation Corps. In addition to completing the trail, they installed 14 posts marking stations of natural interest. An interpretive guide to the trail and its stations was once published by the Department of Conservation and Natural Resources. I found a copy several years ago at the DCNR office in Harrisburg, though I have been unable to locate one since. The trail remains pretty much the same, though several of the posts have been removed. In particular, the original trail used to include a side spur to the summit of Rocky Knob. That spur has been closed in recent years, perhaps because of incidents that have occurred along it and difficulty of maintenance—it was extremely steep and rugged.

From the beginning of the loop, turn left leaving the CCC road behind. The hike walks much better clockwise than it does counterclockwise. The trail continues along mostly level terrain through a forest of oak with the thick understory of mountain laurel, sassafras, and blueberry. You'll pass several stations along the way. Station number 2 provides an orientation to forest strata, calling attention to the diverse understory. Station number 3 was marked to call attention to examples of tropisms, how trees and plants grow in response to the available light that makes its way through the forest canopy. Station number 4 is a fairly obvious one pointing out a colony and mound built by Allegheny mound-building ants, one of several such mounds alongside the trail.

As the trail continues, you will contour around the edge of Sier Hill. During the fall and winter you'll have nice views to the east across Birch Run Hollow. At 1.4 miles, you'll reach station number 9, an overlook that offers an excellent view to the southeast of Lone Pine Run Reservoir and the South Mountain countryside. From there, the trail continues along a ridge until a set of double blazes marks the beginning of a descent to the saddle between Sier Hill and Rocky Knob. The descent is short, but rather steep and requires care. Upon reaching the saddle, the terrain levels out and at station number 10 you will be at a point just below the large quartzite boulder field that forms the north shoulder of Rocky Knob. The boulders are huge. This is a nice place to take a break in the shade.

Continue from the saddle down the trail toward the west. The arrangement of station posts gets a little confusing here as the next two posts you pass will be numbered 7 and 8. About 50 yards beyond them is the junction with the old summit spur. Please refrain from exploring as the terrain is closed and quite hazardous. At about 2.4 miles, you will reach the lower end of the CCC road at station 13. To complete the hike, turn right and follow the road up a steady but gentle hill for nearly 2 miles back to the trailhead.

A worthwhile side trip begins at station 13 and follows the recently constructed footpath down the hollow out to Birch Run Road at the Lone Pine Run Reservoir. The walk through this lower part of the hollow is quite beautiful as it is filled with thick rhododendrons growing along the banks of the creek. The trail stays to the left (east) of the creek for most of the way before crossing it a couple of hundred yards shy of Birch Run Road. It is marked for its length with prolific orange blazes. Walking the lower section adds about a mile to the loop hike.

You might alternately begin the excursion from Birch Run Road rather than from Ridge Road. The trailhead is located about 50 feet past the guardrail to the west on Birch Run Road.

NEARBY ACTIVITIES

Pine Grove Furnace State Park on PA 233 to the north has two lakes with swimming areas, picnic area, biking and hiking trails, and the site of the old Pine Grove Furnace. It also has a wonderful campground. Your best bet is to stop by the park office at the intersection of PA 233 and Pine Grove Road for a park map and information on current events.

55 ROCKY RIDGE COUNTY PARK

KEY AT-A-GLANCE INFORMATION

LENGTH: 4.8 miles

CONFIGURATION: Loop

DIFFICULTY: Moderate

SCENERY: Nice walk through the woods, 2 nice views at park overlooks

EXPOSURE: More shade than sun

TRAIL TRAFFIC: Moderate

TRAIL SURFACE: Dirt and cinders, some sections of paved

HIKING TIME: About 2.5 hours

DRIVING DISTANCE: About 3 miles from US 30 and PA 24 east of York

ACCESS: 8 a.m.–dusk

MAPS: USGS York Haven; a park map of the trails is available at parking areas.

FACILITIES: Toilets and water available at parking area

WHEELCHAIR TRAVERSABLE: No

SPECIAL COMMENTS: A good hike for warbler-watching in the spring

IN BRIEF

This hike follows several of the park trails along the south perimeter of the park before visiting the north overlook and returning to the car.

DESCRIPTION

Located on a ridgetop just a few miles northeast of York, the 750-acre Rocky Ridge County Park is a popular location for local bird-watchers. During the spring, it is visited by a variety of warblers, including black and white warblers, ovenbirds, chestnut-sided warblers, redstarts, blue warblers, yellow throats, and green warblers. In both the fall and spring, the two park overlooks provide excellent vantage points from which to view the seasonal hawk migrations. And the woods are home to a variety of woodland species, including scarlet tanager, thrushes, nuthatches, yellow-billed cuckoo, blue jays, downy woodpeckers, and flycatchers. It is a popular park that can be crowded on weekends, though you can always find some degree of solitude on the many trails that traverse its pretty oak forest.

This hike begins from the parking lot for the Wildlife Picnic Area, the first area on the right as you enter the park. Walk out of the back of the parking lot by a NO PARKING sign

GPS Trailhead Coordinates

UTM Zone (WGS84) 18T

Easting   358122

Northing   4429977

Latitude   N 40° 00′ 29.09″

Longitude   W 76° 39′ 44.19″

Directions

From US 30 east of York, take the Mount Zion (PA 24) exit and follow PA 24 north for 1.25 miles to Deininger Road. Turn right on Deininger Road and follow it into the park. Park in the Wildlife Picnic Area parking lot, the first picnic area on the right.

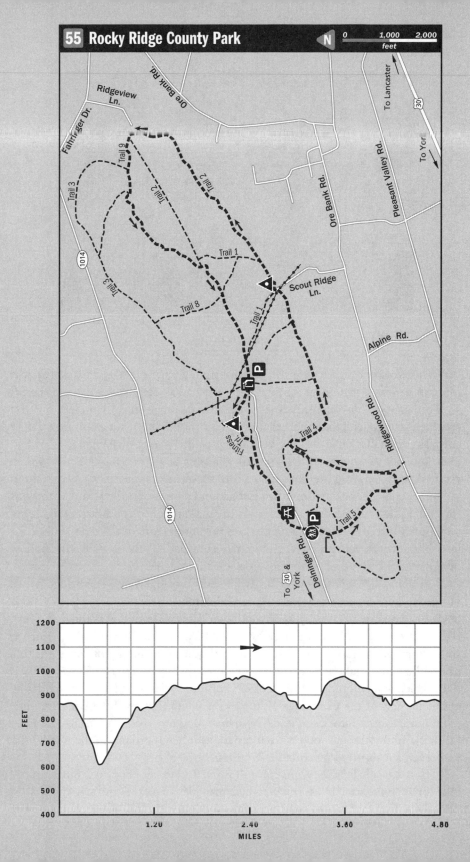

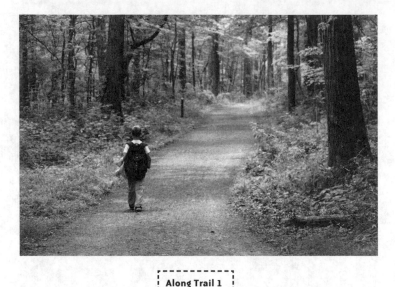

Along Trail 1

between two spruce trees onto the obvious trail, a wide old logging path. Follow the trail to where it forks at a bench and turn left. Green-fiberglass signposts for Trail 5 mark both directions. In a short distance, another Trail 5 goes left, but you continue straight, and then another trail heads off to right. Again, continue straight and pass through a small clearing with many wildflowers growing in it.

At about 0.25 miles, you'll come to a half-log bench at a trail junction where you will veer left. You are now on Trail 6. Descend a rather steep, washed-out section of hillside, passing some water bars and another trail junction with signs for Trail 6. Just beyond that intersection, the main roadbed continues straight, but our route on Trail 6 goes left at an obvious turn onto more of a footpath. Traverse into a hollow just above a creek and join a major path. Walk up the scenic hollow on a nice dirt trail passing some lovely rock outcrops.

At about 0.9 miles, Trail 6 turns left and crosses over a footbridge by an old pump house. Stay to the right here and climb for a short distance to a foot-bridge across a small creek. Just beyond, you'll reach Trail 4, a major path. Turn right and cross another footbridge by a bench. Continue along Trail 4, which is smooth and level, staying right at all the trail junctions, until you come out to a power line and a junction with a major gravel path (1.8 miles). This is Trail 1, onto which you will turn right. An observation deck lies ahead and it provides an excellent view of the Conestoga Valley to the south. Follow Trail 1 for a couple of hundred yards into the woods to a dirt footpath that departs to the right (Trail 2). Turn right and follow the footpath as it bends around to the north until you reach a major trail junction (2.75 miles).

Trail 2 heads left here. You can follow that (and cut about 0.2 miles off the hike) or continue straight on Trail 9, which provides a nice trek through the woods. Following Trail 9, you will soon pass the junction with Trail 3, descending quite

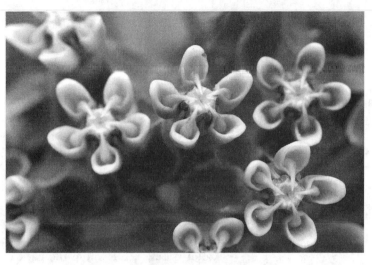

Common milkweed

precipitously to the right. Continue straight, traversing the hill first descending and then ascending. Soon Trail 9 reaches the ridge again where it joins the wide gravel path of Trail 1, just 100 feet west of where that trail and Trail 2 come together. Turn right on Trail 1, and follow it to the large parking area (3.9 miles).

Walk through the lot angling toward its northwest corner, near some restrooms. Pick up the gravel path leading to the north observation deck, and walk out to the deck past some cherry trees. You'll have a view from the observation deck that will give you a good idea of how the park got its name. From the observation deck, follow the Fitness Trail straight into the woods. (Don't follow the path that heads downhill!) Hike along the Fitness Trail to a trail junction. Turn right and follow the path alongside the park road for a couple of tenths of a mile until you reach the pavilions at the Hidden Laurel Picnic Area (4.6 miles). Walk through the picnic area, across the parking lot, and then across the park road into the Wildlife Picnic Area parking lot to your car.

NEARBY ACTIVITIES

With its picnic pavilions, playgrounds, volleyball court, and trails, the park is the obvious location for additional activities. However, if you want a real treat, take a tour of the Harley-Davidson motorcycle factory just a few miles away in York. Information on tours is available at **www.harley-davidson.com.**

56 SAMUEL S. LEWIS STATE PARK LOOP

KEY AT-A-GLANCE INFORMATION

LENGTH: 1.3 miles

CONFIGURATION: Loop

DIFFICULTY: Easy

SCENERY: Nice views of York and Lancaster counties

EXPOSURE: More sun than shade

TRAIL TRAFFIC: Heavy

TRAIL SURFACE: Dirt with stretches of paved trail

HIKING TIME: 45 minutes–1 hour

DRIVING DISTANCE: 2.8 miles from US 30 at Wrightsville

ACCESS: Dawn–dusk

MAPS: USGS Red Lion; park map

FACILITIES: Restrooms, water, picnic facilities

WHEELCHAIR TRAVERSABLE: No, but the park roads and summit of Mount Pisgah are accessible by wheelchair.

SPECIAL COMMENTS: The meadow in the center of the park is popular with kite-flying enthusiasts.

GPS Trailhead Coordinates

UTM Zone (WGS84) 18S

Easting 367670

Northing 4428479

Latitude N 39° 59′ 46.10″

Longitude W 76° 33′ 0.53″

IN BRIEF

Following the established Hill Top Trail, this pleasant hike makes a loop around the perimeter of Samuel S. Lewis State Park just below the top of Mount Pisgah, finishing on the hilltop.

DESCRIPTION

Samuel S. Lewis State Park is located atop the 885-foot Mount Pisgah in east central York County. Lewis, for whom the park is named, served as Secretary of the Pennsylvania Department of Forest and Waters from 1951 to 1954. He also served as Secretary of Highways under Gifford Pinchot during his term as governor.

The park was opened in 1954 and was initially cobbled together from three tracts of land: some farmland owned by Lewis, an arboretum owned by Walter Stine that is still part of the park, and an additional tract of farmland owned by a local family. The park is located on an upland layer of the Piedmont Physiographic Province in Pennsylvania, consisting mostly of rolling farmland, south of the Cumberland Valley and east of South Mountain. The park is part of the Pennsylvania Trail of Geology and a comprehensive guide to its geology and the surrounding countryside is available at the park.

This short hike provides a loop around the park and to the top of Mount Pisgah. The park tends to be rather busy, especially on weekends, but it is a lovely place for a picnic and a walk. This hike is a great outing with the

Directions ────────────────→

From US 30 east of York, take the Wrightsville exit and head south on Cool Creek Road about 1.5 miles. Turn right on Mount Pisgah Road. The park entrance will be ahead on your left.

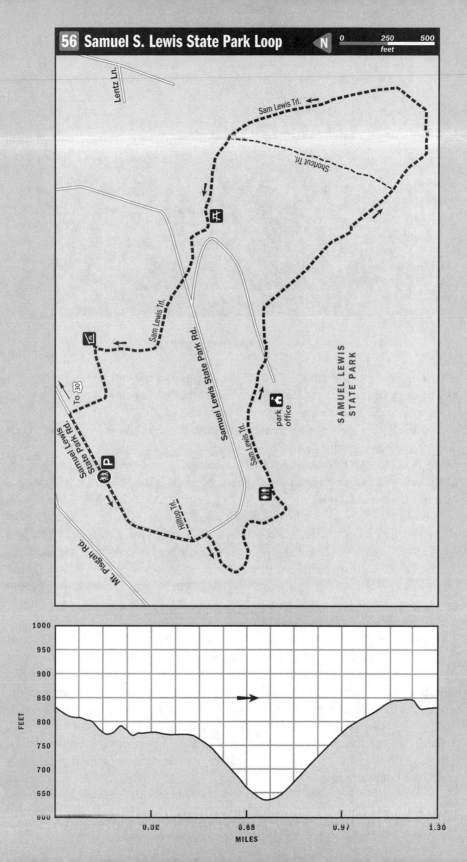

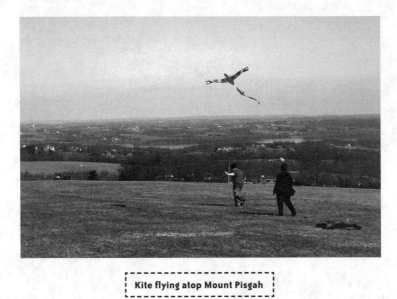

Kite flying atop Mount Pisgah

kids, and the views toward the Susquehanna River and the east are expansive. On a clear day you can see as far as Governor Dick Hill in Lebanon County, 18 miles to the northeast, and the Safe Harbor Dam to the south.

Being higher than the surrounding terrain, the park always seems to have a nice breeze blowing through it, even in the summer. Be sure to bring a kite for flying from the top of Mount Pisgah. The hilltop's exposure, however, does subject it to some rather high winds at times. Much of the arboretum, in fact, has suffered from wind damage.

Begin this hike by walking out of the main parking area west and south along the park road. In about 200 yards, you'll come to a sign for the Hill Top Trail entering the woods on the right. Turn right and follow the orange blazes through a beautiful stand of old fir trees with an understory of mountain laurel and holly bushes. At the end of the fir trees, you'll pass some restrooms and then cut downhill across a large meadow toward the park maintenance building and office.

Cross the road by the park office and follow the trail along the shoulder of the park road south toward a playground. When you reach the playground, turn right on the path and follow it downhill into the woods. Before it descends, a dirt road departs to the right. That road leads a couple of hundred yards back into the woods before ending at private property.

After about 0.7 miles, you'll pass the junction with the Short Cut Trail, departing to the left. If you don't feel like doing the lower part of the loop to see a beautiful stand of pine trees, turn left here; you'll reach the Hill Top Trail in a couple of hundred yards, saving about 0.3 miles. Otherwise, continue downhill for a short distance farther. The trail bends left across the hillside and enters a meadow with a beautiful grove of mature pine trees. Walk across the field, turn

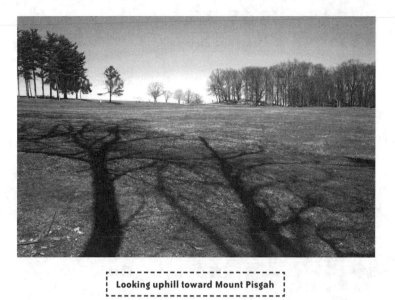

Looking uphill toward Mount Pisgah

left and follow the fence line and the pine grove uphill for about 0.25 miles to the upper junction with the Short Cut Trail, entering from your left.

From the junction, angle left toward the rock outcrop and pass it to its right. At the end of the rocks, you'll find some picnic tables near the park road. Cross the road and make a beeline for the pavilion in the middle of the large meadow on the top of the hill. The park arboretum will be to your left as you make your way up the hill and is worth a walk over to visit. Several trees are marked with plaques identifying them. European beech, persimmon, English yew, among other trees can be found there.

The pavilion atop Mount Pisgah offers shade and picnic benches, and the meadow surrounding it offers the best views and best kite-flying in the park. You'll find an interpretive sign that identifies some of the points on the distant landscape at the pavilion. To return to your car, walk along the paved path from the pavilion back to the parking area.

NEARBY ACTIVITIES

Aside from the attractions of hiking and kite-flying, the park has many picnic tables and a ball field. The hilltop is a wonderful place for viewing the stars, and local clubs often organize stargazing events in the park. Contact the park for information: (717) 432-5011.

57 STRAWBERRY HILL NATURE PRESERVE

KEY AT-A-GLANCE INFORMATION

LENGTH: 4.5 miles

CONFIGURATION: Loop

DIFFICULTY: Moderate

SCENERY: Beautiful woodlands

EXPOSURE: Shade

TRAIL TRAFFIC: Light

TRAIL SURFACE: Dirt

HIKING TIME: 2–3 hours

DRIVING DISTANCE: About 13 miles from US 15 and US 30 east of Gettysburg

ACCESS: Dawn–dusk

MAPS: USGS Iron Springs; a trail map is available at the trailhead.

FACILITIES: Portable toilets and pump water

WHEELCHAIR TRAVERSABLE: No

SPECIAL COMMENTS: The nature preserve is a wonderful place for kids, and many shorter variations of this hike can be made as needed.

GPS Trailhead Coordinates

UTM Zone (WGS84) 18S

Easting 293302

Northing 4408721

Latitude N 39° 48′ 12.09″

Longitude W 77° 24′ 52.03″

IN BRIEF

This hike follows the Nature Trail out of the parking area to the Swamp Creek Spur and the Swamp Creek Trail, east of the creek. Near the confluence of Swamp Creek's east and west forks, the hike picks up the 4-mile Foothills Trail loop, which circumnavigates private land before rejoining Swamp Creek Trail west of the creek.

DESCRIPTION

I learned about the Strawberry Hill Nature Center from Audubon Pennsylvania's *Susquehanna River Birding and Wildlife Trail Guide*. It is a little-known gem of an area well worth the trip. Located just 9 miles from Gettysburg in a valley in the southeast section of South Mountain, the center and preserve are oriented toward the interests of nature lovers. It has more than 12 miles of trails that wind through mature forest and wetlands. The nature center has an exhibit on the local flora and fauna, and provides educational programs for school groups and the public

The tract of land on which the center is located was established in 1986 by Hans and

Directions ————————————→

From US 15 east of Gettysburg, follow US 30 west through the center of town. At the traffic circle, head south on Business 15 to PA 116 west (one block south of the circle). Turn right onto PA 116 and follow it south for 7.2 miles to Bullfrog Road on the right. Turn right on Bullfrog Road and follow it to a stop sign (1 mile). After the stop sign, Bullfrog Road turns to Mount Hope Road. The parking area is about 2 miles along Mount Hope Road on the left. The trailhead is directly across the street next to a small pond and cabin.

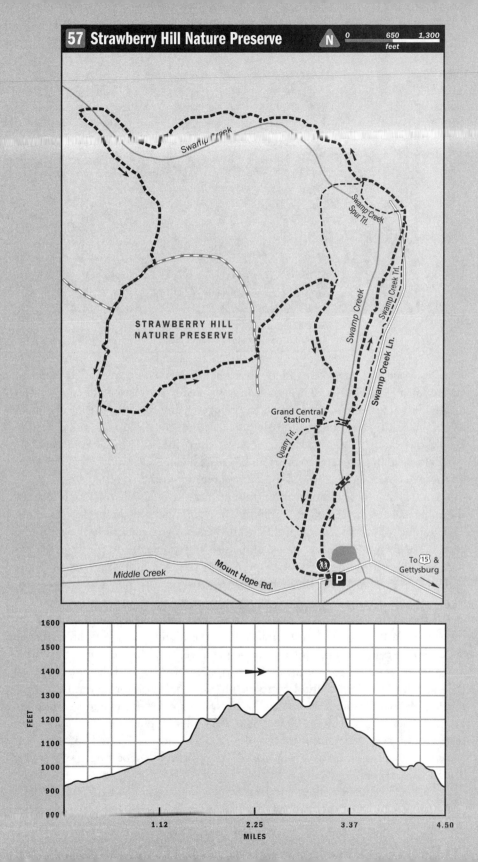

N

| 0 | 650 | 1,300 |

feet

Swamp Creek

Swamp Creek Spur Trl.

Swamp Creek

Swamp Creek Trl.

Swamp Creek Ln.

**STRAWBERRY HILL
NATURE PRESERVE**

Grand Central
Station

Quarry Trl.

Middle Creek

Mount Hope Rd.

To 15 &
Gettysburg

P

FEET

1600
1500
1400
1300
1200
1100
1000
900
900

MILES

1.12   2.25   3.37   4.50

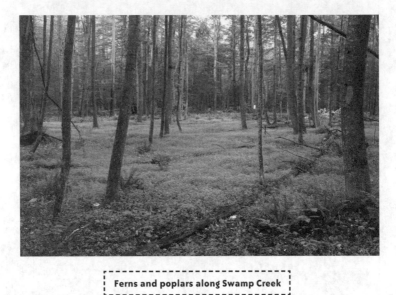

Ferns and poplars along Swamp Creek

Frances Froelicher, who sought to preserve its natural beauty and to support environmental education. The Froelichers originally purchased the small pond located just across the road from the nature center. In order to preserve the quality of the pond water, they gradually purchased much of the land along Swamp Creek, the watershed that feeds the pond, creating the 500 plus-acre preserve.

This hike links several of the trails to create a nice loop around the perimeter of the nature preserve. From the parking area, cross the street toward the log cabin and hiking information station (trail maps are available here). Continue past the cabin and follow the Nature Trail into the pines next to the preserve's pond. The Nature Trail is marked by prolific white blazes. Cross a footbridge over to the east side of Swamp Creek in a forest of mature tulip poplars, and continue following the wide path aside the creek. You'll soon see pink blazes, which mark the path of the Swamp Creek Trail. Just before crossing a second footbridge, turn right onto the Swamp Creek Trail, which follows the old Fort Chamber Road.

After about 200 feet, the Swamp Creek Spur (also blazed in pink) heads to the left while the Swamp Creek Trail follows the roadbed to the right. The spur is the most recent addition of trails to the preserve, and it passes through what is arguably the prettiest part of the preserve as it hugs the bank of the creek. Follow the spur through the beautiful bottomlands for a half mile or so until it reconnects with the Swamp Creek Trail in an area of thick ferns and tall poplars (1 mile). Turn left, and after 100 feet or so the trail and spur split again for a short distance. Stay on the trail this time, and in 100 yards or so the trail and spur join again by junction with the green-blazed Foothills Trail, departing to the right. A trail sign marks the junction.

Turn right onto the Foothills Trail, which follows an old haul road initially and then departs from the roadbed to avoid private property. The trail gets rather rugged for a short distance as it winds through some swampy and rocky woods, crossing several boards. The green blazes are abundant, however, so finding your way should be no problem. Soon the trail becomes more distinct, and it makes a sharp right turn uphill and then joins with a good road heading left and passing beneath some clear areas.

Follow the path as it wanders through the upper part of the hollow in a beautiful forest of huge tulip poplars, beech trees, and carcasses of old pine trees filled with holes that make wonderful nesting places for owls, woodpeckers, and squirrels. At about 2 miles, you'll reach a small clearing at a gated road. Turn left and cross the creek. Shortly thereafter, the trail makes a sharp left turn into the woods at a turn marked by double green blazes. Follow the path left, traversing the top of the hollow. If you come to this area in July, be ready to spend some time sampling the wild raspberries.

After passing through the hollow, you'll reach a significant dirt road (2.5 miles) onto which you'll turn right. Follow that past an old cabin to an intersection where the main road goes to the right. Continue straight at the intersection, following the green blazes downhill on an old roadbed for a fair distance until you come to a junction with another dirt road, marked by green blazes (2.9 miles). Turn left and climb for a ways, passing some private property on the right before crossing over a ridgetop. The trail descends quite steeply from the ridge for a short distance before meeting up with another significant dirt road below. Turn left on this road and follow it for about 50 feet to a place where the green blazes head off to the right downhill along a smaller road. Turn right and follow the path around to the right, dropping into Swamp Creek. Soon you'll reach the Swamp Creek Trail again (3.7 miles), at which point you will turn right.

Continue walking along the trail above the creek until you reach a major junction of trails, called Grand Central Station. It is marked by a sign and has a nice bench where you can rest your weary feet. From Grand Central Station, continue straight following white blazes past the red-blazed Quarry Trail on the right. Shortly afterward, you'll reach the parking area and the log house.

NEARBY ACTIVITIES

You can take in the scenery at the pond, which has a platform for turtles to sun themselves, or visit the nature center. Gettysburg National Military Park is 9 miles to the northeast. Visiting there after a hike at Strawberry Hill makes for a reasonable and full day.

58 SUNSET ROCKS

KEY AT-A-GLANCE INFORMATION

LENGTH: 8.1 miles

CONFIGURATION: Balloon

DIFFICULTY: Moderate hiking with some difficult scrambling on Little Rocky Ridge

SCENERY: Forest, Toms Run, excellent views of South Mountain area

EXPOSURE: Mostly shade

TRAIL TRAFFIC: Generally light

TRAIL SURFACE: Dirt

HIKING TIME: 4–5 hours

DRIVING DISTANCE: 7.3 miles from Interstate 81 and PA 233 south of Carlisle

ACCESS: Open

MAPS: USGS Dickinson; Michaux State Forest public-use map; *Appalachian Trail, PA Route 94 to US Route 30 (Sections 12 and 13)*

FACILITIES: Water and restrooms near trailhead in Pine Grove Furnace State Park

WHEELCHAIR TRAVERSABLE: No

SPECIAL COMMENTS: The scrambling over Little Rocky Ridge can be time-consuming and is not a good place for young children. A good pair of boots is useful for this hike. Walk the loop section of this hike counterclockwise.

IN BRIEF

This popular hike follows the Appalachian Trail from Pine Grove Furnace State Park for several miles to the Toms Run Shelters. Just beyond the shelters, it picks up the Sunset Rocks Trail and follows that over Sunset Rocks and Little Rocky Ridge back to the Appalachian Trail, about 1.5 miles from the parking area.

DESCRIPTION

Aside from passing through some extraordinarily beautiful forest and by the ruins of Camp Michaux, this hike offers some of the best views in South Mountain from the Little Rocky Ridge. You'll want to take extra care on the ridge, as traversing it requires scrambling over and among several large rock outcrops.

Begin this hike at the parking area next to the general store at Pine Grove Furnace State Park. Walk past the front of the store and turn right onto the first road and follow it out to PA 233 following the white Appalachian Trail blazes. At the stop sign, turn left and walk along the shoulder for about 0.25 miles. Turn right and cross the road at the A.T. sign and follow the blazes along a dirt road, past private property, through a forest of pine trees and tall oak trees. The trail is lined with a thick understory of rose hips and honeysuckle.

GPS Trailhead Coordinates

UTM Zone (WGS84) 18T

Easting 303205

Northing 4433909

Latitude N 40° 1′ 56.88″

Longitude W 77° 18′ 23.25″

Directions

From Interstate 81, take Exit 37 (Newville/ PA 233). Follow PA 233 south for 7.8 miles to the intersection with Hunters Run Road at Pine Grove Furnace State Park. After PA 233 turns right, turn left toward the campground, furnace stack, and general store. Park in the large parking area on the right, next to the general store.

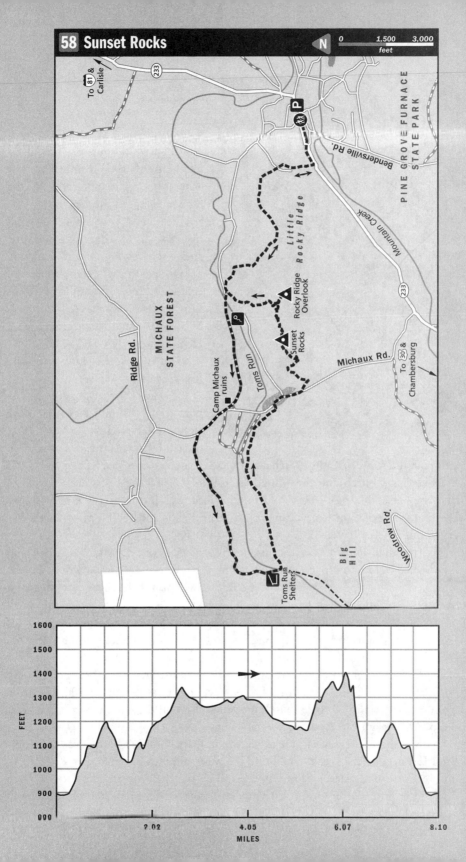

58 Sunset Rocks

N

0   1,500   3,000
feet

To 81 &
Carlisle

233

PINE GROVE FURNACE STATE PARK

P

Bendersville Rd.

Mountain Creek

Little Rocky Ridge

233

Rocky Ridge Overlook

Sunset Rocks

Michaux Rd.

To 30 &
Chambersburg

MICHAUX STATE FOREST

Ridge Rd.

Toms Run

Camp Michaux ruins

Woodrow Rd.

Big Hill

Toms Run Shelters

Elevation Profile

FEET	
1600	
1500	
1400	
1300	
1200	
1100	
1000	
900	
000	

2.02   4.05   6.07   8.10

MILES

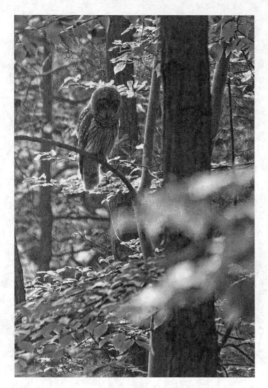

Barred owl

Soon you'll cross a little creek and then wind your way through a lovely forest to the footbridge over Toms Run. The east end of the Sunset Rocks Trail departs to the left here, and you can follow that directly up to the ridge and the rocks, making an out-and-back trip of about 3 (very steep!) miles. To follow our hike, though, cross Toms Run and follow the A.T. along a hillside to a significant gravel road. Head to your left on the road and follow that past the Halfway Spring (on the left).

Follow the road for a distance until the A.T. leaves it to the right under some telephone lines (2.3 miles). In 100 yards or so, you will pass the ruins of Camp Michaux. Once a church camp shared by the United Presbyterian Church and the United Church of Christ, the ruins are unusual in that they resemble more of an old military outpost. Interestingly, it served as a Civilian Conservation Corps camp during the 1930s and then a prisoner of war camp during World War II.

After admiring the scenic ruins, follow the A.T. out to Michaux Road and then to the right and along the road to where the trail reenters the woods on the left (2.65 miles). Upon entering the woods, you will pass through some of the most beautiful fern-filled forest you can imagine. Saunter your way through this small paradise. In another mile, you'll cross a small, shallow, sandy creek with a NO CAMPING AREA sign. Just beyond, you'll reach the Toms Run Shelters (3.85 miles).

When I did this hike, the first thing that I noticed upon reaching the shelters was a healthy population of chipmunks. When I sat down for a break, I had the good fortune of seeing a beautiful barred owl land in a tree about 100 feet away from me. The sighting made sense, of course. With all the chipmunks in the area, the owl had plenty to feed on.

From the shelters, continue along the A.T. for 100 feet or so, crossing Toms Run. Just beyond the creek, you'll find the west terminus of the Sunset Rocks Trail on your left (blue blazes). Turn left and follow that path over some rocky terrain through an unusual hollow filled with saplings of what appear to be red birch trees. You'll pass two small clearings, the second of which you'll skirt to the right.

At the far end of it, look to your left and you will see one of the largest ant mounds you can imagine. Also note: I found both of the clearings to be populated by an inordinately large number of bees. I didn't get stung, but if you have allergies, you should bear this in mind.

Follow the trail through a swampy area, over some decrepit boardwalks, and past a large forest management area on the right. This is an excellent place to see pileated woodpeckers. Continue past the clearing until you come out to Michaux Road. Turn right and follow the shoulder over the crest of a hill for about 0.3 miles. The trail reenters woods on the left, just beyond the crest by a private drive numbered 111 (5.25 miles). You'll find double blazes on a tree to the right of the drive.

Follow the trail back into the woods, passing a nearby private residence on the left. Continue uphill into the woods until you reach the Little Rocky Ridge by a couple of boulders. This is a good rest spot and it offers a nice view to the south.

Follow the blazes along the ridge uphill to the east. As you progress farther along the ridge, the going gets more rugged and you'll need to be prepared to do some scrambling and some route finding. It is an amazing ridge, however, with quartzite rock outcrops among hickory, oak, black gum, and pine trees. Mountain laurel grows from the crevices, and the views are incredible.

Working your way across the ridge is a rather time-consuming proposition, and at times the blazes can be a little mystifying. Just continue your way among the rocks, resisting the temptation to descend some inviting deer path too soon. Follow the ridge to a prominent saddle with blazes and a *very obvious* and well traveled descent path to the left (6 miles). From the saddle, a small side path takes you farther out on the Little Rocky Ridge to a wonderful, vertiginous overlook after about 200 yards. The walk to the overlook is worth every bit of effort and is a great place for a long rest. It has arguably the nicest view in South Mountain and definitely on the hike.

From the overlook, return to the saddle and follow the descent trail downhill to the north for about 0.6 miles, at which point you will reach the eastern terminus of the trail at the Toms Run crossing on the A.T. Turn right and follow the A.T. back to your car at Pine Grove Furnace.

NEARBY ACTIVITIES

Pine Grove Furnace State Park on PA 233 to the north has two lakes with swimming areas, picnic areas, biking and hiking trails, and the site of the old Pine Grove Furnace. It also has a wonderful campground. Your best bet is to stop by the park office at the intersection of PA 233 and Hunters Run Road for a park map and information on current events.

59 WHITE ROCKS AND CENTER POINT KNOB

 KEY AT-A-GLANCE INFORMATION

LENGTH: 3.25 miles

CONFIGURATION: Out-and-back

DIFFICULTY: Easy–moderate

SCENERY: Quartzite outcrops and nice views of South Mountain area

EXPOSURE: Mostly shade

TRAIL TRAFFIC: Moderate

TRAIL SURFACE: Dirt

HIKING TIME: 2 hours

DRIVING DISTANCE: About 22 miles from US 11 and PA 641 west of Harrisburg

ACCESS: Open; on state-forest land

MAPS: USGS Mechanicsburg and Dillsburg

FACILITIES: None

WHEELCHAIR TRAVERSABLE: No

SPECIAL COMMENTS: Be cautious about loose rocks when passing over the outcrops, because rock climbers may be below you.

GPS Trailhead Coordinates

UTM Zone (WGS84) 18T

Easting 322083

Northing 4444569

Latitude N 40° 7′ 57.48″

Longitude W 77° 5′ 17.84″

IN BRIEF

This pleasant hike follows the White Rocks Trail from Kuhn Road up to and over White Rocks to the Appalachian Trail below Center Point Knob. A short walk along the A.T. takes you to the top of the Knob before retracing the route back to the car.

DESCRIPTION

This hike offers some lovely scenery, with large quartzite rock outcrops (popular with area rock climbers), a beautiful understory of mountain laurel, and great views. It is the only place that I have seen a gray fox, which makes it distinctive in my mind. It would be a nice hike to do with older kids, though some care needs to be taken passing the rock outcrops.

The hike begins at the prominent blue-blazed trail, about 100 feet uphill and along the shoulder of Kuhn Road from a yellow forest gate. You may begin from the gate. If you

----

Directions ⟶

From US 11 west of Harrisburg, take PA 641 (Trindle Road) west toward Mechanicsburg. Follow PA 641 for 7 miles to PA 174 (Boiling Spring Road). Turn left and follow PA 174 for about 12 miles to Boiling Springs. Keep your eyes open for the Allenberry Resort and Playhouse on the left just before Boiling Springs. After passing the Allenberry, look for Bucher Hill Road on the left. Turn left and follow that alongside the pond and town park. Turn left onto Mountain Road at the stop sign before crossing the pond. Cross over Yellow Breeches Creek and turn left onto Ledigh Drive. Follow Ledigh Drive for 1.8 miles to Kuhn Road. Turn right. The parking area is about 0.7 miles along Kuhn Road on the right by a yellow gate. The main trailhead is about 100 feet farther up the road. It has a sign and a set of blue blazes.

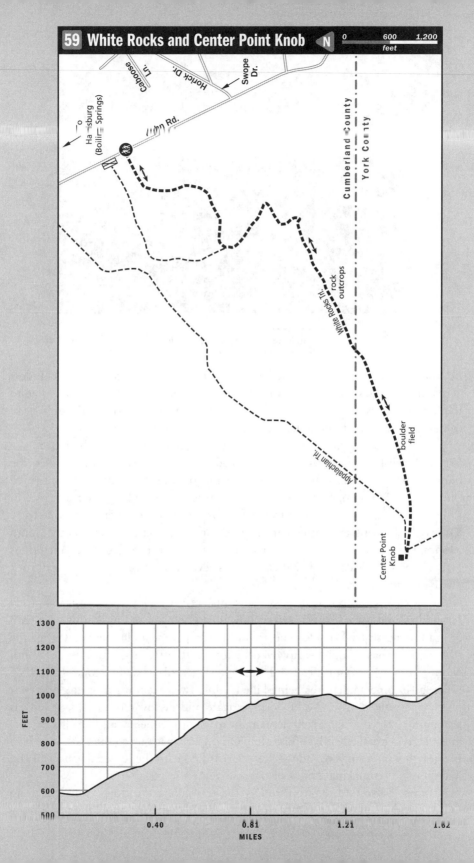

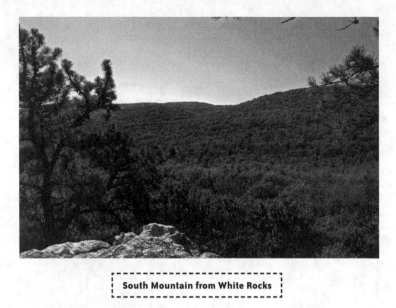

South Mountain from White Rocks

do, follow the dirt road behind it for about 200 feet or so to three large boulders across an old track to your left, turn left, and in another 100 feet or so come to the blue-blazed trail. Turn right. If you continue past those boulders, you'll need to make some route-finding decisions and pass by private land.

If you begin at the blue-blazed trail (a sign indicating that it is indeed the White Rocks Trail is located at the trailhead), simply follow the trail. Follow the blue blazes as the trail winds steadily, but not too steeply, uphill until you reach the ridge (0.75 miles). Follow the trail to the right (west) along the ridge, and in a short distance you will come to the first of the two prominent rock outcrops. The rock outcrops are formed from hard quartzite characteristic of the South Mountain province, and they tower as high as 40 feet in places. The precipitous face on the south side of the rocks provides several practice routes for local rock climbing enthusiasts.

The first outcrop may be passed over its crest, which requires some exposed scrambling and use of hands. Alternately, it can be bypassed by following a path around its north (right) side. The second outcrop appears immediately after the first, and it is passed quite easily over the top. Both offer beautiful views of South Mountain. On the morning I did this hike, I heard an awful, loud screeching noise, as if some animal was being killed, while I was standing atop the first rock outcrop. I walked around a bit to investigate and discovered a nest of squirrels screaming like wildcats. I had actually heard squirrels behaving like this before, but it is so unusual that I had forgotten. On my way back up to the trail, I ran into the gray fox snooping around the area. Perhaps it heard the screeching as well and had its mind on making a meal of the squirrels.

From the second outcrop, follow the trail along the ridge. You'll have no more scrambling until you return. If you do this hike in early June, the blossoming

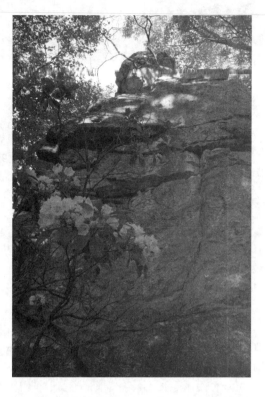

Mountain laurel and first outcrop

mountain laurel in this area is outstanding. At about 1.4 miles, you'll pass by a small boulder field, and then not far beyond that you'll reach a small saddle where the A.T. enters from the south. You'll find a campsite here and a sign that points the way to Center Point Knob, 1,060 feet, north along the A.T. It is worth the 0.25-mile hike up to the top for the view it offers to the north, especially during the fall and winter.

Follow the A.T. to the top, which is marked by a sign. After a nice rest, retrace your route back to the car. Be sure to keep track of the blazes on the descent from the ridge, as the path splits in several places.

NEARBY ACTIVITIES

Nearby Boiling Springs is a charming, historic town, which has restaurants and a beautiful park. The Appalachian Trail Conference Mid-Atlantic Regional Office is also located in the heart of town, and is worth stopping by. They have loads of information about the A.T. and the surrounding area.

60 WILLIAM H. KAIN COUNTY PARK LOOPS

KEY AT-A-GLANCE INFORMATION

LENGTH: 6.4 miles

CONFIGURATION: Figure-8

DIFFICULTY: Moderate

SCENERY: Lake Williams and Lake Redman

EXPOSURE: Mostly shaded

TRAIL TRAFFIC: Moderate

TRAIL SURFACE: Dirt

HIKING TIME: 3–3.5 hours

DRIVING DISTANCE: About 3 miles from Interstate 83 and PA 182 south of York

ACCESS: Dawn–dusk

MAPS: USGS York; park map available at parking area and online at ycwebserver.york-county .org/Parks/Kain.htm.

FACILITIES: Water and toilets at parking areas

WHEELCHAIR TRAVERSABLE: No

SPECIAL COMMENTS: Trails in the park are used frequently by mountain bikers and can get busy on weekends.

IN BRIEF

This hike follows Trail 4 as it passes above Lake Williams to the Lake Redman dam. At the top of the dam, it makes a side loop of about 1.9 miles following Trail 1 above Lake Redman. Returning to the dam, this hike drops to the parking area along South George Street, where it picks up Trail 2. It follows this trail the rest of the way around Lake Williams, completing a circuit of the lake.

DESCRIPTION

Walk to the back of the parking loop at the Lake Williams Activity Area, where you will find Trail 4 (identified by a numbered green-fiberglass post). An old roadbed, it heads uphill away from the lake over a large log placed to keep motor vehicles off of the trail. Don't confuse this with a second trail, a footpath without a number beginning about 50 feet or so to its left. It heads over toward the lakeshore.

Walk up the hill to a clearing with a little bench and a trail crossing. Turn left onto an old carriage path and follow it into the woods and eventually above the shore of the lake. Like most of the trails in this part of the park, this one is popular with mountain bikers and it can get busy especially on the weekends. The path above the lake is pretty among tall

GPS Trailhead Coordinates

UTM Zone (WGS84) 18S

Easting   352869

Northing   4416988

Latitude   N 39° 53′ 24.72″

Longitude   W 76° 43′ 15.08″

Directions

From Interstate 83, take Exit 4, PA 182 west. Follow 182 to South George Street. Turn left. Follow South George Street south, past the Lake Redman Dam, into the town of Jacobus. Turn right on Water Street. The entrance to the Lake Williams Activity Area is about 1 mile on the right.

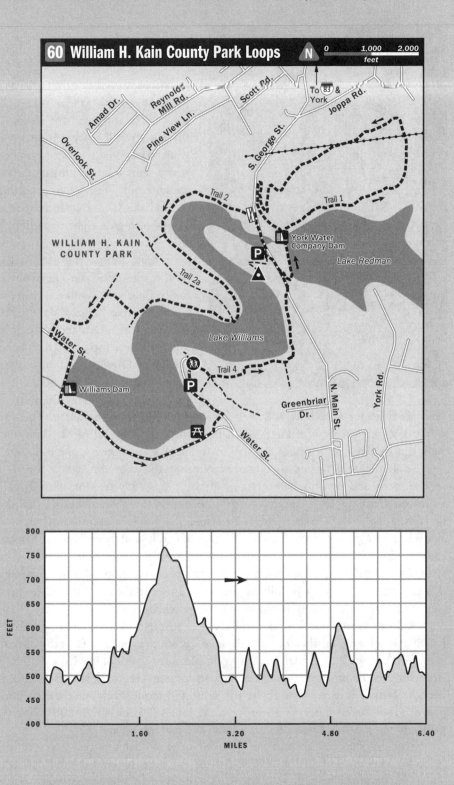

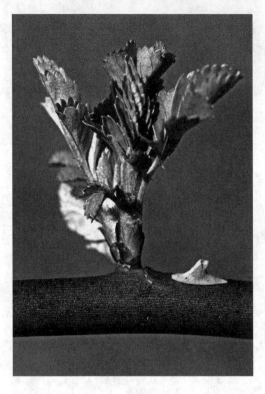

pine trees and the walking is on a pleasant smooth grade. When the trail drops to near the level of the lake, you'll reach a junction of trails marked with several numbers that seem a bit confusing. Head straight on Trail 4 to continue around the lake. (*Note:* A spur of Trail 4 also goes right and uphill at this point.)

Walk around the eastern end of the lake until you come out to South George Street by a gate across from the Lake Redman dam. Cross the street, turn left, and walk up to and across the top of the dam heading north. From the end of the dam, you'll take a short secondary loop hike of 1.9 miles along the shore of Lake Redman for a distance and then back over a hill from the north. The dam offers a wonderful view of Lake Redman. From the north end of the dam, turn right onto a nice open carriage road, Trail 1. The walking here is quite pleasant.

Soon the trail begins to climb away from the lake through a forest of spruce trees, and near the top of the hill you'll pass the junction with Trail 7. Continue climbing Trail 1 until you pass beneath some power lines that extend above the highway to your right. Just beyond the power lines, the trail makes a sharp left turn, passes through a short section of forest, and then proceeds beneath the power lines heading east. After about 0.25 miles, follow the path into the woods to the left of the power lines. The trail becomes more of a footpath as it descends around the edge of hill. As you circle closer to the dam, the hillside gets steeper and the trail makes a couple of long switchbacks.

Follow the trail out the dam, walk back across its top, and then down to the parking area by the outflow of Lake Redman. From the south edge of the parking area, you can walk up a path to a viewing platform overlooking Lake Williams. According to the information sign at the parking area, the park is rich in cultural history. Native Americans lived in the area and stone tools have been found nearby. The creek supported 16 mills in the late 1700s to early 1800s. The old gristmill was located across the creek from the parking area.

Much of the land around the shore of Lake Williams is characterized as a wetland. This means that for at least part of the year the land is saturated with water, it has typically dark soil, and it is populated by plants that enjoy a wet habitat. Just across the creek, you can see a stand of cattails and black willows, both wetland species. Ospreys and bald eagles both nest in the area, and the lake is home to wood and black ducks as well as scads of frogs and turtles who can be seen sunning themselves on logs in the spring.

From the parking area, cross the creek and walk along the road for about 50 yards in front of the yellow house. At the drive to the house, turn left through a gate and pick up Trail 2, another carriage road. You'll follow this trail most of the way around Lake Williams. About a mile from the parking area, you'll come to a bench on the shore of the lake at the point of a peninsula. Trail 2a enters here from atop the peninsula. Continue along the shore of the lake for another 0.3 miles, enjoying the excellent views, to a marshy area and a junction with a trail heading uphill to your right. Leave the shore of the lake and follow that trail for a short distance until it ends at a T-intersection. Turn left and follow the trail downhill past some horse farms to an area that, at the time of this writing, was being developed.

Route finding gets a little complicated at this point as the area is currently under construction. In effect, you simply want to get out to Water Street only a couple of hundred feet to the southwest. The easiest way to do so is to get on the main development road and follow it out of the development. Bear in mind that the trail may be rerouted in the future.

When you reach Water Street, turn left and you will see a sign welcoming you to William H. Kain County Park. Follow the road down to the dam at the outflow of Lake Williams, about 0.25 miles. Walking along the road is not unpleasant. Cross the dam and follow Water Street as it climbs up and around the lake. At 0.75 miles from the dam (6.14 miles total), you'll pass a picnic area on the left. Just beyond the picnic area, a trail enters the woods to the left. Turn left, walk through the woods for a short distance to the day-use access road. Turn left and walk back to your car.

NEARBY ACTIVITIES

The park offers moonlight boat rides on Lake Redman led by an amateur astronomer. The York County Parks Department has built a 350-foot ADA-accessible walking deck at the Lake Redman Activity Area, located near the Iron Stone Hill Road parking lot. For maps and information, check the Web site at **ycwebserver.york-county.org/Parks/Kain.htm**.

Richard M. Nixon County Park is located just across Water Street from the Lake Williams Activity Area. It has its own system of trails and an environmental-education center (**ycwebserver.york-county.org/Parks/Nixon.htm**).

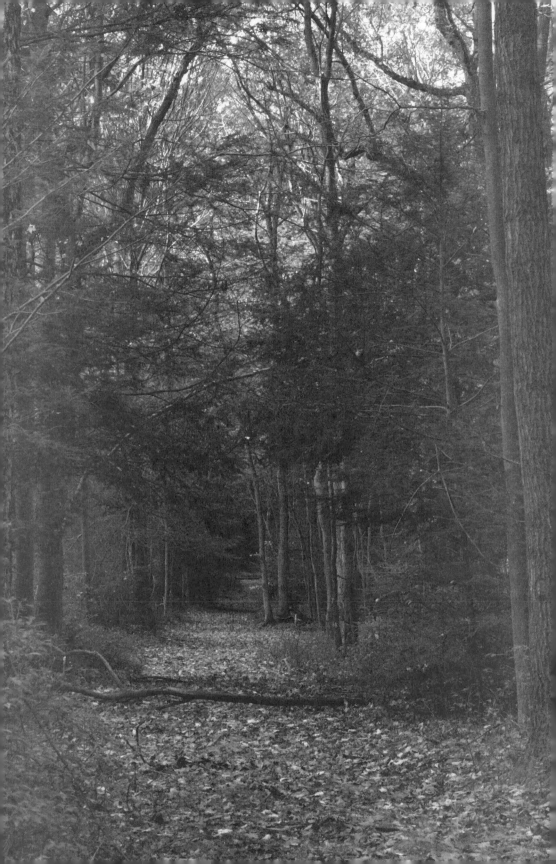

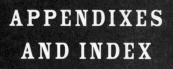

APPENDIXES
AND INDEX

APPENDIX A:
SOME USEFUL MAPS AND GUIDES

Appalachian Trail in Pennsylvania, Sections 1 through 6: Delaware Water Gap to Swatara Gap. Published by Keystone Trails Association, Cogan Station, PA.

Appalachian Trail in Pennsylvania, Sections 7 and 8: Swatara Gap to Susquehanna River. Published by Keystone Trails Association, Cogan Station, PA.

Appalachian Trail, Susquehanna River to PA Route 94 (Sections 9, 10, and 11). Published by the Potomac Appalachian Trail Club, Inc., Vienna, VA.

Appalachian Trail, PA Route 94 to US Route 30 (Sections 12 and 13). Published by the Potomac Appalachian Trail Club, Inc., Vienna, VA.

Guide to the Horse-Shoe Trail. Published by the Horse-Shoe Trail Club, Inc.

The Pennsylvania Atlas and Gazetteer. Published by DeLorme, Yarmouth, ME.

A Public Use Map for Michaux State Forest. Published by Pennsylvania Department of Conservation and Natural Resources, Bureau of Forestry.

A Public Use Map for Tuscarora State Forest. Published by Pennsylvania Department of Conservation and Natural Resources, Bureau of Forestry.

Susquehanna River Birding and Wildlife Trail Guide. Published by Audubon Pennsylvania, Harrisburg, PA.

Tuscarora Trail, Map J, Appalachian Trail, PA, to PA Route 641. Published by the Potomac Appalachian Trail Club, Inc., Vienna, VA.

APPENDIX B:
LOCAL HIKING AND OUTDOOR-EQUIPMENT STORES

Harrisburg
Bass Pro Shop
3501 Paxton Street
Harrisburg, PA 17111
(717) 565-5200

Dick's Sporting Goods
5086 Jonestown Road
Harrisburg, PA
(717) 652-3174

Gander Mountain
5005 Jonestown Road
Harrisburg, PA 17112
(717) 671-9700

Wildware Backcountry
995 Peiffers Lane
Harrisburg, PA
(717) 564-8008

Lancaster
Eastern Mountain Sports
541 Park City Center
Lancaster, PA 17601
(717) 397-8120

York
Dick's Sporting Goods
Route 30 and Kenneth Road
York, PA 17404
(717) 848-1696

Dunham's Sporting Goods
411 Eisenhower Drive
Hanover, PA 17331
(717) 630-0074

Gander Mountain
1880 Loucks Road
York, PA 17404
(717) 767-2002

APPENDIX C:
HIKING CLUBS AND NATURE PRESERVATION/CONSERVATION ORGANIZATIONS

Central Pennsylvania Conservancy
www.centralpaconservancy.org

Cumberland Valley Appalachian Trail Club
www.geocities.com/cvatclub

Friends of Wildwood Nature Sanctuary
www.wildwoodlake.org/support/
membership-application.aspx

Keystone Trails Association
www.kta-hike.org

Lancaster County Conservancy
www.lancasterconservancy.org

Lancaster Hiking Club
community.lancasteronline.com/
lancasterhikingclub

Mason Dixon Trail System
www.masondixontrail.org

Ned Smith Center for Nature and Art
www.nedsmithcenter.org

Pennsylvania Department of Conservation and Natural Resources
www.dcnr.state.pa.us

Potomac Appalachian Trail Club
www.potomacappalachian.org

Susquehanna Appalachian Trail Club
www.satc-hike.org

York Hiking Club
www.yorkhikingclub.com

INDEX

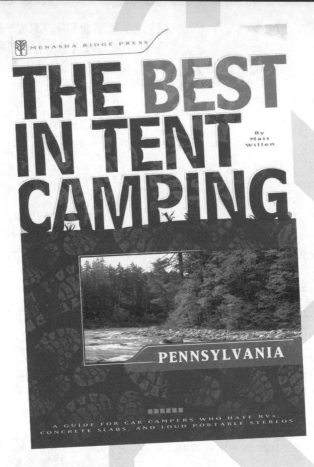

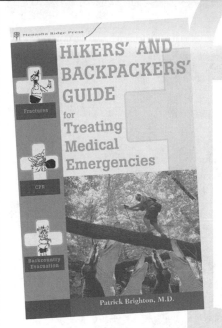
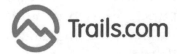

AMERICAN HIKING SOCIETY

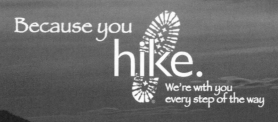

Because you **hike.**
We're with you every step of the way

American Hiking Society gives voice to the more than 75 million Americans who hike and is the only national organization that promotes and protects foot trails, the natural areas that surround them and the hiking experience. Our work is inspiring and challenging, and is built on three pillars:

Volunteerism and Stewardship: We organize and coordinate nationally recognized programs – including Volunteer Vacations, National Trails Day® and the National Trails Fund –that help keep our trails open, safe and enjoyable.

Policy and Advocacy: We work with Congress and federal agencies to ensure funding for trails, the preservation of natural areas, and the protection of the hiking experience.

Outreach and Education: We expand and support the national constituency of hikers through outreach and education as well as partnerships with other recreation and conservation organizations.

Join us in our efforts. Become an American Hiking Society member today!

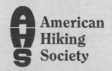

American Hiking Society

1422 Fenwick Lane · Silver Spring, MD 20910 · (301) 565-6704
www.AmericanHiking.org · info@AmericanHiking.org

DEAR CUSTOMERS AND FRIENDS,

SUPPORTING YOUR INTEREST IN OUTDOOR ADVENTURE, travel, and an active lifestyle is central to our operations, from the authors we choose to the locations we detail to the way we design our books. Menasha Ridge Press was incorporated in 1982 by a group of veteran outdoorsmen and professional outfitters. For 25 years now, we've specialized in creating books that benefit the outdoors enthusiast.

Almost immediately, Menasha Ridge Press earned a reputation for revolutionizing outdoors- and travel-guidebook publishing. For such activities as canoeing, kayaking, hiking, backpacking, and mountain biking, we established new standards of quality that transformed the whole genre, resulting in outdoor-recreation guides of great sophistication and solid content. Menasha Ridge continues to be outdoor publishing's greatest innovator.

The folks at Menasha Ridge Press are as at home on a white-water river or mountain trail as they are editing a manuscript. The books we build for you are the best they can be, because we're responding to your needs. Plus, we use and depend on them ourselves.

We look forward to seeing you on the river or the trail. If you'd like to contact us directly, join in at www.trekalong.com or visit us at www.menasharidge.com. We thank you for your interest in our books and the natural world around us all.

SAFE TRAVELS,

Bob Sehlinger

BOB SEHLINGER
PUBLISHER